Patient Care
in Neurosurgery

DATE DUE

APR 2 1993	
OCT - 9 1993	
OCT 25 1996	
NOV 1 2 1996	
NOV 2 6 1996	
APR 2 1 2005	
JUL 2 0 2005	

Patient Care
in Neurosurgery

Third Edition

Nelson M. Oyesiku, M.D.
Resident in Neurosurgery, Emory
University School of Medicine, Atlanta,
Georgia

A. Loren Amacher, M.D.
Attending Neurosurgeon, Department of
Neurosurgery, Geisinger Medical Center,
Danville, Pennsylvania

Foreword by
George T. Tindall, M.D.
Professor and Chairman, Division of
Neurosurgery, Emory University School of
Medicine, Atlanta, Georgia

Little, Brown and Company
Boston/Toronto/London

Contents

Foreword

Neurosurgery has grown into an expanding and exciting specialty. Its training programs reflect the growth that has occurred but also demand acquisition of a fundamental knowledge base. Providing the core to its strong educational foundation are the basic and clinical neurosciences, as well as the basic principles of surgery.

The many fine trainees who are attracted to neurosurgical training programs will find this third edition of *Patient Care in Neurosurgery* of particular use, as should surgical residents and students rotating on a neurosurgical service. The material presented follows a logical course; the early chapters deal with pertinent aspects of clinical neurosurgical physiology, and later chapters present diagnostic and therapeutic outlines for commonly encountered neurosurgical problems. The authors have created an effective framework that trainees can use to organize a rational approach to patient management.

This excellent edition brings the unique insights and range of expertise of its authors to the special needs of the neurosurgical house officer. Nelson Oyesiku is a resident in the neurosurgical training program at Emory University, and Loren Amacher has extensive experience in training residents in neurosurgery. Together, they have written a valuable guide for the neurosurgical trainee, one that will ensure a firm foundation in the basic principles of neurosurgical patient care.

George T. Tindall, M.D.

Preface

When, in the spring of 1985, Nelson Oyesiku appeared in my office as a candidate for Clinical Fellow in neurosurgery at Hartford Hospital, it took but a few seconds for me to recognize a young man of exceptional promise and quality. Since then, my intuition has been vindicated in every respect. The writing of this book has been a pleasure for me because of my collaboration with him. For Nelson, the effort and discipline of producing this work has been arduous—what with forging ahead with his own training—and a priceless learning experience.

This text, with its procedural notes and illustrations, is intended for the perusal and aid of house staff not yet initiated into the routines and mysteries of neurosurgery. It is informative and understandable for most who must or who wish to gain more insight into that rather intimidating black box that is the subject and object of what, after all, is the Queen of Surgeries.

We express respects to Dr. James R. Howe, author of the first two editions. We have retained his overall outline. Deeply felt gratitude is extended to Susan F. Pioli, Senior Medical Editor at Little, Brown, for asking us to write this edition; to Lisa Peñalver for her excellent artwork; to Dr. George Tindall for graciously providing the Foreword; to Drs. Dan Barrow, Suzie Tindall, and Austin Colohan for reviewing parts of the manuscript; and to Wendy Barringer for reviewing the page proofs.

A. L. A.

I. Clinical Neurosurgical Physiology

1. Cerebral Blood Flow and Metabolism

The human brain is the most complex of organs. In it we live and have our being. The basic functional unit of the central nervous system (CNS) is the neuron and its array of supporting glial cells. Phylogenetically the neuron has adapted itself to the role of information gathering, processing, and forwarding by electrical, chemical, and humoral means. Certain neurons have efferent processes (axons) up to 1 m long, and many neurons can process perhaps 25,000 bytes of incoming information more or less simultaneously. Such activities demand continuous metabolic input, since the neuron cannot store a significant energy supply.

Each neuron contains organelles specifically designed to carry out the multitude of biochemical processes required to transmit and store information. The neuron is responsible for the best (and worst) in human conduct and culture; the neuron makes the brain unique in its extraordinary circulatory and metabolic demands.

Anatomy
Arterial Anatomy

Approximately 850 ml of oxygenated blood is delivered from the heart to the brain each minute through paired carotid and vertebral arteries, which arise as major branches from the aortic arch and right subclavian artery.

The common carotid arteries bifurcate in the neck. The external carotid artery supplies the face, scalp, and cranial meninges. The internal carotid artery penetrates the skull base and supplies the brain. Approximately 80 percent of the brain's blood supply arrives through the internal carotid artery, distributed principally to the frontal, temporal, and parietal lobes through branches of the anterior and middle cerebral arteries.

The vertebral arteries ascend from the aortic arch through the foramina transversaria of the cervical vertebrae. They enter the skull through the foramen magnum and join at the rostral anterior margin of the medulla to form the basilar artery. Branches of the vertebral and basilar arteries supply the brainstem and cerebellum. The terminal branches of the basilar artery are the posterior cerebral arteries, which irrigate the inferior portions of the occipital and temporal lobes (Fig. 1-1).

Collateral Circulation

Figure 1-1 shows the anatomic situation that allows for collateral blood flow if one or more major conduits are interrupted. The circle of Willis,

3

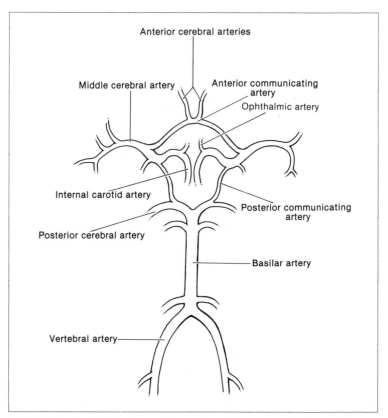

Fig. 1-1. Circle of Willis. The anterior and posterior communicating arteries are important potential channels of collateral circulation.

as it has come to be known, is only a potential mechanism for collateral flow, because one or more of the three major communicating arteries are either rudimentary or missing altogether in approximately 35 percent of patients studied by angiography. Therefore many clinicians speak of the anterior circulation (internal carotid and major branches) versus the posterior circulation (vertebral-basilar system) as if they were physiologically distinct.

In patients whose circle of Willis is anatomically incomplete, acute occlusion of either a carotid or vertebral artery (owing to atherosclerotic thrombosis or trauma) may result in an ischemic neurologic deficit. Redistribution of arterial flow may obviate a potential ischemic injury when there is an anatomically complete circle of Willis. If a major extracranial vessel (carotid or vertebral artery) becomes occluded, anastomoses may form between the external carotid circulation and the

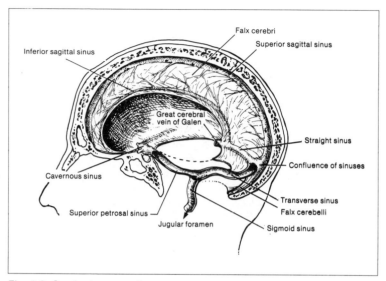

Fig. 1-2. Cerebral venous sinuses.

surface arteries of the brain. For example, collateral blood flow in atherosclerotic disease is often the result of anastomoses arising between the external carotid and ophthalmic arteries. Intracerebral collateral channels are meager at best, and thrombosis of a parenchymal artery may be followed by very little shunting of flow to the ischemic region. Therefore some degree of infarction usually occurs in such a situation.

Venous Anatomy

The cerebral venous system is a valveless series of vessels that can be divided into two groups. The superficial and deep veins drain the parenchyma of the brain. The major venous sinuses are large conduits located within the major dural reflections.

The superficial and deep cerebral veins drain into the venous sinuses, which in turn empty into the internal jugular veins. The sagittal sinus is the main site for reabsorption of cerebrospinal fluid (CSF) into the bloodstream (Fig. 1-2). Occlusion of small superficial cerebral veins is usually well tolerated but occlusion of a large vein, deep or superficial, may produce venous infarction or local tissue edema. The venous sinuses are resistant to collapse because they are held open by the leaves of dura; when occlusion does occur, effects may range from raised intracranial pressure (ICP) to major cerebral infarction.

Input

The brain receives 20 percent of cardiac output, although it accounts for only 2 percent of total body weight, about 1400 gm. This input represents an average *regional cerebral blood flow (rCBF) of 55 ml/100 gm of brain tissue each minute*, varying between 65 and 75 ml/100 gm/ min in gray matter and 15 and 20 ml/100 gm/min in the white matter and from one region to the next. Cerebral blood flow (CBF) is higher in the frontal lobes, followed by the parietal and the temporal lobes. Recent studies of brain metabolism with positron emission tomography (PET) have shown that CBF varies significantly even in the same area.

Cerebral oxygen uptake is similarly quite exacting, consuming some 20 percent of the body's total oxygen uptake, equal to a *cerebral metabolic rate of oxygen ($CMRO_2$) of 3.5 ml of O_2/100 gm of brain tissue each minute* or 50 ml of O_2/min. This supply of blood and oxygen must be virtually uninterrupted to ensure satisfactory organ function.

Complete arrest of the cerebral circulation leads to unconsciousness (depression of neuronal activity) within seconds and to irreversible damage (depletion of energy stores and deterioration of ionic homeostasis, culminating in cell death) within minutes [1]. This traditional concept of cerebral ischemia is being modified, however, since experimental evidence suggests that the brain is more tolerant of ischemia than previously realized, at least under certain conditions [2].

Modulation of Cerebral Blood Flow

Perfusion Pressure and Autoregulation

The driving force in the maintenance of CBF is the cerebral perfusion pressure (CPP). The perfusion pressure is a mathematical function of the mean systemic arterial pressure (MAP) and the ICP:

$$CPP = MAP - ICP$$

The intracranial pressure is readily measurable and closely approximates cerebral venous pressure. It is obvious that the pressure in the veins must slightly exceed the ICP or the extravascular pressure to prevent their collapse. Venous pressure is in fact about 2 to 5 mm Hg higher than ICP.

The CPP in turn determines CBF according to:

$$CBF = \frac{CPP}{CVR}$$

where CVR is the cerebral vascular resistance.

The large and medium-size arteries (carotid arteries and principal branches) divide into the principal resistance vessels, the small arteries and arterioles. These vessels together constitute the precapillary resistance vessels, which with the capillaries account for about 80 percent of CVR. The residual 20 percent is a function of the venules and veins.

The resistance of a blood vessel is inversely proportional to the fourth power of its radius:

$$CVR \; \alpha \; \frac{1}{r^4}$$

For example, halving the radius would reduce CVR by a factor of 16. Thus small changes in vessel size lead to substantial alterations in CBF.

Under normal conditions, and despite fluctuations in CPP, the brain can maintain a constant level of CBF by modifying CVR. This ability, known as *autoregulation*, is a vascular response resulting in vasodilatation at low perfusion pressures and vasoconstriction at high perfusion pressures. These compensatory changes in vessel diameter secondary to transmural pressure maintain a constant flow—a phenomenon known as the *Bayliss effect* [3].

Autoregulation has limits. At a CPP of approximately 50 mm Hg, CBF begins to fall off precipitously and symptoms of cerebral ischemia begin to appear. Conversely, a CPP of 150 mm Hg or greater causes CBF to increase rapidly and can lead to blood-brain barrier disruption and edema formation. This may present clinically as hypertensive encephalopathy (Fig. 1-3).

The limits of autoregulation are not inflexible. They are modified or reset by the tone of the vessels, which can be altered by hypocapnia or hypercapnia, decreased sympathetic tone or sympathomimetics, acidosis or alkalosis, hypermetabolism or hypometabolism, and various drugs. Thus the autoregulation curve may be "left-shifted," allowing for increased CBF at lower values of CPP, or "right-shifted," permitting a greater CPP without necessarily causing a breakthrough of CBF (see Fig. 1-3).

In patients with chronic hypertension the autoregulatory curve is displaced to the right, representing a vascular adaptation that enables such patients to tolerate higher arterial perfusion pressures. This adaptation takes time and is probably secondary to hypertrophy of the vessel wall.

Of the various theories to explain autoregulation, the *myogenic* hypothesis is probably the strongest. It proposes that smooth muscle contraction or relaxation results from the distending intramural pressure through an intrinsic local reflex [3]. The response is rapid, being initiated within seconds and essentially complete in about 15 to 30 seconds. The integrity of the reflex may also depend on hypothalamic influences.

Neurogenic Control

The cerebral vessels large and small, are supplied with vasomotor nerves (nervi vasorum)—sympathetic and parasympathetic. The num-

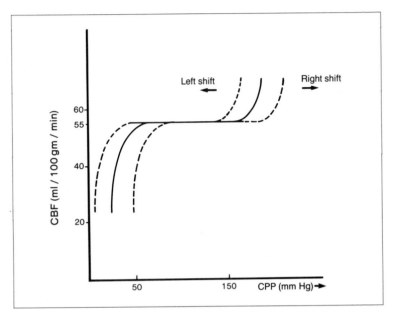

Fig. 1-3. Cerebral autoregulation curve. Cerebral blood flow (CBF) remains virtually constant between cerebral perfusion pressure (CPP) of 50 and 100 mm Hg. Interrupted lines show right and left shift of the curve, resulting from modifications of vasomotor tone (see text).

ber of nerves diminishes with decreasing vessel size although nerve density remains unchanged. The veins are not as well innervated as the arteries. Autonomic innervation has been shown to be associated with various neurotransmitters and peptides.

Sympathetic nerve fibers arise mainly from the ipsilateral superior cervical ganglion and contain norepinephrine. Norepinephrine may react with alpha- or beta-receptors on cerebral vessels to induce vasoconstriction and vasodilatation, respectively [4].

An intracerebral "intrinsic" system, arising from the locus ceruleus, is believed to provide noradrenergic input to the cerebral microvasculature. A peptide, neuropeptide Y, is known to coexist with norepinephrine in cerebral nervi vasorum, where it mediates relatively prolonged cerebral vasoconstriction.

The parasympathetic cholinergic system has recently been shown to originate in the sphenopalatine ganglion [5]. Acetylcholine causes vasodilatation through muscarinic receptors. Two peptides, vasoactive intestinal polypeptide (VIP) and peptide histidine isoleucine (PHI), reach the cerebral vasculature by fiber systems that are closely associated; both mediate vasodilatation [6].

The sensory ganglion of the trigeminal nerve is a relay station for a large number of fibers that innervate the cerebral vessels. It contains many peptides. The trigeminocerebrovascular system is probably involved in the perception of nociceptive stimuli of vascular origin; by releasing vasodilators it may mitigate some of the effects of pronounced vasoconstriction after such events as subarachnoid hemorrhage [7]. Maximal stimulation of sympathetic nerves reduces CBF by 5 to 10 percent. A similar vasodilator response has been shown for the parasympathetic system [8, 9].

The role of neurogenic control may be modulation of cerebral blood volume or resetting of the autoregulatory curve. Despite intense research in this area, more questions have been raised than answered.

Functional/Metabolic Control

Increased neuronal activity obligates an increased metabolic rate, leading to increased demand on blood supply to provide substrate and oxygen. This coupling of metabolism to blood flow operates under various conditions that have been quantified during experimental rCBF measurements [10]. The relationship between CBF and metabolism can be described as follows:

$$CMRO_2 = \frac{CBF \times AVDO_2}{100}$$

where $CMRO_2$ is the cerebral metabolic rate of oxygen, CBF is the cerebral blood flow, and $AVDO_2$ is the arteriovenous oxygen difference.

Normally the $AVDO_2$ is 4.0 to 8.5 vol% at a pCO_2 of 40 mm Hg. It is a measure of oxygen extraction by the tissue, which in turn is an estimate of the rate of metabolism.

Where $CMRO_2$ is constant and CBF varies, $AVDO_2$ measurements provide a good estimate of CBF, with a high $AVDO_2$ implying a lower CBF and vice versa. To determine $CMRO_2$, one must measure CBF directly, then calculate $CMRO_2$ from the equation. Methods of measuring CBF are outside the scope of this text, and the reader is referred to the suggested readings.

Increased metabolic activity leading to increased CBF occurs classically in seizures. The opposite situation is observed in dementia, in cerebral depression from barbiturates, and in many types of coma. Precisely what factor(s) couple CBF to metabolism is the subject of current investigation. Likely candidates include adenosine and the hydrogen and potassium ions [11].

Chemical Control

CBF is exquisitely sensitive to changes in the partial pressure of CO_2 (pCO_2). Carbon dioxide is the product of brain metabolism and is freely

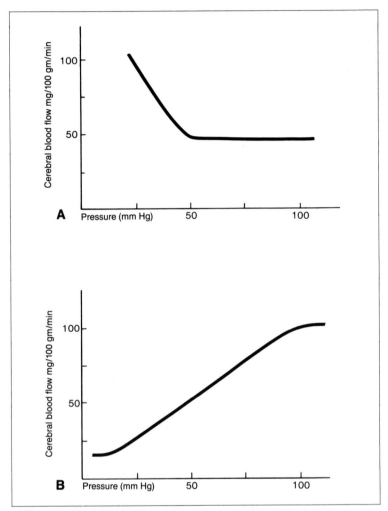

Fig. 1-4. A. Relationship between arterial oxygen tension (pO₂), and cerebral blood flow. B. Relationship between arterial carbon dioxide tension (pCO₂) and cerebral blood flow.

diffusible between blood and CSF. It is therefore in a unique spatial position to provide homeostatic regulation of CBF [12].

In the pCO_2 range of 25 to 60 mm Hg, the relationship of CBF to pCO_2 is exponential. For each mm Hg change in pCO_2, CBF changes by approximately 4 percent, assuming that autoregulation is intact (Fig. 1-4B). Hypocapnia causes cerebral vasoconstriction, and this vasoconstriction significantly reduces *cerebral blood volume (CBV)*. Consequently, hyperventilation (HV) is a powerful tool for lowering ICP, by lowering CBV.

Hypercapnia induces cerebral vasodilatation, increases CBV, and elevates ICP. For these reasons, hypercapnia should be avoided in clinical settings where raised ICP is likely to be present.

Carbon dioxide reactivity is thought to be mediated by pH variations in the periarteriolar CSF. Exactly how pH variations influence the tone of smooth muscle is not known. However, changes in Ca^{2+} are a possible mechanism. The effect of changes in CO_2 occurs within minutes and is maximal at 12 minutes. Adaptation generally occurs within 48 hours, with a return of CBF to normal. Accordingly, clinical use of HV may not remain effective in lowering ICP indefinitely, but it may continue to provide benefit by preventing the adverse effect of hypercapnia in areas of focal damage and by helping to maintain compliance of the brain.

To a lesser extent, changes in pO_2 are also responsible for altering CBF [13]. Moderate variations in oxygen tension cause only slight changes in CBF. Presumably this is due to the fact that the dissociation curve for oxyhemoglobin is almost horizontal at normal pO_2, thus allowing for little change in O_2 content of arterial blood or cerebral oxygen delivery. Marked reduction of pO_2 causes vasodilatation and increases in CBF. This increase appears at about a pO_2 of 50 mm Hg, doubles at 30 mm Hg, and becomes maximal at 20 mm Hg, below which a switch to anaerobic glycolysis occurs [14] (Fig. 1-4A).

The vasodilatory effect of hypoxia is probably secondary to lactic acidosis, although there is increasing evidence that the nucleoside adenosine is responsible for hypoxic vasodilatation [15]. When energy supply is low, adenosine triphosphate (ATP) is formed at the expense of adenosine diphosphate (ADP). The adenosine monophosphate (AMP) generated is dephosphorylated to yield adenosine and inorganic phosphate (P_i) as:

$$ADP + ADP \rightarrow ATP + AMP \rightarrow ADENOSINE + P_i$$

Ordinarily adenosine is recycled by phosphorylation reactions to nucleotides, but it may accumulate under ischemic conditions. Adenosine has been shown to be a potent dilator of cerebral vessels and may effect augmentation of CBF when CPP is low.

This action of adenosine is probably mediated by adjustments in free calcium flux, which alters smooth muscle reactivity [15, 16]. Moreover, like CO_2, it is a by-product of cerebral metabolism and is readily diffusible, making its putative role in cerebrovascular homeostasis a logical one.

Hematocrit and Blood Viscosity

CBF is low with a high hematocrit. More O_2 is carried per unit volume of blood, and a lower CBF is required to maintain the same O_2 delivery.

Furthermore, blood viscosity rises with increasing hematocrit. Conversely, CBF increases at lower hematocrit. Under normal circumstances the cerebral vessels compensate for changes in viscosity, for example, vasodilatation in response to increased viscosity. However, if the circulation is already maximally dilated in compensation for ischemia, increased viscosity would be decidedly deleterious. This is observed clinically in stroke patients, in whom a larger infarct and a more severe neurologic deficit may be seen when the hematocrit is high. Hemodilution mitigates this to some degree [17]. A hematocrit of about 33 percent has been advocated as optimal for the ischemic brain [18].

In addition to the hematocrit, blood viscosity is also influenced by plasma proteins, erythrocyte deformability, platelet aggregation, and blood velocity.

Cerebral Metabolism: Basic Concepts

Energy for neural function comes from splitting energy-rich molecules of ATP. The majority of ATP is produced by the oxidative metabolism of glucose. For this the brain uses about 20 percent of the body's total O_2 consumption—a $CMRO_2$ of about 50 ml of O_2 per minute or 3.5 ml of O_2 per 100 gm/min. This demand for O_2 is continuous, since it cannot be stored. Significant hypoxia therefore rapidly results in coma within a few minutes.

To feed its metabolic machinery, the brain also requires glucose. It uses some 77 mg/min, or *5.5 mg/100 gm of brain tissue each minute—the rate of cerebral metabolism of glucose (CMRglu)*, which is 25 percent of all the glucose used by the body. The respiratory quotient (RQ) of the brain is almost unity, implying an almost total dependence on carbohydrate for energy production.

Neurons require tremendous quantities of energy to keep membrane pumps operating, particularly those for sodium. To maintain electrical conductive efficiency, sodium with its attached water moieties must be pumped out of the cell continuously; at the same time, the neuron must recover its potassium ions, which tend to leak out down a concentration gradient.

Other crucial energy requirements of the cell are those for neurotransmitter and protein synthesis, internal membrane stabilization (especially the potentially autodigestive lysosomes), and messenger RNA synthesis. Most of the brain's high metabolic demand comes from neurons. The cerebral metabolic rate is higher in gray matter than in white matter. Cerebral metabolism increases with neuronal activity, and as regional cerebral metabolism increases, so does rCBF. Part of the membrane pump's function is to rid the cell of excess intracellular H^+. This ion is released rapidly as metabolism increases. As H^+ reaches the extracellular environment, it acts locally on capillaries and small arterioles to induce vasodilatation, thereby increasing CBF [11].

Glucose reaches neurons through a facilitated transport mechanism across the blood-brain barrier. The initial breakdown of glucose to pyruvate occurs along the Embden-Meyerhof pathway by glycolysis. In the presence of adequate O_2, pyruvate then forms acetyl CoA, which enters Krebs' (citric acid) cycle to generate H^+ atoms. By H^+ acceptors, mainly nicotinamide-adenine dinucleotide (NAD) and the electron transport cytochrome oxidase chain, glucose is converted to useful energy:

1 glucose + 6 O_2 + 38 Pi → 6 CO_2 + 44 H_2O + 38 ATP

For each molecule of glucose, 38 molecules of ATP are generated through the aerobic glycolytic pathway, a process that depends almost entirely on healthy mitochondria.

In the absence of sufficient oxygen, glycolysis would stop through lack of NAD. However, pyruvate then becomes the hydrogen ion acceptor, yields lactate, and recovers NAD. Lactic acid accumulates, and lactic acidosis results. Anaerobic glycolysis is a poor harvest, reaping only 2 moles of ATP per mole of glucose. Insufficient ATP is produced to keep membrane pumps operating at required efficiency. Consequently, glucose consumption must increase during hypoxia to meet demands. Unfortunately, this leads to an increase in lactate load that may have a direct toxic effect on the neuron. In normal situations about 5 percent of glucose used follows an anaerobic pathway.

Another pathway for the oxidation of glucose is the hexose monophosphate shunt. This yields 36 moles of ATP for each mole of glucose, using NADPH as H^+ acceptor and producing $NADPH_2$, (needed for synthesis of fatty acids for membranes and organelles) and pentoses (needed for synthesis of nucleic acid).

The brain has a small energy store of phosphocreatine (PCr) that is in equilibrium with ATP:

PCr + ADP + H^+ → Cr + ATP

In the absence of glucose the brain metabolizes ketone bodies, byproducts of fatty acid oxidation. Ketone bodies gain the brain's metabolic pool through carrier-mediated transport and are oxidized by acetyl CoA, entering Krebs' cycle. A certain amount of glucose consumption is required to facilitate ketone metabolism. Consequently, ketones per se cannot entirely substitute for the brain's energy supply. During fasting they provide up to three-fourths of the energy supply, and gluconeogenesis maintains the requisite amount of glucose to fuel the system.

The brain receives amino acids from the systemic pool by facilitated transport and synthesizes the rest. It has a particularly high concentration of glutamic and aspartic acids. The rate of protein turnover in the brain is rather high and increases with physiologic stimulation [19]. The nitrogen balance of the brain is approximately zero.

Table 1-1. Flow Thresholds in Cerebral Ischemia

CBF (ml/100 gm/min)	Physiologic Derangement
16–17	EEG flattening (synaptic transmission failure)
15	Evoked potentials abolished
10	Membrane failure
<10	Structural cell damage

From this very brief summary of the events of cerebral metabolism it is obvious that O_2 is essential to the efficient production of energy. It is equally true that glucose is essential to the safe intracellular detoxification of O_2, one of the most active and toxic chemicals in all of nature. This delicate, vital machinery depends on adequate cerebral perfusion.

Clinical Aspects

Flow Thresholds

Neuronal activities such as energy metabolism, ionic pumps, and synaptic transmission depend on CBF. Certain levels of CBF, called *flow thresholds* have been correlated with specific derangements (Table 1-1). Clinical studies during carotid endarterectomy [20, 21] and on experimental animal models [22] have demonstrated that reversible failure of *neuronal electrical activity (synaptic transmission)* occurs at a CBF of *15 to 17 ml/100 gm/min*, evidenced by electroencephalogram (EEG) flattening or loss of cortical evoked potential responses (EPs).

A reduction of CBF to *10 ml/100 gm/min* results in *membrane failure*, evidenced by increased extracellular K^+. The threshold of membrane failure is closely associated with the development of structural cell damage after a variable time delay (Table 1-1).

The status of the ischemic brain between the two thresholds, namely, the upper threshold of electrical failure and preserved viability and the lower threshold of ionic pump failure and threatened viability, can be described as functional inactivation with structural integrity. The term *zone of penumbra* or *ischemic penumbra* has been coined to describe these idling neurons [1]. The metaphor has its origin in the celestial event during which a zone of partial obscurity girdles a tenebrous sun. This zone of penumbra surrounds a central core of ischemic tissue.

Therapeutically, this zone represents potentially salvageable tissue. Restoration of CBF to normal levels (as with embolectomy, revascularization, endarterectomy, or pharmacotherapy) may allow for functional restitution of still viable neurons. The ischemic penumbra is often manifest as a neurologic deficit that resolves spontaneously or following therapy.

Derangements

An understanding of the clinical derangements of CBF and cerebral metabolism will be improved by a familiarity with the terms in contemporary use by clinical neuroscientists.

Luxury Perfusion

The brain's functional and metabolic state is a prime determinant of CBF. When this coupling of flow and function is lost, one possible result is a state of relative hyperemia, or *luxury perfusion*, where CBF is in excess of metabolic demand [23, 24]. Such impairment of metabolic regulation frequently occurs in cerebral ischemia. The mismatch may be due to the accumulation of mediators (e.g., H^+, adenosine, lactic acid) that cause vasodilatation. Luxury perfusion is observed in regions surrounding areas of ischemia.

Vasoparalysis

Adaptations in the cerebral vasculature are active phenomena, at least under normal conditions. They occur in response to changes in perfusion pressure (autoregulation) and chemical concentrations (e.g., H^+, lactate, O_2). Blood vessel unresponsiveness may occur to both autoregulatory and pCO_2 changes, a condition known as *complete vasoparalysis*. CBF is then "pressure-passive" (Fig. 1-5). Sometimes vasoparalysis involves only loss of autoregulation while CO_2 responsiveness is maintained, a condition referred to as *dissociated vasoparalysis*. Vasoparalysis may occur in areas of brain damaged by ischemia or trauma. Vasoparalysis may be responsible for a state of luxury perfusion.

Intracerebral Steal

Ischemic tissue adjacent to normal parts of the brain is at risk. Any situation that causes the normally reactive vessels to dilate (e.g., hypercapnia or hypotension) will shunt blood away from the already ischemic area, which is less able to respond to a similar vasodilator impulse because its vessels are already maximally dilated or in vasoparalysis. Obviously, this situation can exacerbate the effects of ischemia [25].

Inverse Intracranial Steal

As suggested, this is the opposite of intracerebral steal. This situation may occur following a vasoconstrictor stimulus (e.g., hypocapnia or hypertension), CBF falls in normal autoregulated vessels, shunting blood into adjacent ischemic brain in the so-called Robin Hood effect, after the charitable outlaw of Sherwood Forest.

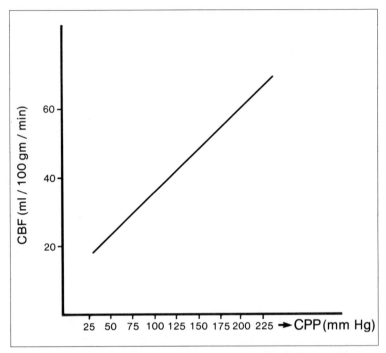

Fig. 1-5. Cerebral autoregulation curve from an area of brain damaged by ischemia. CBF is pressure dependent or pressure passive.

Normal Perfusion-Pressure Breakthrough

This phenomenon was initially described by Spetzler et al. [26] in connection with arteriovenous malformations (AVMs). The AVM is a low-resistance circuit relative to nearby vessels that have normal vascular resistance. With time, the vasculature of the surrounding brain becomes more dilated, to compete more favorably with its gluttonous neighbor that steals from the regional cerebral circulation. This area of surrounding normal brain can eventually lose autoregulatory capacity and even undergo structural change.

When the AVM is obliterated by surgery or endovascular techniques, the regional flow then preferentially enters the surrounding vessels, which are by now ill-equipped to mount a vasoconstrictor response to the increased CBF entering at a normal perfusion pressure. This condition may then lead to a breakthrough in the capillary bed, with resultant edema or hemorrhage.

Anticipation of this phenomenon when treating large, high-flow AVMs located on distal vessels may suggest the wisdom of staged procedures. In addition, meticulous attention to control of blood pressure in the postoperative period will reduce the likelihood that normal perfusion-pressure breakthrough will occur [26].

False Autoregulation

Severely injured brain may have areas where autoregulation is in abeyance from vasoparalysis, yet the "pressure-passive" phenomenon does not always occur. In some areas CBF is chronically depressed, and elevation of arterial pressure may fail to increase blood flow; however, reduction of perfusion pressure results in a sharp drop in CBF. The term *false autoregulation* has been applied to this phenomenon [27–29]. The precise mechanism is unknown but the clinical importance is clear. Elevation of blood pressure in such patients to increase CBF may be misdirected zeal. The desired result may not occur; instead, the brain insult may be exacerbated from enhanced edema and increased ICP. Experimental data indicate that high levels of CPP may in fact worsen edema in areas of blood-brain barrier disruption when ICP is controlled at low normal levels [30].

Conversely, disregard for hypotension may drastically curtail CBF, setting the stage for secondary ischemic events in an already compromised circulation.

Stroke/Cerebral Ischemia

Stroke is a frequent cause of cerebral ischemia, and atherosclerotic occlusive disease is the most common cause of stroke. The usual site of this lesion is the extracranial carotid artery.

When a cerebral vessel becomes progressively narrowed from atheroma, one of two mechanisms can cause ischemia: (1) the lumen may be so narrowed that blood flow falls precipitously, or (2) emboli from the atheroma may temporarily or permanently obstruct small distal channels. In either case, rCBF falls and focal ischemia occurs. Short-lived focal ischemia produces a transient ischemic attack (TIA); a permanent occlusion may result in an infarct.

Stroke causes heterogenous shifts in CBF and metabolism. In the central zone of dense ischemia, energy metabolism falls to near zero. The result is a metabolic cascade progressing through energy depletion to membrane failure.

Failure of the ATP-dependent Na^+-K^+ ionic pump leads to increased extracellular potassium and intracellular sodium. Glial uptake of extracellular K^+ and Cl^- ions causes glial swelling and cerebral edema that worsens ischemia by increasing the diffusion distance of O_2 to the neurons, typically 150 Å in the physiologic state. Furthermore, the extracellular accumulation of potassium stimulates brain metabolism at a time when cells can ill-afford an increase in metabolic demands. This worsens lactacidosis and further compromises energy balance [31].

Intracellular sodium accumulation causes membrane depolarization and interalia uncouples flow and metabolism. Voltage-dependent Ca^{2+} channels open, leading to Ca^{2+} influx. This free Ca^{2+} load in time overwhelms the neuron's Ca^{2+} clearing mechanisms and activates phospholipases, which cleave free fatty acids (FFA) from lipid molecules in the cell. This at once increases cell permeability due to structural damage and provides substrate, arachidonic acid (FFA), to combine with O_2 along one or the other of two prostaglandin-synthesis pathways: the *lipooxygenase pathway*, which produces leukotrienes that induce increased membrane permeability, or the *cyclooxygenase pathway*, which produces thromboxane A_2 (TXA_2) and prostacyclin (PGI_2). The former (TXA_2) causes vasoconstriction and platelet aggregation; the latter (PGI_2), vasodilatation and inhibition of platelet aggregation. Under normal conditions the balance is physiologic; however, ischemia alters the equilibrium in favor of TXA_2, further jeopardizing an already beleaguered microcirculation.

By-products of the arachidonic cascade are "active O_2 species" or "O_2-derived free radicals," believed to be the final common pathway in the initiation of destructive chain reactions in biologic membranes [32].

Another pathway in the derangement of cellular metabolism in ischemic conditions involves *excitatory neurotransmitters*, particularly glutamate. In ischemia, release of this neurotransmitter and its action on postsynaptic receptors causes an influx of Na^+, Ca^+, and Cl^-. The immediate effect is neuronal swelling, which may cause cell death by lysis. Neurons escaping this osmotic execution are then threatened by the arachidonic cascade triggered by intracellular Ca^{2+} accumulation. Current research in this area is being directed toward inhibition of the neurotransmitter pathway by blocking the postsynaptic receptor. Some investigators have demonstrated the efficacy of this approach using the N-methyl-D-aspartate (NMDA) receptor blocker 2-amino-7-phosphoheptanoic acid (APH) to ameliorate the effects of cerebral ischemia [33].

Aneurysmal Subarachnoid Hemorrhage

Rupture of an intracranial aneurysm may severely disrupt intracranial vascular dynamics. As blood is liberated into the subarachnoid space, ICP rises dramatically [34]. In severe cases, or if there is associated intracranial hematoma, the neurologic deficit may be profound. Usually the ICP correlates with the patient's clinical state, varying between 15 mm Hg in good-grade patients and 45 mm Hg in poor-grade patients [35, 36].

Regional CBF measurements show reductions that are closely related to the patient's clinical grade. Reductions in rCBF by 25 to 50 percent have been demonstrated. Critically low CBF values are seen in patients with severe vasospasm or intracranial hypertension.

Similarly, cerebral metabolism is altered, with reductions in $CMRO_2$ and

$AVDO_2$. Dissociated reductions between rCBF and $CMRO_2$ are also seen, implying the uncoupling of flow and metabolism. CSF lactic acidosis is also a common feature [36–39].

Blood bathing the subarachnoid cisterns irritates the underlying cerebral vessels. Long-lasting cerebral vasospasm may result, worsening the clinical situation by causing cerebral ischemia.

Tumors

CBF may be affected by a tumor in a number of ways. Increased interstitial pressure around the tumor causes veins and capillaries to collapse and the regional blood volume and rCBF to decrease [39].

Autoregulation of CBF and CO_2 reactivity are disordered at the periphery of the tumor and even in remote regions of the brain. Tumor vessels may be free of any autoregulatory control. As the mass grows or as tissue pressure rises intermittently, ischemia increases in the tissue surrounding the tumor. There is then a shift toward anaerobic glycolysis, which results in local acidosis. This may lead to luxury perfusion, increase in blood volume, and increase in local tissue pressure. Edema occurs, and further brain compression and neurologic deficit may result.

The normal relationship between CBF and metabolism can be reestablished by reducing ICP or surgically removing the lesion.

Hypertension

As MAP rises, the upper limit of autoregulation is exceeded and "breakthrough" occurs. There is forced vasodilatation of the cerebral arterioles and increased CBF. The blood vessel wall and blood-brain barrier are ultimately disrupted, and increased vascular permeability, cerebral edema, or hemorrhage results. The clinical presentation is hypertensive encephalopathy, with depressed sensorium, delirium, or seizures. In chronically hypertensive patients without the superimposed acute clinical syndrome, the autoregulation curve is "reset" to the right over a variable period. These patients also have a higher value for the lower limit of autoregulation. Higher CPP must be maintained in these patients to prevent ischemia [41, 42].

Arteriovenous Malformations

An arteriovenous malformation (AVM) is a congenital vascular anomaly in which the normal capillary interface between the venous and arterial systems fails to develop. The result is an abnormal communication that may parasitize rCBF, namely, recruit vessels from the surrounding brain, leading to intracerebral steal. Brain tissue around such a lesion may become ischemic, causing a neurologic deficit or seizures.

Another phenomenon associated with AVMs, normal perfusion-pressure breakthrough (see above), may complicate the surgical excision or embolization of a high-flow AVM. The typical manifestation is edema or hemorrhage.

Seizures

The effects of seizures on cerebral metabolism and CBF have been studied extensively in laboratory animals. During seizures, neurons fire rapidly, and the rate at which they consume both O_2 and glucose increases. CBF rises concomitantly. If seizures continue, anaerobic glycolysis ensues and acidic metabolites are produced. These in turn cause cerebral vasodilatation and a further elevation in local CBF. Of importance is the finding that seizure-induced increases in CBF may occur in homologous areas of the hemisphere contralateral to the seizure focus. These are called *mirror foci*. It is important to abolish seizures as soon as possible with anticonvulsants and to ensure a steady flow of O_2 to offset the brain's heightened metabolic needs. Continuous seizures (status epilepticus) have been shown to produce severe neurologic deficits in the absence of proper, rapid care.

Aging and Dementia

Because it is possible to quantitate CBF by noninvasive methods, the relationship between CBF and natural occurrences such as aging has been studied. A number of investigators have shown that with advancing age, CBF and vascular reactivity show a steady decline [43]. CBF in the gray matter of patients who are 60 years old may be 10 to 20 percent less than that of patients who are in their 20s. Cerebrovascular reactivity to CO_2 (increase in CBF) or O_2 (decrease in CBF) is significantly impaired in the elderly; patients over 80 show little, if any, response. In elderly subjects, activation of regional activity (speech and limb movements) produces less of an increase in CBF than in younger subjects. Patients with dementia show similar reductions in CBF, vascular reactivity, and activated responses. The reductions in CBF from aging or dementia seem to correlate with the amount of cortical atrophy demonstrated on computed tomography (CT) of the brain, suggesting that diminished flow may be a response to the reduction in cell population and overall metabolic demand.

Increased Intracranial Pressure

To better understand how ICP influences CBF and metabolism, recall that:

CPP = MAP − ICP

Normal CPP is about 80 to 85 mm Hg. Cerebral ischemia may occur if CPP falls below 50 mm Hg unless compensatory mechanisms come into play. One such important mechanism is the Cushing response. When the ICP rises and the CPP falls to a critical level, the resulting cerebral hypoxia triggers lower brainstem centers to increase systemic arterial pressure. When ICP continues to rise in the face of a maximal Cushing response, CPP may fall to a point where CBF ceases. Oxygen and glucose metabolism ceases, and brain death occurs.

Head Trauma

With trauma, CBF may increase, decrease, or remain the same. Clinical outcome may, with certain limitations, be determined by the CBF response [44]. Results of CBF measurements in head trauma patients show some distinct patterns. In one group CBF is high despite normal metabolic demand, indicating luxury perfusion or the hyperperfusion syndrome. Here, elevated CPP may induce vasogenic edema and ICP may rise because of increased CBV and diffuse vasogenic brain swelling. This situation tends to occur in children [45]. Another group of patients have reduced CBF; here there is correlation between CBF and CMRO$_2$, indicating intact metabolic regulation. The clinical course usually parallels the change in CBF. If CBF continues to fall, outcome is poor. Normal CBF usually but not always indicates a favorable outcome. Long-term follow-up of severely brain-injured patients characteristically shows low CBF and CMRO$_2$ values [45].

References

1. Astrup J., Siesjö B. K., Symon L. Thresholds in cerebral ischemia. The ischemic penumbra. *Stroke* 12:723, 1981.
2. Hossmann K-A., Zimmerman V. Resuscitation of brain after one hour of complete ischemia. I. Physiological and morphological observations. *Brain Res.* 81:59, 1974.
3. Bayliss W. M. On the local reaction of the arterial wall to changes of internal pressure. *J. Physiol.* (London) 28:220, 1902.
4. Edvinsson L., Owman C. Pharmacological characteristics of adrenergic α- and β-receptors mediating the vasomotor responses of cerebral arteries in vitro. *Circ. Res.* 35:835, 1974.
5. Hara H., Hamill G. S., Jacowitz D. M. Origin of cholinergic nerves to the rat major arteries: Coexistence with vasoactive intestinal polypeptide. Brain Res. Bull. 14:179, 1985.
6. Suzuki Y., McMaster D., Lederis K., et al. Characterization of the relaxant effects of vasoactive intestinal peptide (VIP) and PHI on isolated brain arteries. *Brain Res.* 322:9, 1984.
7. McCulloch J., Uddman R., Kingman T. A., et al. Calcitonin gene-related peptide: Functional role in cerebrovascular regulation. *Proc. Natl. Acad. Sci. USA* 83:5731, 1986.
8. Kobayashi S., Waltz A. G., Rhoton A. L. Effects of stimulation of cervical sympathetic nerves on cortical blood flow and vascular reactivity. *Neurology* 21:297, 1971.
9. Salanga V. D., Waltz A. G. Regional cerebral blood flow during stimulation of seventh cranial nerve. *Stroke* 4:213, 1973.
10. Sokoloff L. Influence of functional activity on local cerebral glucose utilization. In Ingvar D. H., Lassen N. A. (eds.). *Brain Work: The Coupling of*

Function, Metabolism and Blood Flow in the Brain. Copenhagen: Munksgaard, 1977. Pp. 385–398.

11. Siesjö B. K. Cerebral circulation and metabolism. *J. Neurosurg.* 60:883, 1984.
12. Sokoloff L. The action of drugs on the cerebral circulation. *Pharmacol. Rev.* 11:1, 1959.
13. Siesjö B. K., Berntman L., Rehncrona S. Effect of hypoxia on blood flow and metabolic influx in the brain. *Adv. Neurol.* 26:267, 1978.
14. Kogure K., Scheinberg P., Reinmuth O. M., et al. Mechanisms of cerebral vasodilatation in hypoxia. *J. Appl. Physiol.* 28:223, 1970.
15. Winn H. R., Rubio G. R., Berne R. M. The role of adenosine in the regulation of cerebral blood flow. *J. Cereb. Blood Flow Metab.* 1:239, 1981.
16. Fenton R. A., Bruttig S. P., Rubio G. R., et al. Effect of adenosine on calcium uptake by intact and cultured vascular smooth muscle. *Am. J. Physiol.* 242:H797, 1982.
17. Strand T., Asplund K., Eriksson S., et al. A randomized control trial of hemodilution in acute ischemic stroke. *Stroke* 15:980, 1984.
18. Kee D. B. Jr., Wood J. H. Rheology of the cerebral circulation. *Neurosurgery* 15:125, 1984.
19. Minderhoud J. M. *Cerebral Blood Flow: Basic Knowledge and Clinical Implications.* Amsterdam: Excerpta Medica, 1981.
20. Trojaborg W., Boysen G. Relationship between EEG, regional cerebral blood flow and internal carotid artery pressure during carotid endarterectomy. *Electroenceph. Clin. Neurophysiol.* 34:61, 1973.
21. Sundt T. M., Sharbrough P. W., Anderson R., et al. Cerebral blood flow measurements and electroencephalograms during carotid endarterectomy. *J. Neurosurg.* 41:310, 1974.
22. Branston N. M., Symon L., Crockard H. A., et al. Relationship between the cortical evoked potential and local cortical blood flow following acute middle cerebral artery occlusion in the baboon. *Exp. Neurol.* 45:195, 1974.
23. Lassen N. A. The luxury perfusion syndrome and its possible relation to acute metabolic acidosis localized within the brain. *Lancet* 2:1113, 1966.
24. Olsen T. S., Larsen B., Skriver E. B., et al. Focal cerebral hyperemia in acute stroke. *Stroke* 12:598, 1981.
25. Symon L. The concept of intracerebral steal. *Int. Anesth. Clin.* 7:597, 1969.
26. Spetzler R. F., Wilson C. B., Weinstein P., et al. Normal perfusion pressure breakthrough theory. *Clin. Neurosurg.* 25:651, 1978.
27. Enevoldsen E. M., Jensen F. T. Autoregulation and CO_2 response of cerebral blood flow in patients with acute severe head injury. J. Neurosurg. 48:689, 1978.
28. Miller J. D., Garibi J., North J. B., et al. Effects of increased arterial pressure on blood flow in the damaged brain. *J. Neurol. Neurosurg. Psychiatry* 38:657, 1975.
29. Overgaard J., Tweed W. A. Cerebral circulation after head injury. I. Cerebral blood flow and its regulation after closed head injury with emphasis on clinical correlations. *J. Neurosurg.* 41:531, 1974.
30. Durward Q. J., Del Maestro R. F., Amacher A. L., et al. The influence of systemic arterial pressure and intracranial pressure in the development of cerebral vasogenic edema. *J. Neurosurg.* 59:803, 1983.
31. Hertz L. Features of astrocyte function apparently involved in the response of the central nervous system to ischemia-hypoxia. *J. Cereb. Blood Flow Metab.* 1:143, 1981.
32. Fridovich I. The biology of oxygen radicals. *Science* 201:875, 1978.
33. Simon R. P., Swan J. H., Griffiths T., et al. Blockade of N-methyl-D-aspartate

receptors may protect against ischemic damage in the brain. *Science* 226:850, 1984.
34. Nornes H., Magnaes B. Intracranial pressure in patients with ruptured saccular aneurysm. *J. Neurosurg.* 36:537, 1982.
35. Voldby B., Enevoldsen E. M. Intracranial pressure changes following aneurysm rupture. I. Clinical and angiographic correlations. *J. Neurosurg.* 56:186, 1982.
36. Voldby B., Enevoldsen E. M. Regional cerebral blood flow, intraventricular pressure and cerebral metabolism in patients with ruptured intracranial aneurysm. *J. Neurosurg.* 62:48, 1985.
37. Grubb R. L., Raichle M. E., Eichling J. O., et al. Effects of subarachnoid hemorrhage on cerebral blood volume, blood flow and oxygen utilization in humans. *J. Neurosurg.* 46:446, 1977.
38. Voldby B., Enevoldsen E. M. Intracranial pressure changes followng aneurysm rupture. II. Associated cerebrospinal fluid acidosis. *J. Neurosurg.* 56:197, 1982.
39. Penn R. D., Kurtz D. Cerebral edema, mass effects and regional blood volume in man. *J. Neurosurg.* 46:282, 1977.
40. Endo H., Larsen B., Lassen N. A. Regional cerebral blood flow alterations remote from the site of intracranial tumors. *J. Neurosurg.* 46:271, 1971.
41. Enevoldsen E. M. Autoregulation of cerebral blood flow in patients with malignant hypertension and hypertensive encephalopathy. *Acta Med. Scand.* (Suppl.) 678:43, 1983.
42. Fein J. M. Hypertension and the central nervous system. *Clin. Neurosurg.* 29:666, 1982.
43. Yamamoto M., Meyer J. S., Sakai F., et al. Aging and cerebral vasodilator responses to hypercarbia. *Arch. Neurol.* 37:489, 1970.
44. Bruce D. A., Raphaely R. C., Goldberg A. I., et al. Pathophysiology, treatment and outcome following severe head injury in children. *Childs Brain* 5:174, 1979.
45. Obrist W. D., Gennarelli T. A., Segawa H., et al. Relation of cerebral blood flow to neurological status and outcome in head injured patients. *J. Neurosurg.* 51:292, 1979.

Suggested Readings

Bes, A., Braquet P., Paoletti R., et al. (eds.). Cerebral ischemia. *Proceedings of the Third International Symposium on Cerebral Circulation* (Toulouse, France, 1983). Amsterdam: Excerpta Medica, 1984.
Hartmann A., Hoyer S. (eds.). Cerebral blood flow and metabolism measurement. *Proceedings of the International Symposium on Cerbral Blood Flow and Metabolism Measurement in Man* (Heidelberg, Germany, 1983) Berlin: Springer-Verlag, 1985.
Hartmann A., Kuschinsky W. (eds.). Cerebral ischemia and hemorheology. *Proceedings of the International Symposium on Cerebral Ischemia and Hemorrheology* (Germany, 1987). Berlin: Springer-Verlag, 1987.
Minderhoud J. M. *Cerebral Blood Flow: Basic Knowledge and Clinical Implications.* Amsterdam: Excerpta Medica, 1981.
Raichle M. E. The pathophysiology of brain ischemia. *Ann. Neurol.* 13:2, 1983.
Siesjö B. K. *Brain Energy Metabolism.* New York: John Wiley & Sons, 1978.
Wood J. H. *Cerebral Blood Flow: Physiologic and Clinical Aspects.* New York: McGraw-Hill, 1987.

2. Intracranial Pressure

The intracranial pressure (ICP) is determined by the volume of blood, cerebrospinal fluid (CSF), and brain tissue within the intracranial space and is referenced to atmospheric pressure. The skull is a rigid, fixed-volume container. Intracranial volume (ICV) may range between 1000 and 1600 ml. Normal ICV constituents include brain tissue (cellular volume), 70 percent; CSF and extravascular water, 23 to 25 percent; and blood, 5 to 7 percent. Of these constituents, the cerebral blood volume (CBV) is the most easily and rapidly altered.

Physical Properties

The adult brain weighs 1.3 to 1.5 kg and is about 70 to 80 percent water. The brain is at once *elastic* and *plastic.* An elastic substance resists deformation from stress and returns to its original shape and position when the stress is removed; a plastic substance is easily deformed and does not regain its original shape. The brain may react in either fashion depending on the nature and duration of the underlying stress.

Intracranial blood volume resides mostly within the venous sinuses, venules, and cerebral veins. Intracranial blood volume is about 2 to 4 ml/100 gm of brain tissue, with higher values in the gray than in the white matter. CSF is distributed between the ventricles and the subarachnoid spaces.

Intracranial Compartments

The intracranial space is divided into the *supratentorial* (anterior and middle fossae) and *infratentorial* (posterior fossa) compartments by the tentorium cerebelli. The supratentorial compartment is separated incompletely into right and left compartments by the falx cerebri. The posterior fossa communicates with the spinal canal at the foramen magnum and with the supratentorial space at the tentorial incisura. The brain is a compliant substance with a limited capacity for movement within and between the various compartments.

The term *compartmentalization* refers to a relative lack of communication between compartments, usually due to obstruction of CSF flow; this may lead to pressure gradients and shifts of brain tissue.

Mechanics of Intracranial Pressure

The *Monro-Kellie doctrine* [1, 2] identified two components in the cranium that were considered noncompressible—brain and blood. The skull was seen as a rigid, fixed-volume container, and any change in one of the components was offset by a reciprocal change in another. This the-

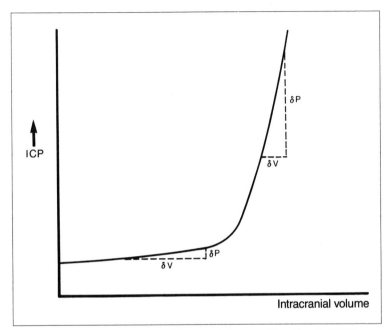

Fig. 2-1. Pressure/volume curve of intracranial space. The slope is δP/δV. Note difference in the slope on the left side compared with the right side of the curve.

ory was later modified by Burrows [3] to include CSF as a component. The concept can be expressed mathematically as [4]:

$$V_{brain} + V_{blood} + V_{CSF} + V_{lesion} = V_{intracranium}$$

An increase in the volume of one constituent can be balanced by a decrease in that of another, at least temporarily. CSF and blood are the principal spatial buffers in the intracranial space. Translocation of CSF or blood and brain tissue shifts make it possible for a lesion to expand. However, if expansion is unlimited or rapid, compensatory mechanisms may fail, resulting in intracranial hypertension.

This relationship is expressed in the *pressure-volume (P/V) curve* of the intracranial contents (Fig. 2-1), expounded ably by Langfitt et al. [5–7]. The curve is hyperbolic. Initially the slope is almost horizontal, but it becomes progressively steep as volume increases.

Elastance

Elastance, a measure of the brain's *stiffness* or *rigidity*, is expressed as:

$$Elastance = \frac{\delta P}{\delta V}$$

Normally, elastance is low. In the initial segment of the curve (see Fig. 2-1), the slope $\delta P/\delta V$ (elastance) is small. The steep part of the curve shows large increases of ICP in response to small increments in volume. This situation represents a failure of intracranial adaptive responses, resulting in exponential rises in $\delta P/\delta V$. Elastance can be assessed by the *volume-pressure relationship (VPR)*.

Compliance

Compliance is the reciprocal of elastance. It is defined as:

$$\text{Compliance} = \frac{\delta V}{\delta P}$$

Normally, compliance is high, allowing for volume increments without necessarily elevating intracranial pressure.

Effect of Time

Adaptations in CSF volume and CBV to accommodate an expanding intracranial lesion are more efficient with a slowly expanding lesion than with one that is expanding rapidly.

A family of P/V curves can be constructed to demonstrate the effect of time on the evolution of intracranial hypertension. Figure 2-2 graphically illustrates the urgency of different clinical neurosurgical conditions. A rapidly expanding epidural hematoma from a bleeding middle meningeal artery approximates curve t, while a slowly growing meningioma more closely resembles curve 4t. Urgency of treatment depends on such relationships. An epidural hematoma usually requires immediate attention because of rapidly increasing intracranial pressure. A meningioma may be managed electively in the majority of cases.

Location

The location of a mass lesion is of major import in determining its effect on ICP. A critically positioned mass may obstruct CSF pathways but only contribute a small amount to ICV. The effect on ICP is then magnified by obstructive hydrocephalus. A colloid cyst of the third ventricle is a good example.

The effects on ICP of adding equivalent amounts of volume to the epidural or CSF space further illustrate the point. Volume increments in the epidural space incite greater elevations in ICP than do equal increments into the ventricles [8]. Thus a single P/V curve does not apply to the entire intracranial space.

Intracranial Hypertension

Etiology

Pathologic elevations of ICP may occur in association with a vast number of intracranial events and derangements. In general, one or more of the following situations may arise:

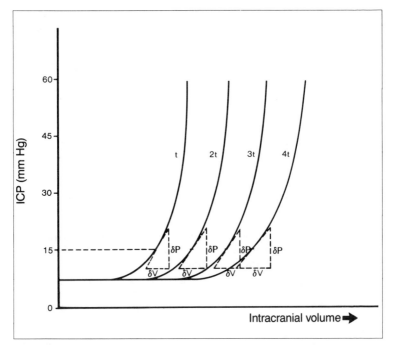

Fig. 2-2. Pressure/volume curves showing the influence of time on the evolution of intracranial pressure. At a given point on the curve the slope shows the progression t > 2t > 3t > 4t. t is a rapidly expanding mass, with 4t being the slowest.

1. Uncompensated additional focal mass in the intracranial space that slowly or rapidly exceeds a critical volume; tumors or intraparenchymal hemorrhages are good examples.
2. Cellular swelling exceeding the buffering capacity of the intracranial space; examples here include the cytotoxic edema of metabolic encephalopathies, hypoxia and infarction, trauma, and meningoencephalitides.
3. Extracellular edema may occur with infection, trauma, pseudotumor cerebri, subarachnoid hemorrhage, vasculitides, and hyperthermia.
4. Uncompensated expansions in intracranial blood volume; examples are states of hyperfusion, hypercapnia, volatile anesthetics, and obstructed venous outflow [9].

Sudden short-lived spikes of ICP occur naturally with Valsalva's maneuvers such as coughing or straining, and in pathologic states the hysteresis curve is prolonged. A slow, low-amplitude rise in ICP occurs during sleep; with rapid eye movement (REM) episodes, ICP usually increases by a few mm Hg [10]. Only in patients with borderline ICP-buffering capacity are such events likely to precipitate a crisis.

Clinical Signs

The warning signs of increasing ICP include a decreasing level of consciousness, restlessness and agitation, papilledema, vomiting, cranial nerve palsies (commonly third and sixth), focal paresis, decerebrate-decorticate posturing, and the Cushing response. Once abnormal posturing occurs, the patient is usually on the steep part of the P/V curve, necessitating immediate measures to reduce ICP and increase intracranial compliance.

Effects

Mortality from sustained ICP elevation in one study of head injury was estimated at 100 percent for patients with ICP over 60 mm Hg, 74 percent in those with ICP exceeding 40 mm Hg, and 45 percent for those with ICP between 20 and 40 mm Hg [11].

Cerebral Blood Flow

Recall the relationship (in Chap. 1):

$$CPP = MAP - ICP$$

where CPP is the cerebral perfusion pressure and MAP is the mean systemic arterial pressure.

And:

$$CBF = \frac{MAP - ICP}{CVR}$$

It is clear that any increase in ICP will tend to reduce CPP and the driving force of CBF. This may ultimately affect the critical supply of oxygen and nutrients to the brain (Fig. 2-3). Autoregulation adjusts for the shortfall in CPP until the lower limit is reached. When ICP exceeds 40 mm Hg or CPP is less than 50 mm Hg, CBF begins to fall precipitously [12]. Continuous monitoring of MAP by arterial line and ICP allows CPP to be determined.

Cerebrospinal Fluid Turnover

The rate of formation of CSF remains constant over a wide range of ICP. Only when ICP curtails blood flow to the choroid plexi does the rate of production significantly diminish [13]. The absorption rate of CSF rises in concert with intracranial hypertension. The relationship appears to be exponential as long as the CSF pathways remain open.

Electrical Activity

When ICP exceeds 40 mm Hg, brain electrical dysfunction frequently becomes depressed [14]. It is likely that neurophysiologic dysfunction

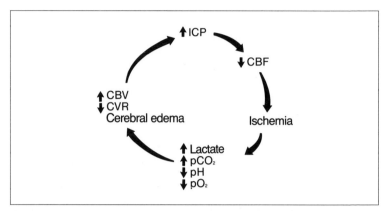

Fig. 2-3. Cycle of interdependence of cerebral blood flow (CBF), metabolism, and intracranial pressure (ICP). CVR, cerebral vascular resistance; CBV, cerebral blood volume.

in intracranial hypertension is related to changes in regional cerebral blood flow (rCBF).

Herniation Syndromes

As focal lesions within the cranial cavity expand, they displace adjacent structures, resulting in well-known herniation syndromes. Brain herniation can initiate vascular and obstructive complications that may aggravate the original expanding lesion and convert a potentially reversible problem into an irreversible one.

Subfalcine (cingulate) herniation occurs when an expanding hemisphere shifts, forcing the cingulate gyrus under the falx cerebri, compressing and displacing the anterior cerebral artery and internal cerebral vein.

Transtentorial herniation of the medial temporal lobe over the tentorial edge causes an impaired level of consciousness, dilatation of the ipsilateral pupil (from compression of the third cranial nerve), contralateral (usually) hemiparesis, or decerebrate posturing. It almost always produces ipsilateral third nerve compression, making pupillary dilatation a frequently reliable localizer of a mass in the ipsilateral hemisphere. Whether the ipsilateral cerebral peduncle becomes compressed (contralateral hemiparesis) before the contralateral peduncle gets jammed into the opposite tentorial edge (ipsilateral hemiparesis) depends on the size of the incisura. During transtentorial herniation up to 30 to 40 percent of patients who develop a hemiparesis will do so ipsilateral to the pathologic condition. Hemiparesis as an indicator of laterality may therefore be a false localizing sign.

Central transtentorial herniation refers to central and downward displacement of the brainstem and basal ganglia, with rostrocaudal compression through the tentorial notch. This type of herniation occurs mainly in response to bihemispheric disease or extracerebral lesions at or near the vertex. Both uncal and central transtentorial herniation may induce occlusion of the posterior cerebral artery, with resultant occipital infarction and swelling.

Tonsillar herniation of the cerebellar tonsils through the foramen magnum results in early symptoms of headache and neck pain and signs of meningeal irritation. Late features include signs of medullary dysfunction, e.g., hypertension, bradycardia, and apnea. Tonsillar herniation is generally the result of an expanding lesion within the posterior fossa. Posterior fossa lesions may cause upward herniation through the tentorial opening.

Cardiorespiratory Effects

Neurosurgeons have been aware of cardiorespiratory responses to intracranial hypertension since the late 1800s [15]. Cushing, at the turn of this century, popularized the concept in his triad of signs: systemic arterial hypertension, bradycardia, and respiratory irregularities [16, 17].

There is evidence that compression or other interference with a region of the medulla is responsible for these cardiorespiratory signs. The Cushing response is triggered earlier by mass lesions producing kinking, distortion, or compression of the brainstem (which may occur at a relatively low ICP elevation) than by lesions causing a more diffuse rise in ICP.

The response in the latter tends to be delayed until the ICP equals or exceeds the diastolic blood pressure. With diffuse traumatic edema, the Cushing response is frequently an agonal event. The increased blood pressure is secondary to increased sympathetic drive, leading to peripheral vasoconstriction and increased cardiac output.

Respiratory irregularities include Cheyne-Stokes respiration, hyperventilation, and ataxic and apneustic ventilation. Neurogenic pulmonary edema (NPE), or noncardiogenic pulmonary edema can occur from increased ICP. It is frequently seen in patients with severe head injury and poor-grade subarachnoid hemorrhage. The underlying mechanism is probably an intense alpha-adrenergic discharge involving both the pulmonary and systemic circuits. Severe vasoconstriction causes shunting of blood from the high-resistance systemic circulation to the relatively low-resistance pulmonary circuit, resulting in elevation of hydrostatic pressure and pulmonary edema [18].

Gastrointestinal Effects

Gastric erosions or ulcers as described by Cushing [19] may occur with intracranial hypertension. Prophylaxis is important to reduce morbidity.

Oral antacids or H_2-receptor antagonists taken on a regular regimen are recommended.

Intracranial Pressure Monitoring

Are the undesirable neurologic effects of intracranial hypertension due to the elevation of ICP per se, or are they due to its effect on CBF and cerebral metabolism? An even more provoking question is whether raised ICP is directly related to a poor outcome. Miller found that in head-injured patients at least, a major cause of mortality was uncontrollable intracranial hypertension [20]. It is axiomatic that elevated ICP can only be addressed if one knows it is elevated. This line of reasoning prompted the evolution of ICP monitoring.

Several techniques have been described for monitoring ICP [21]. Since a comprehensive register is outside the scope of this book, only some of the more important will be discussed. The ideal method should be (1) minimally invasive; (2) easy to use, and reasonably priced; have a low risk of infection; and (3) provide dependable data. Currently used devices include the subarachnoid bolt, ventricular catheter, subdural catheters, epidural transducers-sensors, and fully implantable transducers (telemetric devices). Each has its advantages and disadvantages. The use of each technique carries some risk, which must be weighed against the potential benefit.

Lundberg's pioneering work led to the wide acceptance of ICP monitoring as a useful tool in neurosurgical practice [22]. He studied various waveforms and their clinical correlates using a ventricular catheter for continuous pressure monitoring. Following his publication, more ICP monitoring devices have been studied, and more data have accumulated regarding ICP.

The relative benefits of ICP monitoring are still debated. Although it is difficult to show that this practice has significantly affected patient outcome in large series, there is little doubt that certain patients benefit from its use.

Indications

Neurosurgeons differ in their indications for ICP monitoring. Some instances in which it may be employed include the following:

1. *Head injury.* Severe closed head injury in which the patient is comatose, or less severe head injury in which the patient harbors an intracerebral hematoma and direct surgical attack should be avoided. With coexisting multiple trauma (chest and abdominal), there is frequently a sustained need for assisted ventilation. Muscle relaxants and narcotics for sedation or analgesia may also be necessary. In this situation two valuable indexes of clinical neurologic status—level of consciousness and pupillary response—are ob-

scured. Under these circumstances ICP monitoring can be a valuable parameter, alerting the neurosurgeon to incipient clinical deterioration.

2. *Intracerebral hemorrhage.* Especially if the clot is large but a nonsurgical approach has been elected because the clot is located deep in the brain or in eloquent cortex.
3. *Neoplasm.* Particularly if intracranial compliance is impaired.
4. *Cerebral edema.*
5. *Metabolic encephalopathy.* Liver failure secondary to hepatitis or Reye-Johnson syndrome [23].
6. *Anoxic brain injury.* Secondary to cardiac arrest or near-drowning [24].
7. *Subarachnoid hemorrhage.*
8. *Postoperative craniotomy patients* [25].
9. *Encephalitis.*
10. *Pseudotumor cerebri* (benign intracranial hypertension).

In all these situations the rationale is to measure ICP so that therapy can be tailored accordingly.

Procedures

Virtually all ICP devices can be inserted with the patient supine, brow up, in neutral head alignment. The incision and burr hole are made at least 2 cm anterior to the coronal suture and 2.5 to 3 cm lateral to the sagittal suture. The foramen of Monro is a common reference point for zeroing the external transducer. Various devices and procedures are described below.

Intraventricular Catheter. The intraventricular catheter (IVC) is usually placed in the nondominant lateral ventricle by a frontal-twist drill hole, and ICP is measured by connecting the catheter to a fluid-filled tubing and pressure transducer. The waveform is displayed on the oscilloscope, and hard copies are obtainable on a strip recorder.

Because the IVC dwells in a naturally fluid-filled space, the quality of the recording is high and rapid changes in pressure are readily detectable. Particular indications for ICP monitoring with the IVC include acute hydrocephalus or any situation where it is desirable to remove CSF to control ICP (Table 2-1).

Equipment. Most units provide "ICP trays" containing the following:
1. Sterile towels, gown, and gloves
2. 70% alcohol or povidone-iodine solution
3. 5-ml syringe with 22-gauge × 1½-in. needle
4. 5-ml 1% lidocaine with 1:100,000 epinephrine solution
5. $\frac{9}{64}$-in. twist drill
6. Small curet
7. Silastic ventricular catheter with fitted stylet
8. Three-way stopcock

Table 2-1. Intraventricular Catheter

Advantages	Disadvantages
Allows for drainage of CSF and control of ICP.	Risk of infection
CSF analysis for lactic acid, enzymes, amines, and so on	Technically difficult if ventricles are displaced or small
Volume/pressure response determinations	Risk of brain injury or hemorrhage
High-quality recordings	

  9. Drainage bag and pressure tubing system with transducer assembly
10. Sterile 0.9% NaCl solution (preservative-free)
11. No. 10 and no. 11 scalpel
12. 3-0 nylon suture on curved cutting needle and scissors
13. Needle holder
14. Periosteal elevator
15. Self-retaining Weitlander retractor

The ventricular catheter is made of radiopaque Silastic and has 5-cm markings from the tip. It usually comes with a fitted stylet and a trocar for subcutaneous tunneling.

The drainage system should be equipped with vinyl tubing, clamps, three-way stopcocks, luer lockport for monitoring, and a latex injection-sampling site. There should be a drip chamber with antireflux valve, sterile atmospheric vent, and antimicrobial filter. The drip chamber empties into a graduated collection bag.

A fiberoptic transducer-tipped catheter may be used with the IVC. This device obtains pressure readings at the "source" and does not require leveling because there is no external transducer. A major advantage of this device is that very precise ICP readings can be made while allowing for continuous CSF drainage. The fiberoptic cable can be connected to a digital pressure monitor that provides a constant display of mean ICP or can provide output to other monitors to obtain an oscilloscope display or hard-copy readout (Camino OLM Ventricular Bolt Pressure Monitoring Kit, model 110-4H, Camino Labs, San Diego, CA 92121).

Procedure. The step-by-step procedure is as follows:
1. Generally, the right frontal area is used. Some surgeons prefer to place the monitor over the pathologic hemisphere. Shave a generous area of right frontal scalp, first with an electric clipper and then with a razor.
2. Prepare scalp with 70% alcohol or povidone-iodine solution.
3. Drape with sterile towels.
4. Infiltrate scalp with 1% lidocaine with 1:100,000 epinephrine solution at a point 3 cm anterior to the coronal suture and 3 cm lateral to the midline.

5. Make a 2.0- to 2.5-cm linear parasagittal incision through the full thickness of the scalp to the bone.
6. Loosen the pericranium with a periosteal elevator and place a self-retaining retractor in the incision.
7. Make a twist drill hole.
8. Flush out bone debris with sterile saline irrigation.
9. Make a cruciate incision in the dura with a no. 11 scalpel, taking care not to injure the underlying brain or blood vessels.
10. Free hand technique is as follows: Direct the ventricular catheter with stylet toward the medial canthus of the ipsilateral eye downward in a coronal plane 2 cm anterior to the external auditory meatus. In this trajectory, enter the ventricle at a distance of about 5.0 to 5.5 cm from the skull surface. Feel for a characteristic "give" as the ependyma is traversed. Watch for the egress of one or two drops of CSF from the end of the catheter, and then immediately pinch off the lumen between the thumb and index finger to prevent excess CSF leakage.
11. Inserting a ventricular catheter using the Ghajar guide [26]. The Ghajar guide (Sparta Instrument Corp, Hayward CA 94545) is a rigid pyramidal structure composed of a hollow tube on an equilateral tripod (Fig. 2-4B). It is placed over a burr hole to guide the ventricular catheter in a path perpendicular to the skull surface. Because the contour of the lateral ventricle parallels that of the skull, a catheter passed at right angles to the skull will enter the ventricle in a similar trajectory. The central tube of the guide comes in three sizes, so select the ventricular catheter appropriately to ensure a smooth passage. Hold the ventricular catheter in one hand while steadying the guide over the twist drill hole with the other. Proceed to cannulate the ventricle. Usually at a depth of 5.0 to 5.5 cm a slight "give" is felt and the ventricle is entered. Grasp the catheter through the base of the guide with forceps to prevent dislodgment, then lift guide and stylet in one motion (Fig. 2-4A). The guide provides more accuracy over the free-hand technique, particularly for the less experienced operator.
12. The catheter is brought out through a separate stab wound, 2.5 cm posterior to the incision in a subgaleal tunnel, with a trocar or curved hemostat. If doubt exists regarding catheter location, inject 5 ml of air into the ventricle for contrast and obtain anteroposterior and lateral skull films to confirm catheter placement within the ventricular system. Remember that air injected into a ventricle may expand due to heat absorption. There should be an exchange of fluid for air to prevent a sudden increase in ICP, especially when intracranial compliance is low.
13. The catheter is attached to a leur hub and secured with 3-0 nylon suture. The pressure tubing is connected to one port of the three-way stopcock, and the drainage tubing, reservoir, and bag for CSF collection are connected to the other port. The third port connects to the hub of the ventricular catheter. All connections are luerlock (Fig. 2-5). Ensure that all air bubbles are flushed out of the system.

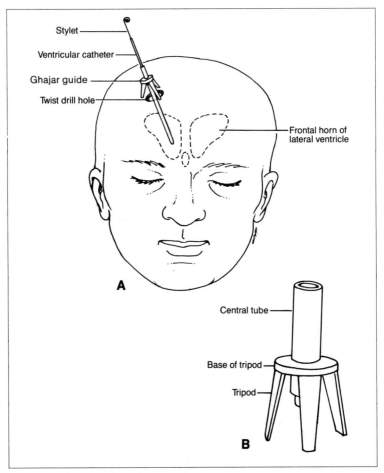

Fig. 2-4. Use of Ghajar guide for ventricular cannulation. A. Placement of guide and passage of ventricular catheter. B. Ghajar guide.

14. Inability to tap the ventricle: occasionally one is unable to enter the ventricle at the first pass. Remove the stylet and slowly withdraw the catheter. *Never redirect* the catheter with stylet while still within brain tissue, since this will almost certainly cause parenchymal injury. Reconnoiter the landmarks and try again. An aggressive attempt at catheter placement after two consecutive misses is misdirected zeal. Ask a senior colleague for assistance.
15. The transducer is zeroed to the level of the foramen of Monro.
16. Set the drip chamber to desired pressure level; position at the appropriate level (in millimeters of water) from the zero point (foramen

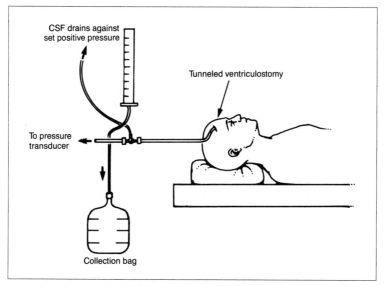

Fig. 2-5. ICP monitoring by intraventricular catheter. CSF, cerebrospinal fluid.

of Monro). This arrangement provides controlled drainage of CSF against positive pressure (i.e., CSF drains when ICP exceeds the set level) [27]. Continuous drainage is possible with recording of ICP through the transducer, although the waveform is somewhat dampened. This setup is desirable because it provides a ready avenue for decompression during episodes of sudden ICP elevations (see Fig. 2-5).
17. When monitoring is discontinued, remove the catheter and close the incision with 3-0 nylon suture.

Subarachnoid Bolt

The subarachnoid screw-bolt (Richmond bolt) has been described by Vries et al. [28]. It consists of a hollow screw inserted through a twist drill hole anterior to the coronal suture, usually over the nondominant hemisphere. The hollow screw, the tip of which sits in the subarachnoid space, is fluid-coupled to a transducer through pressure tubing (Table 2-2). A number of modifications of the original screw are on the market.
Equipment. In addition to those items listed on pp. 33–34, a ¼-in. twist drill and a Richmond bolt are needed. The subarachnoid bolt is a hollow, stainless-steel device with a luer lock connector on the distal end and threads for screwing into the skull on the proximal end. Several subarachnoid bolts are available on the market. They include:

1. The *Philly bolt* (Philadelphia Medical Specialities. Inc., Laurel

Table 2-2. Subarachnoid Bolt

Advantages	Disadvantages
Inexpensive	Risk of infection
Relatively easy to install and less invasive than the intraventricular catheter	Easily clogged with blood clot or brain tissue, and may therefore be unreliable
Can be used regardless of ventricular size or anatomy	CSF cannot be drained in useful quantities

Springs, NJ 08021). This bolt is available in two designs—one with the traditional screw threads and the other with an expanding tip (Kel-F tip) made of plastic, which fits snugly into the outer table of the skull and retains its position by friction. The Kel-F tip is especially suited to infants and children with thin skulls.

2. The *Codman ICP kit* (Codman & Shurtleff, Inc., Randolph, MA) features a user-friendly drill assembly in addition to the other items (Fig. 2-6).
3. The *Camino bolt* is a fiberoptic transducer-tipped catheter for use in the subarachnoid space (Camino OLM Intracranial Pressure Monitoring Kit, Model 110-4B, Camino Labs, San Diego, CA 92121). Subarachnoid pressure can be measured by inserting the transducer-tipped catheter approximately 4.5 cm into the Camino bolt.

The fiberoptic devices can monitor ICP from the subarachnoid space, ventricles (see page 35), or brain tissue itself. However, cost is an important consideration, especially if much monitoring is done.

Procedure. The step-by-step procedure for the subarachnoid bolt is as follows:

1. Follow steps 1 through 9 on pages 34–35.
2. Curet the dural leaves against the bone to ensure an adequate opening. The goal is to establish good communication between the subarachnoid space and the bolt.
3. Screw the bolt perpendicularly into the hole until secure; thread until the tip is 1 mm below the surface of the dura.
4. Suture scalp around the bolt.
5. Flush the bolt with sterile 0.9% NaCl to remove air and debris.
6. Connect the bolt to calibrated transducer system through the stopcock assembly and pressure tubing; flush the tubing and fill it with sterile saline to ensure uninterrupted fluid-coupled transduction.
7. Apply povidone-iodine ointment and dressings.
8. When monitoring is discontinued, remove the bolt and close the scalp with 3-0 nylon sutures.

Subdural Catheter

The subdural cup catheter (*Wilkinson cup catheter*) consists of a ribbonlike Silastic catheter with a central lumen. At the intracranial end

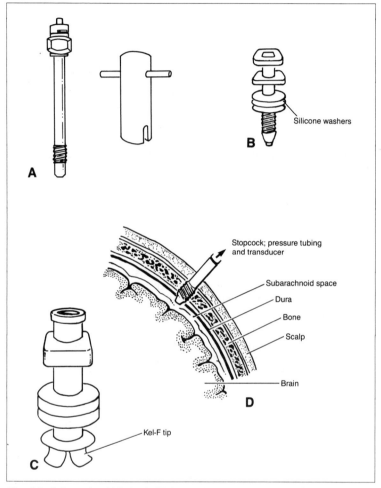

Fig. 2-6. Subarachnoid bolt. A. Richmond bolt and wrench. B. Codman ICP bolt. C. Philly bolt. D. Richmond bolt in situ.

the lumen communicates with a rectangular hole—the cup—on one side of the ribbon at its distal end [29]. It is also possible to monitor ICP with a Silastic intraventricular catheter [30, 31].

The catheter is placed in the subdural space and connected to a pressure transducer through fluid-filled tubing. It is specifically designed for postcraniotomy ICP monitoring but can be inserted through a burr hole without craniotomy.

Table 2-3. Subdural Catheter

Advantages	Disadvantages
Relatively simple and safe to place and remove	Risk of infection
	Fluid leakage and catheter elasticity predispose to artifacts and dampening
	Uncertain reliability

Table 2–3 lists the advantages and disadvantages of the subdural catheter.

Equipment. In addition to the items mentioned on pp. 33–34, either a Wilkinson cup catheter (Cordis Corporation, Miami, FL) [29] or a ventricular catheter, 35 cm by 2 mm, Silastic (Cordis Corp., Miami, FL) [30, 31] is required.

Procedure (Fig. 2-7). The subdural catheter is frequently used after craniotomy, in which case install it before the bone flap is replaced. Thread it horizontally underneath the bone edge so that it exits the bone flap through an established burr hole. The distal cup should be in contact with an area of surgically disrupted arachnoid. Then proceed to step 4 on this page. If the subdural catheter is used in another setting, proceed as follows:

1. Follow steps 1 through 9 on pp. 34–35.
2. Fill the catheter with sterile 0.9% NaCl; thread it carefully into the subdural space to a distance of about 4 cm. When it is in use, inject a small amount of fluid (0.1 to 0.3 ml of sterile 0.9% NaCl) at 2-hour intervals to replace leakage from the distal end.
3. Tunnel the catheter through a subgaleal tunnel to exit the scalp about 2.5 cm posterior to the burr hole site through a separate stab wound.
4. Attach a three-way stopcock and pressure tubing to the catheter; secure catheter to the scalp with 3-0 nylon suture.
5. Connect the tubing to a pressure transducer.
6. Use gentle traction to withdraw the catheter when monitoring is discontinued. Close the incision with 3-0 nylon suture.

Epidural Intracranial Pressure Monitoring

Epidural ICP monitoring is performed by inserting a device under the skull so that its diaphragm-sensor is applied to the dura. Epidural pressures have been shown to be a few mm Hg higher than intradural pressures.

Table 2-4 lists the advantage and disadvantages of epidural monitoring.

Equipment In addition to the items listed on pp. 33–34, the following items are necessary:

1. Hudson brace with perforator and 16-mm burr, or power drill.

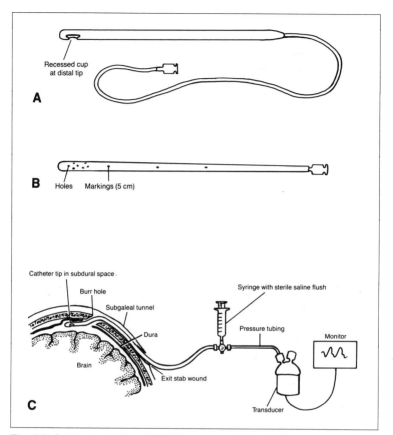

Fig. 2-7. Subdural catheter. A. Wilkinson cup catheter. B. Silastic intraventricular catheter. C. Subdural catheter in situ.

Table 2-4. Epidural Device

Advantages	Disadvantages
Least risk of infection, and if infection does occur, it is outside the meningeal barrier	CSF drainage not possible
Non-fluid-coupled system	Zero-drift may compromise reliability
Least risk of brain injury	Expensive and fragile

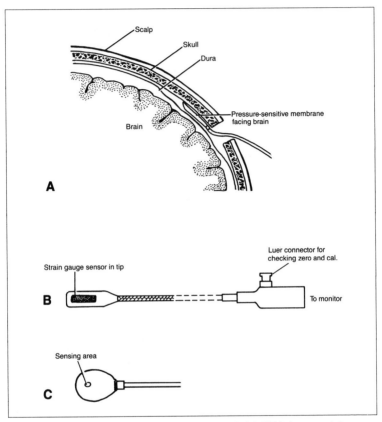

Fig. 2-8. Epidural device. A. Device in situ. B. Model ICT/b intracranial epidural catheter. C. Ladd sensor.

2. Kerrison rongeur.
3. Penfield dissector no. 3.
4. Epidural ICP device consisting of a sensor and monitoring unit. Two such devices in current use are discussed below (Fig. 2-8).

1. Ladd fiberoptic intracranial pressure monitor (Model M1000 Ladd Research Industries, Inc., Burlington, VT 05402). This device employs light to sense the position of a diaphragm that moves in response to external pressure and air. It calibrates pressure by an internal balancing mechanism [32]. The sensor connects to a dedicated monitor-control unit through a pressurized air column that contains three fiberoptic threads. The sensor is easily zeroed and measures a wide range of pressures. It provides a digital readout in 1-mm Hg increments and can be interfaced with a chart strip–chart recorder for continuous recording;

however, there is a small but definable lag in response to ICP fluctuations.

2. Model ICT/b Catheter tip pressure transducer (MMI Gaeltec, Hackensack, NJ 07601). This device [33] consists of a thin-film, strain-gauge pressure sensor at the end of a Silastic catheter with interval markings (Fig. 2-8). It is connected directly from the patient to a pressure monitor. Pressure deflects the sensing diaphragm. It has the advantage of in vivo zeroing capability and calibration, a maneuver accomplished in seconds by adding 0.2 to 0.3 ml of air in a small syringe through a luer lock side port. This raises a Silastic membrane off the transducer and applies equal pressure to both sides of the pressure-sensing diaphragm (zeroing). Calibration is accomplished by attaching a known pressure (mercury manometer) and adjusting the setting on the monitor accordingly. When in use, the luer port is left open to air for reference. It is easily disconnected from the patient for transportation and does not require reference leveling. The lack of fluid-coupling and the catheter's epidural location reduce the risk of infection.

Procedure (see Fig. 2-8). The step-by-step procedure for epidural ICP monitoring is as follows:
1. Follow steps 1 through 6 on pp. 34–35.
2. Place a 16-mm burr hole in the right frontal region. It may be necessary to enlarge it slightly with rongeurs.
3. Remove any overlying slivers of bone with a curet.
4. With a no. 3 Penfield dissector, strip the dura from the inner table for about 3 cm around the burr hole to provide enough room for the sensor to sit without a wedge effect, which may lead to wave dampening or artifactually high ICP readings.
5. Place the transducer in the epidural pocket created, taking care to avoid kinking or crushing it with grasping instruments. Place the device so that the sensing area is in contact with the dura but not indenting it; i.e., it should be coplanar or parallel with the dura, otherwise the dura will be stretched and the pressure recorded will be affected by dural compliance [34]. Ensure that all the active portion of the sensor lies under the bone.
6. Secure the device in place with a suture; apply a dressing.
7. Connect it to the monitor-console.

Patient Care During Intracranial Pressure Monitoring

1. With the IVC, frequent examinations of CSF for Gram's stain, cell count, and cultures are recommended. Withdraw samples from latex aspiration port using sterile technique. Use a 25-gauge × ½-in. needle to avoid lacerating the port. A small amount of CSF may be discarded before the sample is collected.
2. Some groups recommend prophylactic antistaphylococcal coverage while the ICP monitor is in situ. Note that in children, coexisting scalp intravenous infusion with ICP monitoring increases the risk of infection.

3. Monitor functional integrity of the system (CSF pulsations, CSF flow, digital readout). Ascertain that the monitor is on the correct scale. Air bubbles may enter the system and interrupt the fluid column of the IVC, subarachnoid bolt, or subdural catheter and cause inaccurate ICP values or dampened waveforms. They should be flushed out with sterile 0.9% NaCl after the appropriate stopcock adjustments have been made.

4. Set alarms at a suitable upper limit; assess the patient should the alarm trigger. Zeroing of the transducer should be checked as necessary, especially if head position has been altered.

5. Position the patient to avoid kinking of the catheter or tubing. The head may be elevated to 20 to 30 degrees. Children or agitated adults may need sedation or restraints to prevent their tampering with the system.

6. Maintain the relative position between the patient's head and the level of the transducer to ensure consistent data. (Fiberoptic or solid-state systems do not require such attention.)

7. Monitor the patient's vital signs and neurologic status frequently.

8. Inspect the incision site daily; check dressing for CSF leak.

9. Change collection system with IVC as frequently as necessary.

10. Clogging of the IVC, subarachnoid bolt, or subdural catheter, usually with clot or brain tissue, may interrupt monitoring. The device may be cleared by making the appropriate stopcock adjustments, preparing the irrigation port, and flushing with 0.1 to 0.3 ml of sterile 0.9% NaCl in a tuberculin syringe. With the subarachnoid bolt it may occasionally be necessary to reestablish good communication between it and the subarachnoid space.

11. Solid-state or fiber-optic sensors are easily detachable from their monitors, allowing for ease of patient care and transportation. Removal of the patient from the control unit will not disrupt the original calibration. These systems do not require flushing, irrigation, or transducer realignment and thus provide relatively trouble-free use.

Risks of Intracranial Pressure Monitoring

Infection. A review of the literature presents an incidence of infection (ventriculitis or meningitis) varying between 0 and 27 percent with ICP monitoring [35]. In one recent study ICP monitoring was associated with an 11 percent incidence of infection. Of the ICP monitors used, the subarachnoid bolt had the lowest infection rate (7.5%), followed by the subdural cup catheter (14.9%) and the ventricular catheter (21.9%). Regardless of the monitor used, infection was twice as likely in patients with open trauma or cerebral hemorrhage [35]. Similar results were reported by Mayhall et al. in their prospective study; ventriculitis or meningitis developed in 8.9 percent of patients who underwent ventriculostomy. Risk factors included intracerebral hemorrhage, ventricular catheterization for more than 5 days, irrigation of the system, neurosurgical operations, and ICP of 20 mm Hg or more. Based on these findings, they recommend a closed-drainage system, early removal of the catheter, and minimal irrigation [36].

Prophylactic antistaphylococcal coverage in the patient with a ventriculostomy has been advocated [37], and tunneling the catheter in a percutaneous or subgaleal tract has been reported to reduce the risk of infection [38].

When either the IVC or subarachnoid bolt (both fluid-coupled systems) are used, an infection is more likely to be serious because the meningeal barrier is no longer interposed. Epidural monitors have the advantage of dural protection, as the dura is a dependable barrier against infection when intact. This consideration has bearing on the choice of antibiotic therapy should an infection occur during ICP monitoring, since drugs that cross the blood-brain barrier may be necessary in some situations.

With all ICP monitoring systems, watch for fever, leukocytosis, and meningismus.

Hemorrhage–Brain Injury. Intracerebral hemorrhage is more likely with multiple passes of a ventricular catheter. An incidence of 1.4 percent has been reported [39].

False Data. Careful attention must be paid to the dependability of data acquisition. Clinical decisions based on false data may be potentially dangerous. Zeroing and calibration of transducers should be checked regularly, and fluid-coupled systems should remain patent and free of air bubbles or debris. Warning signs such as a dampened ICP waveform, or readings inconsistent with the clinical situation, should be promptly investigated.

Subdural Air. The solid-state catheter tip transducer (Model ICT/b; MMI Gaeltec, Hackensack, NJ 07601) has the useful capability for in vivo zero calibration by injecting air through a side port to distend the diaphragm and then releasing the air slowly. Pneumocephalus secondary to rupture of the diaphragm has been reported. The integrity of the membrane should be ascertained by the method described by Gentleman and Mendelow [40].

Pneumocephalus is also an infrequent complication of placement of a ventricular catheter.

Interpretation and Results

ICP is influenced by other variables such as CSF turnover, systemic arterial pressure, and central venous pressure. Therapeutic decisions should be made only after assessment of all parameters and with knowledge of the existing pathologic state.

Absolute Values of Intracranial Pressure. Normal mean ICP in the recumbent position ranges from 0 to 10 mm Hg. Many neurosurgeons accept an upper limit of 15 mm Hg as normal. In infants the upper limit may be as low as 5 mm Hg. There is substantial fluctuation with coughing, straining, and position.

Intracranial Pressure Waves. There are three varieties of ICP waves as described by Lundberg [22, 41]: A or plateau waves, B waves, and C waves.

Plateau waves occur against a backdrop of raised ICP (more than 20 mm Hg). They have an amplitude of 50 to 100 mm Hg and last 5 to 20 minutes (Fig. 2-9). The term *plateau wave* includes ramp waves and the original A wave of Lundberg [42]. They may occur spontaneously or can be evoked by patient manipulation.

These waves do not have a characteristic frequency, nor do they bear a consistent relationship to cardiorespiratory oscillations. During a series of plateau waves, both pulse amplitude and duration tend to increase, and a terminal wave may follow in which ICP rises to the level of systemic arterial pressure and CBF ceases. Pressure waves are due primarily to changes in CBV secondary to cerebral vasodilatation [42].

Another line of reasoning has been suggested by the work of Rosner et al. [43]. They conclude that plateau waves are induced by an acute fall in the CPP; cerebral perfusion pressures are known to be linearly related to compliance within the autoregulatory range [44, 45]. This implies that cerebral perfusion at the upper limits of autoregulation provides the brain with the maximum buffer against increases in ICP and suggests that a constant and adequate CPP is important in controlling ICP. The clinical implication is that maximal dehydration or head elevation in patients with elevated ICP may diminish blood pressure and CPP, and therefore induce plateau waves [46]. Patients receiving treatment for increased ICP should have central venous pressure (CVP) monitoring and adequate blood volume should be maintained.

Clinical correlates of plateau waves include headache, nausea, vomiting, altered level of consciousness, visual obscuration, pupillary abnormalities, decerebrate or decorticate posturing, systemic arterial hypertension, bradydysrhythmias, and respiratory changes. These waves are ominous; they indicate that compensatory adaptations are failing. Immediate therapeutic intervention is necessary (see the section on management of intracranial hypertension).

B waves have a frequency of 0.5 to 2 Hz and are associated with respirations (see Fig. 2-9). This relationship may be the result of a common brainstem rhythm that alters both respiratory pattern and cerebral vasomotor tone [41]. A significant number of head-injured patients with reduced intracranial compliance demonstrate a close association of B waves with sudden changes in pulmonary vascular compliance. In these patients, pulmonary artery diastolic pressure rises dramatically at the onset of a B wave [47].

C waves have a frequency of 4 to 8 Hz, and may be closely associated with the Traube-Hering-Mayer waves of blood pressure (see Fig. 2-9). Amplitude ranges from 0 to 20 mm Hg.

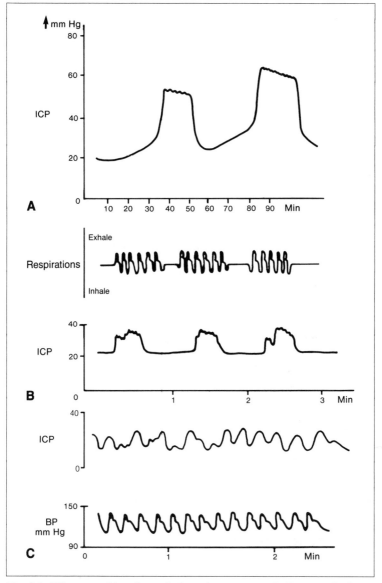

Fig. 2-9. ICP waves of Lundberg. A. A or plateau waves. B. B waves. C. C waves. BP, blood pressure.

A and high amplitude B waves indicate exhaustion of intracranial compensatory mechanisms and frequently antedate clinical deterioration. Low amplitude B and C waves are of lesser clinical significance and may occur in the normal ICP tracing.

Volume-Pressure Response. Miller et al. [48, 49] studied the pressure response following the injection of 1 ml of saline into the lateral ventricle through a ventricular catheter. This relationship is known as the VPR. Expressed in mm Hg/ml; it reflects the brain's elastance. Evaluation of the VPR is easily performed at bedside. An increase in ICP of more than 2 mm Hg following the injection of 1 ml of saline has been shown to be abnormal, indicating reduced intracranial compliance. A value greater than 4 mm Hg should make one suspect a mass lesion [49].

Determination of the VPR may increase the sensitivity of ICP monitoring, particularly in the setting of a normal ICP. An abnormal VPR means a greater value for δP/δV (elastance or "tightness" of the brain) and therefore reduced intracranial reserve.

Studies suggest that the VPR depends on baseline ICP, implying that the P/hr V curve is not of fixed configuration but rather of variable inflection depending on the prevailing situation (Fig. 2-10). The VPR does in fact increase with elevations in ICP, although at very high ICP the VPR decreases.

One clinical study suggests that changes in the VPR frequently antedate changes in mean ICP [50].

Intracranial Pressure Variation. The degree of fluctuation of a mean ICP indicates the amount of compensatory reserve in the intracranial compartment. The greater the variance of ICP, the more likely the system will decompensate [51]. In fact, patients exhibiting a high degree of ICP fluctuation are at risk of developing sustained mean ICP elevations. Thus, analysis of ICP variation, in addition to mean ICP, increases the clinical use of this data.

With elevated mean ICP, secondary increases in ICP (Valsalva's maneuver, agitation, endotracheal suctioning) will tend to be higher and be sustained longer because of the precarious position on the right side of the P/V curve.

Computer-based systems can track ICP variation and perform trend analysis. Simultaneous evaluation of other physiologic variables such as arterial pressure, central venous pressure, pulse rate, respiratory rate, and arterial blood gases can be integrated into the system [52].

Pulse-Pressure Waveform. Study of absolute ICP and the different waves cannot reliably predict future trends on the basis of ongoing events. Pulse-pressure waveform analysis provides additional data in this regard.

The normal ICP tracing is a pulsatile waveform due to arterial and respiratory influences. The integrated arterial pulse surge in the brain is the principal source of the ICP pulse, although still at issue is the exact locus of pulse transmission [53–55].

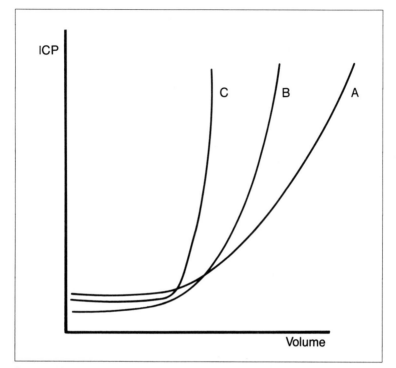

Fig. 2-10. Pressure/volume curves with alternate inflections. A. High degree of compensation. B. Intermediate degree of compensation. C. Precarious degree of compensation that can deteriorate quickly.

Mean ICP is derived from the diastolic pressure plus one-third of the pulse pressure:

$$\text{Mean ICP} = \text{Diastolic ICP} + \frac{\text{Systolic} - \text{Diastolic ICP}}{3}$$

The *intracranial pulse pressure* (*ICP-PP*) widens with increasing mean ICP. The relationship between ICP-PP and mean ICP is virtually linear at ICP values above baseline ICP [56].

The *ICP-PP waveform* (*ICP-PPW*) is composed of at least four peaks (P_1, P_2, P_3, P_4) and a notch (N) [57–59]. The shape of the wave is similar to the arterial pressure but is of smaller amplitude (Fig. 2-11). The origin of all but P_1 remains uncertain. The efficiency of pulse transmission from blood pressure to CSF pulse is influenced by two main factors [55, 60, 61]: elastance of the intracranial system, and cerebral vasomotor reactivity.

A major factor in cerebral elastance seems to be the status of cere-

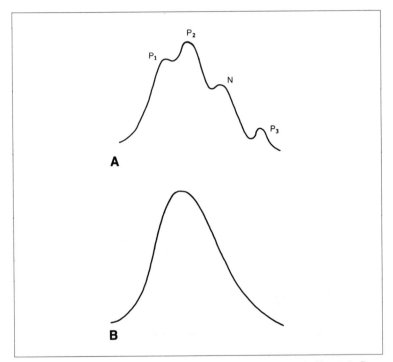

Fig. 2-11. ICP pulse waveform. A. Normal tracing. P_1–P_3, peak; N, notch. B. "Rounding" or "monotonous" tracing with loss of harmonics.

brovascular reactivity. When ICP rises, CPP tends to fall; autoregulation then induces a reduction in CVR (cerebral vasodilatation) to increase CBF.

With progressive cerebral vasodilatation, the transmission of arterial pressure to the brain is increased and the ICP-PPW shows increased amplitude and an arterial shape. This arterialization of the ICP-PPW is also known as "rounding" or "monotonous," since the basic frequency is accentuated while the other harmonics are diminished [58, 59, 62, 63]; thus the respiratory contribution to the ICP-PPW diminishes. A marked elevation of the ICP-PPW amplitude has been observed in raised ICP [64], probably due to altered cerebral elastance.

Morphologic analysis of ICP-PPW by visual inspection is simple but subjective and qualitative. *Spectral analysis* (breaking the complex wave into its component parts) is mathematical, objective, and quantitative [59]. The goal is to identify a point in the evolution of intracranial hypertension at which autoregulatory cerebral vasodilatation occurs before the events of cerebral ischemia are reached [59]. It is possible that therapeutic intervention at this time may be more beneficial.

Management

A rehearsed protocol is most effective in an ICP crisis, as follows:

1. Ensure first that the airway is patent and, if so, if the patient is ventilating. Obtain an arterial blood gas determination immediately.
2. Check vital signs and do a brief neurologic assessment.
3. Ensure that the head is in neutral alignment with the neck.
4. Ensure that the transducer is in the correct position. Level it appropriately and check recordings.
5. Obtain serum electrolyte and osmolality levels.
6. Institute medical therapy (see below).
7. Proceed with computed tomography (CT) scan to exclude a pathologic condition requiring surgery.

Medical Therapy

Respiratory Care. The deleterious effects of hypercarbia and hypoxia on ICP are well recognized. To achieve hyperventilation (HV), initiate a controlled rate of 10 to 12 breaths per minute with a tidal volume of about 15 ml/kg. Frequent blood gas or reliable end-tidal pCO_2 analyses are obtained to ensure a pCO_2 between 25 to 30 mm Hg. Changes in ventilator settings are made to achieve this level of hypocapnia and adequate oxygenation. Further reductions of pCO_2 below 25 mm Hg are counterproductive, since cerebral vasoconstriction and hypoxemia due to increased hemoglobin-oxygen binding may begin to threaten the brain.

HV begins to reduce ICP within a minute of inception. With prolonged HV, CSF pH returns to normal and a new equilibrium is established within 6 to 24 hours [65]. The effects of hypocapnia in reducing ICP may then reduce with time, although a quick return to normocapnia may cause vasodilatation and increase ICP. Therefore the patient should be "weaned" off HV, and ICP should be closely monitored during the withdrawal.

Positive end-expiratory pressure (PEEP) ventilation raises intrathoracic pressure, which is transmitted to the intracranial compartment, thus raising ICP. Lung compliance determines the efficiency of pressure transmission. Patients with poorly compliant lungs (pulmonary edema) will not faithfully transmit intrathoracic pressure; this is fortunate, since these are the very patients who often require high airway pressures for adequate respiration. Cooper et al. found that *PEEP of up to 10 cm of water* was not clinically deleterious to ICP in well-managed patients. They did, however, recommend ICP monitoring in such patients [66].

The abrupt termination of PEEP can elevate systemic blood pressure, which may aggravate intracranial hypertension, especially in areas of impaired autoregulation. For this reason, PEEP should be tapered before it is withdrawn [67, 68]. Although high-frequency ventilation (HFV) produces smaller rises in intrathoracic and mean airway pressure than does conventional ventilation, it holds no advantage in reducing elevated ICP [65].

CSF Drainage. CSF drainage is an extension of a physiologic mechanism to reduce ICP, i.e., the translocation of CSF. If IVC monitoring is in use, CSF can be continuously drained against a *positive pressure of 15 to 20 mm Hg* to control ICP. Aspiration of CSF when ICP elevations occur should be done with caution, since it is possible to precipitate intracranial shifts. When the ventricles are very small, CSF drainage may cause the ventriculostomy to fail from catheter obstruction.

Osmotherapy and Diuretics. Although it is generally believed that hypertonic solutions cause brain volume to shrink by the osmotic extraction of water, no hard data supports this. Mannitol has been shown to decrease blood viscosity by the osmotic extraction of water from body tissues. According to one hypothesis, this reduction in viscosity reduces CVR, with a resultant increase in CBF—a transient hyperemia. Autoregulatory mechanisms now come into play and cerebral vasoconstriction follows, resulting in decreased CBV and ICP [70].

Mannitol is currently the most popular osmotic agent in neurosurgery. It is given as a 20 percent solution (200 mg/ml or 20 gm/100 ml) intravenously over 5–15 minutes. The dose is from 0.25 gm/kg up to 1 gm/kg, with the optimal dose being the smallest amount that reduces ICP [71]. It is effective within 10 to 15 minutes, has a duration of action of 3 to 8 hours, and may be repeated at intervals of 2 to 3 hours [72].

Other osmotic agents such as urea and glycerol [73] have been used to control intracranial hypertension. *Urea* was popularized by Javid [74] but has lost favor because of its penchant for crossing the blood-brain barrier, an undesirable virtue in this setting because of the ensuing rebound effect. *Glycerol* is a naturally occurring trivalent alcohol. As a 50 percent solution given in doses of 0.5 to 1.0 gm/kg by mouth every 4 hours, it effectively reduces ICP [75]. It may also be given intravenously, although this option may be confounded by intravascular hemolysis, nonketotic hyperosmolar hyperglycemia, and oxalic acidemia [75].

Rebound or secondary elevation of ICP can occur from leakage of hyperosmolar solutions into neuronal tissue followed by passive translocation of free water. When it is likely that cerebral swelling is due primarily to hyperperfusion of the brain, osmotic agents that increase CBV even temporarily may worsen the situation.

Osmotic agents evoke a marked diuresis, and a urinary catheter is essential. It may be necessary to monitor fluid status with a central venous catheter. Serum osmolality and electrolyte levels must be frequently checked. It is possible to leach considerable amounts of electrolyte or precipitate a hyperosmolar state, threatening systemic or cerebral homeostasis. A serum osmolality of up to 300 to 310 Osm is well tolerated by most patients.

Diuretics such as *furosemide* (*Lasix*) can be used alone or in conjunction with osmotherapy to reduce ICP. There is some evidence that the combination of furosemide and mannitol is synergistic [76]. The decrease in ICP is due in part to the diuretic effect and possibly to a direct reduction of sodium transport into the brain, decreased CSF production, and a decrease in brain volume [76, 77]. Furosemide may be administered in a dose of 0.1 to 1.0 mg/kg intravenously.

Lidocaine. Lidocaine reduces both the cerebral metabolic rate of oxygen ($CMRO_2$) and CBF and increases CVR. Presumably ICP falls in response to a reduction in CBV. Lidocaine is also an effective cough suppressant. In a dose of 1.5 mg/kg intravenously, it causes a significant but brief drop in ICP [78, 79, 80]. It may be used immediately before endotracheal intubation, surgical stimulation, or nursing procedures when the patient is at risk for developing reactive intracranial hypertension.

Temperature Control. Hyperthermia has been shown to increase cerebral edema, at least in experimental animals, by up to 40 percent [81]. CMR increases about 4 percent per degree centigrade, up to 42°C [82], and this can aggravate intracranial hypertension by increasing CBF and CBV. Temperature should be maintained within physiologic limits by use of antipyretics such as acetaminophen (Tylenol), 650 mg orally or rectally every 4 hours, or cooling blanket. A diligent search for the source of fever should of course be made, and drug fevers should be considered.

Steroids. Steroids are most effective in reducing cerebral edema associated with tumors [83], perhaps by inhibiting a vascular permeability factor expressed by neoplastic cells [84]. The usual regimen is dexamethasone (Decadron), 10 to 20 mg by mouth or intravenously initially, followed by 4 to 6 mg by mouth or intravenously every 6 hours or an equivalent dose of methylprednisolone. It is good practice to prescribe oral antacids or H_2-receptor antagonists simultaneously to prevent steroid-induced gastritis.

Environment. It is well known that triggers such as agitation, suctioning, chest physiotherapy, and painful stimuli can result in elevated ICP [85]. ICP may rise dramatically (80 to 100 mm Hg) during such procedures as endotracheal intubation or suctioning; indeed, in patients with severely compromised intracranial compliance, ICP elevation so induced may persist for a few minutes, seriously compromising CPP. Prevention of such an ICP crisis requires premedication; lidocaine is a good choice [80].

A tranquil environment should be provided for the patient, and nursing procedures should be arranged to minimize discomfort and unnecessary arousal [86].

Positioning. Head elevation and the maintenance of neutral alignment of the head and neck will maximize venous drainage and CSF translocation from the intracranial compartment and lower ICP [88]. Head elevation to 30 to 45 degrees is optimal. Sustained reductions in ICP may be achieved by placing the patient in the sitting or semisitting position [88], but there are some patients in whom intracranial compliance worsens with head elevation [89], particularly of 30 degrees or more (see section on plateau waves). Hip flexion of more than 90 degrees tends to increase intraabdominal and intrathoracic pressure and, hence, ICP.

If ICP is being monitored with an external transducer, it must be realigned when head position is changed.

Barbiturates. Mechanisms of barbiturate action in reducing ICP include (1) reduction in cerebral metabolism, CBF, and CBV and therefore ICP, and, (2) direct vasoconstrictor effect on cerebral blood vessels, particularly the capacitance vessels, leading to a reduction in CBV. Furthermore, the barbiturates, especially thiopental, are believed to be free-radical scavengers; disordered cerebral metabolism and liberation of active oxygen radicals are frequently present with intracranial hypertension, so that there is a further theoretical advantage to their role in control of intracranial hypertension [90].

Barbiturate therapy is generally reserved for a small number of patients with persistent elevations of the ICP not responsive to "conventional therapies," e.g., positioning, hyperventilation, and osmotherapy [92]. An arbitrary but defensible rule of thumb is an ICP exceeding 40 mm Hg for 15 minutes or more after other modalities have failed. *Pentobarbital sodium* (*Nembutal*) is most often used. A total initial dose of 5 to 10 mg/kg is given intravenously in divided doses over 10 to 20 minutes. This may be followed by supplemental doses of 1 to 2 mg/kg at 1- to 2-hour intervals as a bolus or by continuous infusion, depending on ICP response. Dose requirements vary among patients, but generally a serum level of 3 to 5 mg/dl is required to achieve a 20- to 30-second burst suppression pattern on the electroencephalogram (EEG). If ICP cannot be controlled when the EEG shows burst suppression, higher doses are unlikely to be of benefit.

An important side effect of barbiturates administered in this fashion is direct myocardial depression and peripheral vasodilatation, the net effect of which is hypotension. For this reason, monitoring with a Swan-Ganz catheter and arterial line is necessary for optimal management. Volume loading to ensure adequate filling pressures and possibly peripheral vasoconstrictors to maintain a stable mean systemic pressure exceeding 80 mm Hg or a CPP exceeding 60 mm Hg are the cornerstones of therapy. If an adequate blood pressure becomes difficult to sustain, the barbiturate dose should be reduced.

Barbiturate therapy also appears to increase the risk of pneumonia, CNS infection, hypothermia, the syndrome of inappropriate secretion of antidiuretic hormone (SIADH), and sepsis [91].

Therapy may be discontinued when ICP is normalized for at least 24 hours. The dose should be tapered, and if ICP begins to rise, a repeat CT scan and reinstitution of therapy is a logical approach.

The efficacy of barbiturates in modifying patient outcome after head injury remains at issue [91, 92].

Blood Pressure. It has been shown that in intracranial hypertension the undampened transmission of raised systemic blood pressure to a dilated cerebral vascular bed favors the propagation of cerebral edema [67]. This augmentation of vasogenic cerebral edema has led some to advocate antihypertensive therapy for patients with intracranial hypertension when systemic pressure exceeds 160 mm Hg [93]. One must tread carefully, since low perfusion pressure and hypotension may exacerbate brain injury by causing secondary ischemic insult.

Surgical Decompression

It is crucial to exclude a removable mass lesion as a cause of raised ICP. Obtain a CT scan as early as possible to establish this fact. Prompt surgical decompression, when indicated, should be given priority, since little progress can be made if the patient is harboring an expanding mass lesion that is unrecognized or untreated.

References

1. Monro A. *Observations on the Structure and Function of the Nervous System.* Edinburgh: Creech and Johnson, 1783.
2. Kellie G. An account of the appearance observed in the dissection of two of the three individuals presumed to have perished in the storm of 3rd, and whose bodies were discovered in the vicinity of Leith on the morning of the 4th November 1821 with some reflections on the pathology of the brain. *Trans. Med. Chir. Sci. Edinburgh* 1:84, 1824.
3. Burrows G. *Disorders of the Cerebral Circulation.* London: Longman, 1846. Pp. 55–56.
4. Lundberg N. Pathophysiology of intracranial hypertension. In Krayenbuhl H., (ed.). *Advances and Technical Standards in Neurosurgery.* Berlin: Springer-Verlag, 1974. Pp. 4–51.
5. Langfitt T. W., Weinstein J. D., Kassell N. F. Cerebral vasomotor paralysis produced by intracranial hypertension. *Neurology* 15:622, 1965.
6. Langfitt T. W. Increased intracranial pressure. *Clin. Neurosurg.* 16:436, 1969.
7. Langfitt T. W. Pathophysiology of increased ICP. In Brock M., Dietz H. (eds.). *Intracranial Pressure: Experimental and Clinical Aspects.* Berlin: Springer-Verlag, 1972. Pp. 361–365.
8. Sullivan H. G., Miller J. D., Griffith III R. L., et al. CSF pressure transients in response to epidural and ventricular volume loading. *Am. J. Physiol.* 234:R167, 1978.
9. Hulme A., Cooper R. The effects of head position and jugular vein compression on intracranial pressure. A clinical study. In Beks J. W. F., Bosch D. A., Brock M., (eds.). Intracranial Pressure III. Berlin: Springer-Verlag, 1976. Pp. 259–278.
10. Cooper R., Hulme A. Intracranial pressure and related phenomena during sleep. *J. Neurol. Neurosurg. Psychiatry* 29:564, 1966.
11. Miller J. D. Significance and management of intracranial hypertension. In Ishii S., Nagai H., Brock M. (eds.). *Intracranial Pressure V.* Berlin: Springer-Verlag, 1983. Pp. 44–53.
12. Bruce D. A., Langfitt T. W., Miller J. D., et al. Regional cerebral blood flow, intracranial pressure and brain metabolism in comatose patients. *J. Neurosurg.* 38:131, 1973.

13. Cutler R. W. P., Page L. K., Galicich J., et al. Formation and absorption of cerebrospinal fluid in man. *Brain* 91:707, 1968.
14. Greenberg T. A., Mayer D. J., Becker D. P. Correlation in man of intracranial pressure and neuroelectric activity determined by multimodality evoked potentials. In Beks J. W. F., Bosch D. A., Brock M. (eds.). *Intracranial Pressure III.* Berlin: Springer-Verlag, 1976. Pp. 58–62.
15. Spencer W., Horsley V. On the changes produced in circulation and respiration by increase of intracranial pressure or tension. *Philos Trans.* 182:201, 1892.
16. Cushing H. Concerning a definite regulating mechanism of the vasomotor center which controls blood pressure during cerebral compression. *Bull. Johns Hopkins Hosp.* 12:290, 1901.
17. Cushing H. The blood pressure reaction of acute cerebral compression. *Am. J. Med. Sci.* 125:1017, 1903.
18. Theodore J., Robin E. D. Pathogenesis of neurogenic pulmonary oedema. *Lancet* 2:749, 1975.
19. Cushing H. Peptic ulcers and the interbrain. *Surg. Gynecol. Obstet.* 55:1, 1932.
20. Miller J. D., Butterworth J. F., Gudeman S. K., et al. Further experience in the management of severe head injury. *J. Neurosurg.* 54:289, 1981.
21. Jennett B. Techniques for measuring intracranial pressure. In Brock M., Dietz H. (eds.). *Intracranial Pressure: Experimental and Clinical Aspects.* Berlin: Springer-Verlag, 1972. Pp. 365–368.
22. Lundberg N. Continuous recording and control of ventricular fluid pressure in neurosurgical practice. *Acta Psychiatr. Scand.* 36(Suppl.) 149:1, 1960.
23. Venes J. L., Shaywitz B. A., Spencer D. D. Management of severe cerebral edema in the metabolic encephalopathy of Reye-Johnson syndrome. *J. Neurosurg.* 48:905, 1978.
24. Langfitt T. W., Kumar V. S., James H. E., et al. Continuous recording of intracranial pressure in patients with hypoxic brain damage. In Brierley J. B., Meldrum B. S. (eds.). *Brain Hypoxia.* London: Heinemann, 1971. Pp. 118–135.
25. Nakagawa Y., Yada K., Tsuru M. Clinical significance of ICP measurements following intracranial surgery. In Lundberg N., Ponten U., Brock M. (eds.). *Intracranial Pressure II.* Berlin: Springer-Verlag, 1975. P. 350.
26. Ghajar J. B. G. A guide for ventricular catheter placement. Technical note. *J. Neurosurg.* 63:985, 1985.
27. Shapiro H. M., Wyte S. R., Harris A. B., et al. Disposable system for intraventricular pressure measurement and CSF drainage. Technical note. *J. Neurosurg.* 36:798, 1972.
28. Vries J. K., Becker D. P., Young H. R., et al. A subarachnoid screw for monitoring intracranial pressure. *J. Neurosurg.* 39:416, 1973.
29. Wilkinson H. A. The intracranial pressure-monitoring cup catheter. Technical note. *Neurosurgery* 1:139, 1977.
30. Villanueva P. A. Simplified technique for subdural pressure monitoring. Technical note. *Neurosurgery* 16:238, 1985.
31. Sugiura K., Hayama N., Tachisawa T., et al. Intracranial pressure monitoring by a subdurally placed silicone catheter. Technical note. *Neurosurgery* 16:241, 1985.
32. Levin A. B. The use of a fiberoptic intracranial pressure monitor in clinical practice. *Neurosurgery* 1:266, 1977.
33. Roberts P. A., Fullenwider C., Stevens F. A., et al. Experimental and clinical experience with a new solid state intracranial pressure monitor with in vivo

zero capability. In Ishii S., Nagai H., Brock M. (eds.). *Intracranial Pressure V*. Berlin: Springer-Verlag, 1983.

34. Schettini A., McKay L., Mahig J., et al. The response of brain surface pressure to hypercapnic hypoxia and hyperventilation. *Anesthesiology* 36:4, 1972.
35. Aucoin P. J., Kotilainen H. R., Gantz N. M., et al. Intracranial pressure monitors—epidemiologic study of risk factors and infections. *Am. J. Med.* 80:369, 1986.
36. Mayhall C. G., Archer N. H., Lamb V. A., et al. Ventriculostomy-related infection. A prospective epidemiologic study. *N. Engl. J. Med.* 310:553, 1984.
37. Wyler A. R., Kelly W. A. Use of antibiotics with external ventriculostomies. *J. Neurosurg.* 37:185, 1972.
38. Friedman W. A., Vries J. K. Percutaneous tunnel ventriculostomy: Summary of 100 procedures. *J. Neurosurg.* 53:662, 1980.
39. Narayan R. K., Kishore P. R., McWhorter J. M. Intracranial pressure: To monitor or not to monitor. *J. Neurosurg.* 56:650, 1982.
40. Gentleman D., Mendelow A. D. Intracranial rupture of a pressure monitoring transducer: Technical note. *Neurosurgery* 19:91, 1986.
41. Kjallgvist A., Lundberg N., Pontén U. Respiratory and cardiovascular changes during spontaneous variations of ventricular fluid pressure in patients with intracranial hypertension. *Acta Neurol. Scand.* 40:291, 1964.
42. Langfitt T. W. Summary of first international symposium on intracranial pressure, Hanover, Germany, July 27–29, 1972. *J. Neurosurg.* 38:541, 1973.
43. Rosner M. J., and Becker D. P. Origin and evolution of plateau waves: Experimental observations and a theoretical model. *J. Neurosurg.* 60:312, 1984.
44. Gray W. J., Rosner M. J. Pressure-volume index as a function of cerebral perfusion pressure. Part 1: The effects of cerebral perfusion pressure changes and anesthesia. *J. Neurosurg.* 67:369, 1987.
45. Gray W. J., Rosner M. J. Pressure-volume index as a function of cerebral perfusion pressure. Part 2: The effects of low cerebral perfusion pressure and autoregulation. *J. Neurosurg.* 67:377, 1987.
46. Rosner M. J., Coley I. B. Cerebral perfusion pressure, intracranial pressure and head elevation. *J. Neurosurg.* 65:636, 1986.
47. Amacher A. L., Sibbald W. J. Correlation of abnormal intracranial pressure waves with paroxysmal elevations in pulmonary artery diastolic pressure. *Surg. Forum* 38:479, 1977.
48. Miller J. D., Garibi J., Pickard J. D. Induced changes of cerebrospinal fluid volume: Effects during continuous monitoring of ventricular fluid pressure. *Arch. Neurol.* 28:265, 1973.
49. Miller J. D., Leech P. J., Pickard J. D. Volume-pressure response in various experimental and clinical conditions. In Lundberg N., Ponten N., Brock M. (eds.). *Intracranial Pressure II*. Berlin: Springer-Verlag, 1975. P. 97.
50. Miller J. D., Leech P. J. Assessing the effects of mannitol and steroid therapy on intracranial volume-pressure relationships. *J. Neurosurg.* 42:274, 1975.
51. Szewczykowski J., Dytko P., Kunicki A., et al. Determination of critical ICP levels in neurosurgical patients: A statistical approach. In Lundberg N., Ponten U, Brock M. (eds.). *Intracranial Pressure II*. Berlin: Springer-Verlag, 1975. P. 391–392.
52. Janny P., Jouan J. P., Janny L., et al. A statistical approach to long-term monitoring of intracranial pressure. In Brock M., Dietz H. (eds.). *Intracranial Pressure I*. Berlin: Springer-Verlag, 1972. P. 50–64.
53. Adolph R. J., Fukusumi H., Fowler N. O. Origin of cerebrospinal fluid pulsations. *Am. J. Physiol.* 212:840, 1967.
54. Dunbar H. S., Guthrie T. C., Karpell B. A study of the cerebrospinal fluid pulse wave. *Arch. Neurol.* 14:624, 1966.

55. Hamer J., Alberti E., Hoyer S., et al. Influence of systemic and cerebral vascular factors on the CSF pulse waves. *J. Neurosurg.* 46:36, 1977.
56. Avezaat C. J. J., van Eijndhoven J. H. M., de Jong D. A., et al. A new method of monitoring intracranial volume pressure relationship. In Beks J. W. F., Bosch D. A., Brock M. (eds.). *Intracranial Pressure III.* Berlin: Springer-Verlag, 1976. Pp. 308–313.
57. Castel J. P., Cohadon F. The pattern of cerebral pulse: Automatic analysis. In Beks J. W. F., Bosch D. A., Brock M. (eds.). *Intracranial Pressure III.* Berlin: Springer-Verlag, 1976. Pp. 303–305.
58. Hirai O., Handa H., Ishikawa M., et al. Epidural pulse waveform as an indicator of intracranial pressure dynamics. *Surg. Neurol.* 21:67, 1984.
59. Takizawa H., Gabra-Sanders T., Miller J. D. Changes in the cerebrospinal fluid pulse wave spectrum associated with raised intracranial pressure. *Neurosurgery* 20:355, 1987.
60. Hirai O., Handa H., Ishikawa M. Intracranial pressure pulse waveform: Considerations about its origin and methods to estimating intracranial dynamics. *Brain Nerve* 34:1059, 1982.
61. Portnoy H. D., Chopp M., Branch C., et al. Cerebrospinal fluid waveform as an indicator of cerebral autoregulation. *J. Neurosurg.* 56:666, 1982.
62. Portnoy H. D., Chopp M. Cerebrospinal fluid pulse waveform analysis during hypercapnia and hypoxia. *Neurosurgery* 9:14, 1981.
63. Takizawa H., Miller J. D., Sugiura K., et al. Fast Fourier transform analysis of ICP waveform. *ICP J.* 1:38, 1984.
64. Avezaat C. J. J., van Eijndhoven J. M. H., Wyper D. J. Cerebrospinal fluid pulse pressure and intracranial volume pressure relationships. *J. Neurol. Neurosurg. Psychiatry* 42:687, 1979.
65. Horbein T. F., Pavlin E. G. Distribution of H^+ and HCO_3^- between cerebrospinal fluid and blood during respiratory alkalosis in dogs. *Am. J. Physiol.* 228:1134, 1975.
66. Cooper K. R., Boswell P. A., Choi S. C. Safe use of PEEP in patients with severe head injury. *J. Neurosurg.* 63:552, 1985.
67. Schutta H. S., Kassell N. F., Langfitt T. W. Brain swelling produced by injury and aggravated by arterial hypertension. A light and electron microscopic study. *Brain* 91:281, 1968.
68. Aidinis S. J., Lafferty J., Shapiro H. M. Intracranial response to PEEP. *Anesthesiology* 45:275, 1976.
69. Grasberger R. G., Spatz E. L., Mortara R. W., et al. Effect of high frequency ventilation versus conventional mechanical ventilation on ICP in head-injured dogs. *J. Neurosurg.* 60:1214, 1984.
70. Muizellaar J. P., Wei E. P., Kontos H. A., et al. Mannitol causes compensatory cerebral vasoconstriction vasodilatation in response to blood viscosity changes. *J. Neurosurg.* 59:822, 1983.
71. Marshall L. F., Smith R. W., Rauscher L. H., et al. Mannitol dose requirements in brain-injured patients. *J. Neurosurg.* 48:169, 1978.
72. Prockop L. D. The pharmacology of increased intracranial pressure. In Klawans H. L. (ed.). *Clinical Neuropharmacology.* New York: Raven Press, 1976. Pp. 147–171.
73. Grant F. C. The value of hypertonic solutions by mouth, by rectum or by IV injection for the reduction of increased ICP. *Ann. Res. Nerv. Ment. Dis. Proc.* 8:437, 1927.
74. Javid M. Urea in intracranial surgery. A new method. *J. Neurosurg.* 18:51, 1961.
75. Wald S. L., McLaurin R. L. Oral glycerol for the treatment of traumatic intracranial hypertension. *J. Neurosurg.* 56:323, 1982.

76. Pollay M., Fullenwides C., Roberts A., et al. Effect of mannitol and furosemide on blood brain osmotic gradient and intracranial pressure. *J. Neurosurg.* 59:945, 1983.
77. Cotrell J. E., Robustelli A., Post K. Furosemide- and mannitol-induced changes in intracranial pressure and serum osmolality and electrolytes. *Anesthesiology* 47:28, 1977.
78. Bedford R. F., Persing J. A., Probereskin L., et al. Lidocaine or thiopental for rapid control of intracranial hypertension? *Anesth. Analg.* 59:435, 1980.
79. Sakabe T., Naekawa T., Ishikawa T., et al. The effects of lidocaine on canine cerebral metabolism and circulation related to the electroencephalogram. *Anesthesiology* 40:433, 1974.
80. Hamill J. F., Bedford R. F., Weaver D. C., et al. Lidocaine before endotracheal intubation: Intravenous or laryngotracheal? *Anesthesiology* 55:578, 1981.
81. Clasen R. A., Pandolfi S., Laing I., et al. Experimental study of the relation of fever to cerebral edema. *J. Neurosurg.* 41:576, 1974.
82. Meyer J. S., Handa J. Cerebral blood flow and metabolism. During experimental hyperthermia (fever). *Minn. Med.* 50:37, 1967.
83. Galicich J. H., French L. A. Use of dexamethasone in the treatment of cerebral edema resulting from brain tumors and brain surgery. *Am. Practitioner* 12:169, 1961.
84. Stewart P. A., Hayakawa K., Farrell C. L., et al. Quantitative study of microvessel ultrastructure in human peritumoral brain tissue. Evidence for blood-brain barrier defect. *J. Neurosurg.* 67:697, 1987.
85. Mitchell P. H., Mauss N. K., Lipe H., et al. Effect of patient-nurse activity on ICP. In Shulman K. (ed.). *Intracranial Pressure IV.* Berlin: Springer-Verlag, 1980.
86. Shalit N. M., Umansky F. Effect of routine bedside procedures on intracranial pressure. *Israel J. Med. Sci.* 13:881, 1977.
87. Hulme A., Cooper R. The effects of head position and jugular vein compression on intracranial pressure. In Beks J. W. F., Bosch D. A., Brock M. (eds.). *Intracranial Pressure III.* Berlin: Springer-Verlag, 1976. Pp. 259–263.
88. Kenning J. A., Toutant S. M., Saunders R. L. Upright patient positioning in the management of intracranial hypertension. *Surg. Neurol.* 15:148, 1981.
89. Ropper A. H., O'Rourke D., Kennedy S. K. Head position, intracranial pressure and compliance. *Neurology* 32:1288, 1982.
90. Miller J. D. Barbiturates and raised intracranial pressure. *Ann. Neurol.* 6:189, 1979.
91. Ward J. D., Becker D. P., Miller J. D., et al. Failure of prophylactic barbiturate coma in the treatment of severe head injury. *J. Neurosurg.* 62:383, 1985.
92. Eisenberg H. M., Frankowski R. F., Contant C. F., et al. High-dose barbiturate control of elevated intracranial pressure in patients with severe head injury. *J. Neurosurg.* 69:15, 1988.
93. Lundberg N. Non-operative management of intracranial hypertension. In Krayenbuhl H., (ed.). *Advances and Technical Standards in Neurosurgery.* Berlin: Springer-Verlag, 1974. Pp. 3–59.

Suggested Reading

Simon R. H., Sayre J. T. *Strategy in Head Injury Management.* Norwalk: Appleton & Lange, 1987.
Cooper P. R. (ed.). *Head Injury* (2nd ed.). Baltimore: Williams & Wilkins, 1987.
Miller J. D., Teasdale G. M., Rowan J. O., et al. (eds.). *Intracranial Pressure VI.* Berlin: Springer-Verlag, 1986.

3. Brain Water

The adult brain is 70 to 80 percent water. This percentage is higher in fetal brain, and the gray matter has a higher fraction (80%) than the white matter (68%). The water content of the brain is a rough index of its stage of maturation and degree of myelination [1].

Water is present in all four intracranial fluid compartments: intracellular, extracellular, subarachnoid–cerebrospinal fluid (CSF), and intravascular. The cell membrane isolates the intracellular compartment, and the blood-brain barrier insulates the brain from the intravascular space.

Water moves freely from blood to CSF to brain and back in response to osmotic gradients and hydrostatic pressures. Most of the water in the brain arrives there by diffusion. Katzman and Pappius noted that a 1400-gm brain produces metabolic water at the rate of 2.5 ml/hour [1]. In contrast, 20 ml/hour of CSF is formed by a choroid plexus weighing only 2 gm.

Brain osmolality is essentially the same as blood under normal conditions. Generally, when the serum osmolality is decreased the brain imbibes water, and vice versa; this predictable sequence does not hold for chronic alterations in serum osmolality because of brain cells' fortunate tendency to adapt to an osmotic challenge [2, 3].

Cerebrospinal Fluid

Physiology

Production

The main source of CSF (80 to 90%) is the choroid plexus [4–6], composed of specialized tufts of highly vascularized pia mater lined with an epithelium of modified ependyma. It is found on the walls of the lateral ventricles and the roofs of the third and fourth ventricles. The fenestrated capillaries in the core of the choroid plexus produce an ultrafiltrate of plasma by hydrostatic pressure. Under the auspices of an active sodium (Na-K adenosine triphosphatase [ATPase]) pump within the choroidal epithelium, sodium (and perhaps other ions) is secreted into the ventricular space. Water follows passively, and CSF is formed [4].

Current evidence suggests that the cyclic nucleotide cAMP, 3', 5'-adenosine monophosphate, is involved in CSF formation. Cyclic AMP is formed from adenosine triphosphate by activation of the enzyme adenylate cyclase; cAMP is present in the CSF, and adenylate cyclase is present in the choroidal cell membrane. The enzyme is activated by cholera toxin, boosting CSF production. This stimulation of CSF formation by cholera toxin provides an a priori argument for the role of cAMP in CSF production, possibly as a secondary messenger [7].

Other sites of CSF formation (extrachoroidal) are known [8, 9], particularly the brain parenchyma at the capillary endothelium. Again, the proffered mechanism is active transport of ions into the adjacent extracellular space and then passive movement of water into the ventricles and subarachnoid space. Extrachoroidal sources account for approximately 10 to 20 percent of CSF output [10].

CSF is produced at a rate of about 0.35 ml/minute, amounting to 20 ml/hour or 500 ml/day [11]. The total volume of CSF in the adult is estimated at 140 ml. This volume is recycled about every 8 hours.

A number of factors influence the rate of CSF formation:

1. *Intracranial pressure–vascular perfusion*. Under physiologic conditions, CSF formation is independent of pressure [11]. However, with increasing intraventricular pressure, cerebral perfusion pressure (CPP) begins to fall, diminishing capillary pressure and the rate of primary filtration across the choroidal capillaries, the important initial step in CSF formation [12, 13]. For similar reasons, systemic hypotension decreases the rate of CSF production by reducing choroid plexus blood flow [14].
2. *Temperature*. The influence of temperature on CSF formation has been studied experimentally. The effect is linear—a 7 percent increase in secretion rate per degree rise in body temperature [15]. This parallels a similar relationship between cerebral blood flow (CBF) and temperature, presenting prima facie evidence for the dependence of CSF formation on CBF [16].
3. *Hypoxia and hypoglycemia*. Lack of oxygen or glucose, vital elements in all cellular activity, significantly reduces CSF production [17, 18].
4. *Neurogenic control*. Adrenergic and cholinergic nerves supply the choroid plexus. *Adrenergic* stimulation causes a reduction in CSF production. Correspondingly, *cholinergic* stimulation increases CSF production [19–23].
5. *Drugs. Acetazolamide* (*Diamox*), a carbonic anhydrase inhibitor, reduces CSF formation [24]. *Furosemide* (Lasix) also reduces CSF formation by the same mechanism but may also inhibit chloride transport [25]. Agents that reduce CSF formation have not been shown to be of significant use in control of hydrocephalus [10].

Circulation

CSF formed in the ventricles is propelled through pathways by the pulsations of the cerebral and choroidal vessels. Of great importance is the phenomenon of *bulk flow*. Since most of the choroid plexus is in the lateral ventricles, the largest volume of CSF is produced at the distal end of the CSF pathway. Simple volume addition promotes flow throughout the system. From the ventricles, CSF passes through the aqueduct and the foramina of Luschka and Magendie into the subarachnoid space. The fluid bathes the brainstem and continues craniad over the

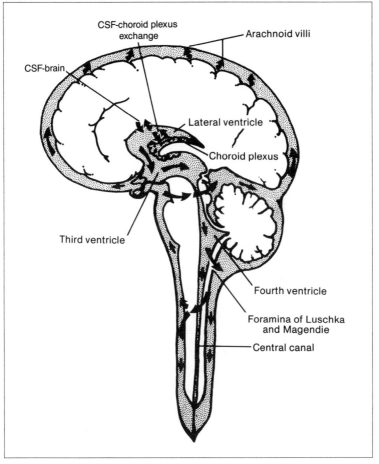

Fig. 3-1. Pathways of cerebrospinal fluid (CSF) circulation.

vertex and caudad into the spinal subarachnoid space and around the ·nerve roots. Other avenues may include the central canal of the spinal cord, the terminal ventricle into the thecal sac and spinal arachnoid villi, and back to the blood (Fig. 3-1). Some CSF may make its way into the extracellular space of the brain and spinal cord, especially when there is increased outflow resistance to CSF.

Absorption

The major sites of CSF absorption into the blood are the arachnoid villi [26, 27]. These structures are herniations of arachnoid membrane through the dura into the lumen of the superior sagittal sinus and other venous structures. Typically, they are found in clusters. There is some controversy regarding the existence of channels connecting the villi to the sinuses. The *open-channel theory* is associated with a pressure-passive CSF efflux. In the *closed-channel model* CSF exits through an active transport mechanism [10]. In any case, CSF flow appears to be a one-way flow from the subarachnoid space to the venous blood. This one-way flow is often referred to as *bulk flow* because all the constituents leave with the fluid.

There is evidence for alternate routes of CSF drainage: lymphatic, bulk flow through the extracellular space of the brain, back flow into the choroid plexus and the arachnoid membrane [28–31].

Function

CSF provides a mechanical cushion, protecting the brain from impact with the bony calvarium during relative movement. Its buoyant action allows for an apparent reduction of brain weight from 1400 gm in air to 50 gm in situ; therefore smaller mechanical vectors are developed during brain motion.

CSF acts as a conduit for the conveyance of some hypothalamic hormones to the hypothalamic-adenohypophysial portal system, e.g., thyroid-releasing hormone (TRH) and luteinizing hormone–releasing hormone (LH-RH). CSF also provides a clearing mechanism for certain substances from the brain, including ions (potassium, iodide), organic acids (penicillin), vitamins, amino acids, and nucleotides. These substances are actively transported across the CSF-blood barrier (choroid plexus and arachnoid villi). The molecular layer of the cortex is nourished by oxygen derived from the CSF. Thus the CSF has an important role in maintaining homeostasis and in metabolism.

Hydrocephalus

Hydrocephalus is a clinical state wherein the production of CSF exceeds its absorption. As a result, CSF accumulates within the ventricles, resulting in ventricular dilatation or increased intracranial pressure (ICP).

Hydrocephalus may be due to an absorptive defect or to CSF overproduction. By far the more common situation is a block in the CSF pathway. When the block is proximal to the foramina of Luschka and Magendie, the hydrocephalus is described as *noncommunicating*, implying a restriction of ventricular fluid access to the subarachnoid space. This type is usually caused by a mass that obstructs the ventricular system or by congenital obliteration of the aqueduct of Sylvius.

Hydrocephalus occurring as the result of a block distal to the foramina of Magendie and Luschka is termed *communicating hydrocephalus.*

Ventricular fluid reaches the subarachnoid space but is not reabsorbed quickly enough to prevent its accumulation. This form of hydrocephalus may be secondary to inflammation (basal meningitis) or hemorrhage in the subarachnoid space. In subarachnoid hemorrhage, blood and its degradation products are swept by bulk CSF flow to the arachnoid villi, impairing the absorption of CSF. Infection and inflammation cause scarring and arachnoid adhesions, obliterating segments of the CSF pathway.

Hydrocephalus may also be the result of oversecretion of CSF by a choroid plexus papilloma. The condition is rare. In this type of hydrocephalus, absorptive capacity is normal but is incapable of handling the increased rate of production, which may exceed 5 liters/day.

Adult-onset communicating hydrocephalus (AOCH), often confusingly termed *normal pressure hydrocephalus (NPH)*, is an entity occurring primarily in the elderly. It presents as a syndrome of dementia, gait disturbance (apraxia or ataxia), and urinary incontinence. The ventricles are dilated, and CSF pressure is usually normal. It is sometimes difficult to distinguish between AOCH and cerebral atrophy of aging (hydrocephalus ex vacuo) on radiologic evidence alone. AOCH is an important, treatable cause of dementia.

Blood-Brain Barrier

The blood-brain barrier denotes a complex anatomic and physiologic phenomenon with many clinical ramifications. Historically, the concept developed from Ehrlich's observations [32]. He injected dyes intravenously into animals and found that although other tissues were stained, the brain remained free of dye.

There are some specialized areas in the brain where the blood-brain barrier is less discriminating or nonexistent. These include the choroid plexus, area postrema, median eminence, hypophysis, tuber cinereum, paraphysis, pineal gland, and preoptic areas [33]. At these loci, blood-CSF interactions occur—CSF production (choroid plexus), transcellular transport (median eminence), and secretion of neurohormonal or neurotransmitter substances. It is well known that many drugs and nutrients are selectively excluded from the central nervous system (CNS), a fact of profound therapeutic importance. A systematic study of various substances repelled by the blood-brain barrier has not revealed any common feature that explains this discretionary action. Molecular size, electrical charge, or lipid solubility do not, per se, account for exclusion from the brain. Similarly, previous hypotheses based on artifactual pathologic evidence from brain tissue itself (lack of extracellular space) are now known to be incorrect [33].

Certain properties facilitate transition of substances from blood to brain. They include: high lipid solubility, a low level of ionization at physiologic pH, and lack of protein binding. Oxygen, carbon dioxide, water, and some drugs appear to enter the brain freely.

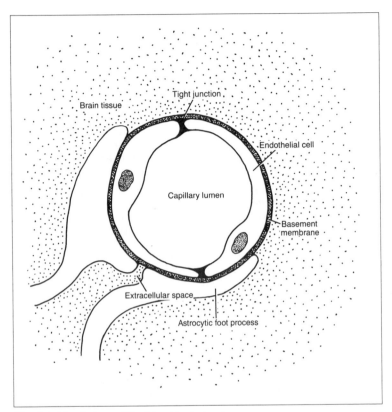

Fig. 3-2. Morphology of the blood-brain barrier.

Morphology

A morphologic description of the blood-brain barrier interface has been developed [34]. Cerebral capillary endothelial cells are united by "tight" junctions (zonulae occludentes). These barriers prevent the passage of protein molecules with a molecular weight of 43,000 or more. Endothelial cells are completely surrounded by a basement membrane. Exterior to this are the foot processes of astrocytes, which wrap themselves around the basement membrane. This glial envelope is incomplete, being separated by intercellular clefts (Fig. 3-2).

Ultrastructurally, the endothelial cells and astrocytic foot processes have many mitochondria, implying a high level of energy use. The endothelial cells also harbor a number of important enzymes associated with carbohydrate, amino acid, and neurotransmitter metabolism [34]. Clearly, if these enzymes metabolize their substrates within the endothelial cell, a diminished concentration will be available for penetration into the brain; conversely, other enzymes actually facilitate the passage of some substances into the brain. Finally, the cerebral capillary has limited pinocytotic activity, at least under normal conditions. Intracytoplasmic vesicles in the endothelial cells, ordinarily sparse, increase during cerebral edema, suggesting a role in the development of vasogenic edema.

Neurochemistry

The blood-brain barrier's essential role is to protect the neuronal environment and thereby maintain homeostasis; this involves various cellular mechanisms that regulate the influx and efflux of substances into the brain.

Lipid Solubility

A high lipid solubility facilitates movement across the cerebral capillary cell membrane. Notable examples include anesthetic agents, nitrosoureas (chemotherapeutic agents for CNS neoplasms), ethanol, and heroin, which notoriously outpaces morphine in traversing the barrier. Known exceptions to this general rule are D-glucose and some amino acids, which gain the brain's metabolic pool primarily by their molecular configuration rather than lipid solubility. Ionized polar (hydrophilic) compounds cross the blood-brain barrier slowly unless there is a specific transport system for the substance.

Carrier-mediated Transport

Carrier-mediated transport may be active or passive. In the former, energy expenditure is required to realize transit against a concentration gradient. The latter, also known as facilitated diffusion, cannot overcome a concentration gradient. Both mechanisms exhibit saturation kinetics and stereospecificity. Compounds that rely on these modalities include amino acids (neutral amino acid transport system), neurotransmitters and purine bases (adenine transport system), D-glucose (hexose transport system), and monocarboxylic acids (monocarboxylic acid transport system) [35].

Clinical Aspects

Hypertension

As previously discussed (see Chap. 1), autoregulation maintains a constant CBF between a range of CPPs (60 to 160 mm Hg). Elevated CPP may increase CBF, causing dilatation and stretching of the cerebral capillary bed. The endothelial tight junctions open and the blood-brain barrier is transgressed, i.e., so-called breakthrough. This may result in cerebral edema [36], which may present clinically as hypertensive encephalopathy. The condition is more often found with acute hypertension, presumably because proliferative vascular adaptive responses occur with chronic hypertension.

Brain Tumors

Cerebral edema associated with brain tumors may be the cause of significant neurological deficit. This form of edema is produced by disruption of the blood-brain barrier with increased vascular permeability and interstitial fluid accumulation. These abnormalities have been variously associated with biochemical mediators [37–39], structural alterations in tumor-induced blood vessels [40], destruction of the cerebral capillary endothelium [41], increased capillary hydrostatic pressure [42], nonspecific tumor secretory products [43], and a vascular permeability factor (VPF) produced and released by malignant glial tumors [44].

Dexamethasone and other glucocorticoids effectively reduce neurological deficits and intracranial hypertension associated with peritumoral brain edema. The suppression of VPF by corticosteroids may account for the efficacy of steroids in reducing symptoms of brain tumor edema [44].

Infection

CNS infections (brain and meninges) may result in breakdown of the blood-brain barrier, although the precise locus of such a defect remains unknown. Protein molecules, leukocytes, and antibiotics (penicillin) readily traverse the barrier in the primal phase of infection. Successful treatment usually restores the barrier.

Seizures

Seizures stimulate cerebral metabolism, and CBF increases to fuel the enhanced activity. The associated acute rise in CPP may exceed autoregulatory limits, resulting in breakthrough and enhanced capillary permeability [45].

Hypercapnia

Hypercapnia results in cerebral vasodilatation, which may cause stretching of the endothelial cells within the cerebral capillary and dehiscence of the tight junctions, with resultant cerebral edema. Fortunately, this phenomenon is frequently reversible [46].

Therapeutic Modification

The blood-brain barrier presents a therapeutic barrier to clinicians seeking to deliver drugs into the brain; consequently, reversible therapeutic modifications of blood-brain barrier permeability are being investigated [47–49]. The major impact has been in the delivery of chemotherapeutic agents (e.g., methotrexate, cyclophosphamide) or specific antibodies in the treatment of CNS neoplasms (i.e., gliomas, lymphomas, metastases).

The technique involves osmotic disruption of the blood-brain barrier using intraarterial mannitol. The barrier opening is monitored by contrast-enhanced computed tomography (CT) brain scan, and the therapeutic agent is delivered. The procedure may be repeated on several occasions in the same patient. The patient is usually given anticonvulsant prophylaxis because of the potential for seizures, and steroids are tapered or discontinued because they may alter barrier modification. Results to date have been encouraging [47–49].

Possible mechanisms for reversible blood-brain barrier disruption include (1) an osmotic shrinkage of the capillary endothelial cell, with retraction of the cell membrane and separation of intercellular tight junctions, and (2) osmotic withdrawal of fluid from the extracellular space into the capillary lumen, with vasodilatation and "unzipping" of the endothelial junctions [50].

Cerebral Edema

Cerebral edema represents an increase in the brain's water content, frequently with an increase in brain volume. The increase in water content is usually proportionally higher in the white matter. Cerebral edema may be focal or generalized. Clinical manifestations include focal neurologic deficits, disturbances of consciousness, intracranial hypertension, and herniation syndromes. Magnetic resonance imaging (MRI) or CT brain scans may demonstrate areas of cerebral edema. The areas of edema appear as low density on the unenhanced CT scan. MRI scans show decreased signal intensity on T1-weighted images and increased signal intensity on T2-weighted images. Positron emission tomography (PET) using rubidium 82 has been used to evaluate loss of integrity of the blood-brain barrier.

Spread of edema fluid is usually by bulk flow. Once developed, cerebral edema may be aggravated by hypercapnia, hypoxia, hyperthermia, hypertension, and volatile anesthetics. Edema may resolve by one of several mechanisms: (1) resorption into the vascular space, (2) transependymal movement into the ventricular space, (3) uptake and degradation of edema fluid protein by glial cells, and (4) pinocytotic transfer of osmotically active particles into the blood from the brain. Klatzo classified cerebral edema into *vasogenic* and *cytotoxic* types [51]. A third form of cerebral edema—*interstitial* or hydrocephalic—was later identified by Fishman [52]. Further study [53] has provided an amplified version of the mechanisms involved in the development of cerebral edema.

Pathophysiology

Vasogenic Edema

Vasogenic edema is the commonest form of cerebral edema encountered clinically. It occurs in response to trauma, tumors, inflammation, lead encephalopathy, and in the later stages of cerebral ischemia. Experimentally, this form of edema may be evoked by a cryogenic lesion in the brain. It is due to increased permeability of brain capillary endothelial cells (disruption of the blood-brain barrier), which then allows water, protein, and sodium to enter and expand the extracellular space. The white matter is particularly vulnerable to vasogenic edema, probably because its lower capillary density and blood flow, and the parallel orientation of the white matter tracts, allow for greater tissue compliance.

Cytotoxic Edema

In cytotoxic edema, the cellular elements (neurons, glia, and endothelial cells) imbibe water and swell, with a corresponding reduction in the extracellular space. Cytotoxic edema is due to a derangement in cellular metabolism, specifically, a failure of the ATP-dependent Na-K pump, allowing sodium and therefore water to accumulate intracellularly. Clinical examples include the early phase of cerebral ischemia, asphyxia, cardiac arrest, and Reye's syndrome. It may be induced experimentally by triethyltin or hexachlorophene poisoning. Cytotoxic edema develops quickly, and may resolve rapidly once the energy supply is restored.

Interstitial (Hydrocephalic) Edema

Interstitial edema is a result of obstructive hydrocephalus [52]. There is an increase in the water and sodium content of the periventricular white matter due to the transependymal movement of CSF. On CT scans this appears as periventricular hypodensity, and on MRI scans it appears as an area of altered signal intensity. Clinically, the manifestations of interstitial edema are minor unless the changes are advanced. Interstitial edema from obstructive hydrocephalus may be reversed by CSF shunting procedures. This type of edema may be seen in patients with severe pseudotumor cerebri.

Hydrostatic Edema

Hydrostatic edema is produced by increases in intravascular pressure that are transmitted directly to the capillary bed without a compensatory increase in cerebral vascular resistance (CVR). There follows an extravasation of water into the extracellular space. The capillary endothelium is not specifically damaged, and the edema fluid is a protein-free ultrafiltrate of plasma [54]. Hydrostatic edema is generally diffuse rather than focal. Severe acute arterial hypertension is one example.

Hypo-osmotic Edema

Hypo-osmotic edema results from a reduction in plasma osmolality by water intoxication or the syndrome of inappropriate secretion of antidiuretic hormone (SIADH). The osmotic gradient developed favors the entry of water into the brain across an intact blood-brain barrier [55]. The edema is generally diffuse.

Treatment and Procedures

Generally, the principles and modalities described in Chapter 2 for the treatment of patients with intracranial hypertension are applicable to the treatment of those with cerebral edema. The procedures for obtaining cerebrospinal fluid are explained below.

Lumbar Puncture

Corning is generally credited with the first lumbar puncture, performed in 1885 for the injection of cocaine for local anesthesia [56]. Quincke in 1891 was able to record and reduce intracranial pressure by lumbar puncture. Queckenstedt described his test of CSF manometrics in 1916.

Indications
1. Investigation of CSF for infections, subarachnoid hemorrhage, multiple sclerosis, and so on.
2. Instillation of contrast material and other pharmaceuticals for radiologic studies or chemotherapy.
3. Withdrawal of CSF to decrease intracranial pressure.

Contraindications
1. Intracranial mass lesions can be excluded by a preliminary CT or MRI scan of the head. In the presence of an intracranial mass, a sudden reduction of CSF pressure by subarachnoid puncture below the mass may lead to shift of intracranial contents and transtentorial or transforaminal herniation.
2. Local pathology—skin infections in the lumbar area. Consider alternate routes of access (see the sections on lateral C1–C2 and cisternal puncture).
3. Coagulopathy is a relative contraindication, since it may result in spinal epidural hematoma [57].

Positioning and Landmarks. Lumbar puncture may be performed with the patient recumbent or sitting. If the recumbent position is chosen, left lateral is preferable for right-handed operators. The patient is urged to flex the spine and bring the knees up to the chest and flex the head.

A line joining the highest point of both iliac crests (Tuffler's line) usually marks the level of the L4 spinous process. In the lumbar spine there is a relatively wide space between the horizontally directed spinous processes. In adults, virtually any interspace below L2 is safe to use, since the lowest part of the cord, the conus medullaris, is at the level of L1–

L2. The caudal limit of the subarachnoid space is about S2. In infants it is safer to stay below L3, since the caudal limit of the conus is lower than in adults. The long axis of the spine should be horizontal; correct sagging by positioning pillows appropriately to avoid being thrown off the midline.

Equipment
1. Sterile gloves and towels.
2. 18- or 20-gauge × 3½-in. spinal needle.
3. 25 gauge × ⅝-in. and 22-gauge × 1½-in. infiltration needles with 5-ml syringe.
4. Three-way stopcock and manometer.
5. 70% alcohol or povidone-iodine solution.
6. Sterile specimen tubes.
7. Band-Aid.

Procedure
1. Shave any hair in the area; prepare the skin with 70% alcohol or povidone-iodine solution.
2. Raise a skin wheal by infiltrating the epidermis with 1% lidocaine & 1:100,000 epinephrine through a 25-gauge needle. Infiltrate the deeper tissues similarly with a 22-gauge needle.
3. Palpate the interspace (usually L4–L5); indent skin with firm thumbnail pressure to mark the interspace.
4. For adults, select an 18- or 20-gauge × 3½-in. spinal needle; in children a 20-gauge × 2½-in. needle is preferable. In infants, use a 22-gauge × 1½-in. needle. In newborns and infants, neck flexion is usually unnecessary and local anesthesia is rarely needed.

Introduce the needle with stylet, exactly in the midline in the interspace, slightly inclined craniad about 30 degrees. Pass it through the intervening tissues, ensuring that the bevel is in the sagittal axis so that the dura is pierced along rather than across its fibers (Fig. 3-3). This promotes closure of the puncture and less likelihood of a postspinal headache from CSF leak.

The ligamentum flavum has a characteristic feel of resistance, and the dura has a "give" or a "snap." Remove the stylet and confirm CSF flow. If flow is sluggish, a nerve root may be in the way; gently rotate needle. Replace the stylet. If the tap is traumatic, observe for clearing of CSF as fluid is collected. If CSF does not clear, abort and repeat the tap at the next higher level.

A further refinement is the *hanging drop* technique. When the needle has entered the interspinous space, remove the stylet and squirt some sterile 0.9% NaCl into the hub of the needle so that a drop hangs at the orifice. Continue to push the needle through deliberately with both thumbs, keeping a close eye on the drop balanced at the hub of the needle. As soon as the epidural space is entered, the drop of saline is sucked in by the negative pressure of the epidural space.

Complete the procedure by advancing the needle 2 mm, puncturing

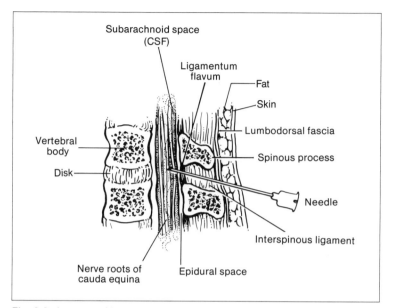

Fig. 3-3. Anatomy of lumbar puncture. Midsagittal section shows lumbar spine with spinal needle in place. Note trajectory and structures traversed.

the dura. This technique is particularly valuable when it is vital to identify the epidural space to introduce material into it (see the section on epidural blood patch). It also prevents overpenetration of the needle.

5. If bone is encountered on the way in, encourage further flexion. If this fails, withdraw the needle and reposition at a more craniad or caudad angle. Employ the *lateral approach* if there is difficulty entering the interspinous space, which can happen in older patients with lumbar spondylosis or calcified interspinous ligaments.

Introduce the needle lateral to the spinous process so that it is inclined toward the midline and cephalad, its tip reaching the sagittal plane at a distance of about 6 cm, where the spinal canal is found. In obese patients, it may be difficult to establish the midline by palpation in the recumbent position; furthermore, the spinal axis tends to sag from the horizontal plane. In this situation the *sitting position* may be preferable. Have the patient sit on the edge of the bed, leaning over a bedstand positioned at nipple level and supported by an assistant. The spine should be flexed with this arrangement. The same principles apply. Having entered the subarachnoid space, do not remove the stylet; have the patient slowly resume the lateral recumbent position and then proceed to perform manometrics and withdraw fluid. In this way one can guard against rapid CSF decompression.

6. Measure CSF opening pressure by connecting the needle to a three-way stopcock and manometer assembly with or without an intervening short length of tubing. The patient should be relaxed with legs extended and head neutral at this point. CSF rises in the manometer and then settles.

7. Collect samples of CSF for analysis.

8. Reinsert the stylet and withdraw the needle and stylet as a unit. Do not withdraw the needle without the stylet in place, since a nerve root may be pulled out.

9. Place a small dressing over the puncture site.

Interpretation and Results. CEREBROSPINAL FLUID PRESSURES. The patient should be relaxed with legs outstretched, head neutral, and breathing normally (not hyperventilating). In healthy adults the pressure in the lateral recumbent position is 70 to 180 mm of water. The pressure tends to be lower in infants, ranging between 70 and 120 mm of water. In the sitting position the fluid column should not rise above the foramen magnum. Very low pressure may suggest spinal block or needle obstruction by nerve roots or meninges. The closing pressure is only important if serial punctures are being performed to lower ICP; a comparison between the closing pressure of the previous tap and the opening pressure of the next tap may provide some estimate of the effect of fluid withdrawal on the reduction of pressure.

TESTS OF CEREBROSPINAL FLUID DYNAMICS. Although the need for ritual performance of various *tests to determine CSF dynamics* has been reduced by the availability of myelography and, lately, MRI of the spine, there is the occasional patient who is unable to undergo either of the above. It is here that the resourceful house officer can make use of "old tricks" when a spinal block is in question:

1. *Queckendstedt test.* With the needle still in place and connected to the manometer, compress the jugular veins by hand for 15 to 20 seconds to occlude venous drainage. With free flow of CSF in the subarachnoid space, jugular compression increases the CSF pressure some threefold. When compression is discontinued, the CSF pressure immediately falls to the original level. This is a positive Queckendstedt test; i.e., there is no block of CSF flow in the subarachnoid space.

2. *Stookey test.* With the needle still in place and connected to a manometer, compress the abdominal wall with the hand over the umbilicus. The abdominal muscles should be relaxed. There should be a pressure rise of about twofold; again, releasing the compression allows the pressure to fall instantly to initial levels.

Using the above two tests of CSF dynamics: the combination of a negative Queckendstedt and a positive Stookey is consistent with a block in the cervical or upper thoracic region. If the block is in the lower thoracic region, Stookey's test shows only a partial rise and Quekenstedt's is negative. Both tests are negative if there is a block in the lumbar region. Sometimes absolutely positive results are not obtained after either test. A partial rise followed by slow fall indicates partial block of CSF flow.

APPEARANCE. The spinal fluid should appear clear and colorless, comparable to water in a similar tube. Turbid CSF may indicate a cell count of at least 500 cells/μl.

XANTHOCHROMIA. Yellow discoloration, or xanthochromia, is usually due to one of the following pigments: bilirubin, oxyhemoglobin, or methemoglobin. When a subarachnoid hemorrhage is suspected, the CSF may be examined for xanthochromia. It takes about 4 to 6 hours following hemorrhage for blood to lyse and release pigments. Bleeding from any source may cause a protein elevation of 1 mg per 1000 red blood cells; elevated protein values out of proportion to this ratio indicate that the hemorrhage antedated the spinal puncture. Jaundiced patients may show xanthochromic CSF.

CYTOLOGY. Cells encountered in the normal spinal fluid include small and large lymphocytes and mononuclear cells. White blood cells should number 0 to 5 cells/μl. Polymorphonuclear leukocytes in the spinal fluid should be regarded as pathologic until proved otherwise, as should eosinophils, which are frequently associated with parasitic infections, subarachnoid hemorrhage, and postmyelographic irritation.

GLUCOSE. Normal glucose values range between 45 and 80 mg/100 ml. This value is strongly influenced by the blood sugar; typically, CSF glucose is two-thirds that of the blood. Hypoglycorrhachia is associated with meningitis, subarachnoid hemorrhage, and meningeal carcinomatosis. Hyperglycorrhachia per se is of no diagnostic significance and is frequently secondary to hyperglycemia.

PROTEIN. Normal protein level is between 15 and 45 mg/100 ml. It is lowest in fluid obtained from the ventricles. Higher levels are associated with meningitis, tumors, and cerebral degenerations. Very high levels may cause the CSF to clot. Immunoglobulin analysis is of use in the diagnosis of multiple sclerosis. The IgG fraction is increased and can be demonstrated in oligoclonal IgG bands; these bands can also appear in other disorders. High levels of myelin basic protein have been shown to correlate with acute exacerbations of multiple sclerosis.

Complications

1. *Post-lumbar-puncture headache* (*PLPH*). Headache may occur if ambulation is resumed too early following the procedure or if too much CSF has been removed or multiple punctures have been performed. It has been related to the size of needle used, occuring less frequently with 22-gauge needles than with 18-gauge ones. It is more common in women [58]. Initial treatment is to encourage fluid intake, bedrest, and a mild analgesia. If the PLPH is very severe, place the patient in the Trendelenburg position and begin intravenous fluids. Most PLPHs are self-limiting. Occasionally it is necessary to perform an epidural blood patch.
2. *Traumatic Tap*. This is usually due to trauma to epidural veins, re-

sulting in bloody CSF that tends to clear as more is drained. Epidural blood contamination occurs more frequently in children. Rarely, an epidural hematoma may develop. This is most likely in patients taking anticoagulants [57]. It is important to distinguish between spontaneous and iatrogenic subarachnoid bleeding. Crenated red blood cells and xanthochromia are common with the former state and absent with the latter one.

3. *Nerve root injury.* This is very rare.
4. *Herniation.* Lumbar puncture in the face of an intracranial mass lesion, especially in the posterior fossa or temporal lobes, may lead to transforaminal or transtentorial herniation. Very rarely, spinal cord shifting may occur in patients with spinal cord tumors. Lumbar puncture may aggravate cord compression by decreasing intraspinal pressure below the tumor and cause neurologic deterioration (spinal coning); the risk is about 14 percent in the presence of a complete block [59].
5. *Epidermoid tumors.* These have been reported to occur many years after a lumbar puncture. They may be prevented by using the stylet to avoid implantation of epidermal tissue [60].
6. *Infection.* Its exact incidence is unknown but is very low. If the needle is pushed too far, one may traumatize or infect a disk space. Ensuring that the needle is directed cephalad will cause it to strike the vertebral body above if the needle is too deep.

Postprocedural Care. It is well to keep the patient in bed for a few hours and to encourage liberal amounts of fluid by mouth. This will reduce the occurrence of PLPH and promote the formation of CSF. Neurologic checks should be performed following the procedure.

Continuous Lumbar Drainage

Continuous lumbar drainage was introduced by Vour'ch in 1960 [61]. It temporarily reduces CSF volume or pressure, and by temporarily diverting the flow of CSF, it facilitates the healing of CSF fistulas [62–64].

Indications
1. CSF fistulas of posttraumatic or postoperative origin (see below). The lumbar drain may also be left in place following the repair of a CSF leak to facilitate closure of the leak and healing of the repair.
2. Intraoperatively to facilitate brain retraction and exposure for aneurysms, transsphenoidal adenomectomy for macroadenoma, or craniofacial surgery.
3. Incisional leak of CSF or subgaleal CSF accumulation underneath a craniotomy flap. Drainage may be used if other methods have failed to prevent the reaccumulation of fluid.

Contraindications. Contradications include those for lumbar puncture. In addition, with persisting CSF fistulas into air-containing sinuses, there is a danger of reversing the fistula flow, thereby allowing air or bacteria into the intracranial cavity.

Equipment. Commercial kits are readily available. These usually contain a drainage system, consisting of:

1. Vinyl tubing equipped with clamps, stopcock, Luer's lockport for monitoring, and a latex injection-sampling site.
2. Drip chamber with antireflux valve and sterile atmospheric vent.
3. Graduated collection bag.
4. Silastic lumbar catheter (Pudenz-Schulte Medical, Santa Barbara, CA) or No. 5 French Stamey ureteral catheter (American Latex Corp., Sullivan, IN) [65].

Procedure
1. Introduce 14-gauge × 3½-in. Tuohy needle with Huber tip (Pudenz-Schulte Medical, Santa Barbara, CA) at the L4–L5 or L5–S1 interspace in the standard fashion for a lumbar puncture. Direct the bevel of the needle cephalad. It is easier if a small stab wound is made in the skin with a no. 11 blade before introducing the Tuohy needle, since it has a blunt tip.
2. Once CSF appears, replace the stylet to interrupt flow and gently thread the lumbar catheter through the needle into the subarachnoid space (ensure that the catheter will fit through the needle before performing the puncture).
3. Advance the catheter 3–5 cm cephalad in the subarachnoid space. Withdraw the needle, taking care to prevent shearing of a portion of the catheter in situ. If there is undue resistance, try again. Connect the proximal end of the catheter to a luer lock adapter, sterile tubing, three-way stopcock, and collecting system.
4. Anchor the catheter and tubing to the patient with adhesive tape. Suspend the drainage bag from bedside or intravenous pole.
5. Tests of CSF dynamics can be applied to check for satisfactory placement of the catheter within the subarachnoid space.
6. Maintain a pressure gradient between the intracranial and intraspinal space. Head elevation of 10 to 15 degrees is optimal. Generally, the reservoir is kept at the level of the lumbar spine with the patient in the recumbent position. The rate of drainage can be varied by changing the relative position of the reservoir or by changing the degree of head elevation.
7. A modification of the conventional *pressure-regulated* system has been described by Swanson et al. [66], providing *flow-regulated* drainage of CSF by attaching the catheter to intravenous tubing that is passed through an IVAC 530 continuous infusion pump. The system is controlled by setting the pump at a set rate. This maintains some accuracy in the rate and amount of drainage independent of patient position. Further, the continuous flow may help maintain tubing patency. The system, as originally described, incorporates two sensors and two pumps. A flow-regulated system with one pump and one sensor in line has been suggested by Graf [67]. A pressure-safety valve has been suggested as an added safeguard against generating excessive negative pressure inside the spinal canal [67].
8. For intraoperative lumbar subarachnoid drainage, an alternate

method is use of an 18-gauge and split mattress if the patient is positioned supine (Lemon technique). Drainage is more rapid with this assembly, perhaps an advantage in the operating room.

Interpretation and Results. Estimated CSF production is about 18 to 21 ml/hour, 0.3 ml/minute, or 500 ml/day. Only about 120 ml of CSF is actually circulating at any given time. The rate of therapeutic CSF drainage varies between 60 to 600 ml/day in reported series [63]. Successful treatment of postoperative CSF fistulas with this procedure has been reported by several authors [62–64]. This technique may be used to record CSF pressures over 24 to 72 hours when searching for diagnoses such as AOCH or pseudotumor cerebri without papilledema.

Complications
1. *Pneumocephalus.* Usually this is due to excessive drainage of CSF and too much head elevation, resulting in negative pressure in the intracranial space. Early signs include altered level of consciousness, nausea and vomiting, headaches, or seizures. Drainage should be discontinued. Place the patient in the Trendelenburg position or flat, begin intravenous fluids, and obtain a CT brain scan for diagnosis [68]. Air entering the subarachnoid space at room temperature will expand when heated to core temperature and may compromise intracranial compliance.
2. *Injury to nerve roots* or spinal cord. This occurs due to traumatic insertion.
3. *Infection.* Staphylococci or mixed flora are most likely.
4. *Herniation.* Usually downward and more likely in the presence of an intraaxial mass lesion within the posterior fossa.
5. Overdrainage of CSF, which may cause low-pressure *headaches* or a *subdural hematoma*.
6. *Catheter blockage* from debris or high viscosity of CSF with elevated protein. *Leakage* of spinal fluid around the catheter may be secondary to blockage of the catheter.
7. *Malpositioned catheter.* If the catheter has been placed into the epidural or subdural space, it will not maintain its functional integrity and CSF will not drain.

Postprocedural Care
1. Change collection system as frequently as needed. Do not allow the drip chamber to fill completely because this predisposes to vent wetting, which entraps air within the bag and possibly alters pressure relationships. If this occurs, simply change the tubing and drainage bag promptly using sterile technique. Close the stopcock to the patient before proceeding.
2. Collect CSF frequently for cell count, Gram's stain, cultures, and biochemical studies. Before puncturing the port, clean site with 70% alcohol or povidone-iodine solution.
3. Prophylactic antibiotics, directed against staphylococci, are recommended by some; their value has not been proved.

4. Check functional integrity, hourly drainage, neurologic status, dressings for leakage of CSF, and catheter exit site.
5. Position patient to maintain a constant relationship to the reservoir.
6. Keep valve upright (if one is used) to prevent reflux and infection.
7. When drainage is discontinued, apply Band-Aid to site.

Epidural Blood Patch

PLPH was first described by Corning in 1885. The headaches are due to continued leakage of CSF from the dural puncture site [69]. Most PLPHs can be treated by bedrest, increased fluid intake, and analgesics [70]. The mean duration of PLPH is 4 days, and 80 percent of patients will recover spontaneously within 2 weeks [71]. The epidural blood patch (EBP) has been advocated by anesthesiologists since 1970 for the treatment of refractory PLPH. Nelson theorized that epidural bleeding from a traumatic lumbar puncture might lead to clot formation over the dura, which would seal the leak [69]. Gormley reported successful treatment of PLPH with the injection of 2 to 3 ml of autologous blood into the lumbar epidural space [72]. DiGiovanni popularized the EBP technique for the treatment of PLPH [73, 78].
Indication. The one indication is protracted PLPH not responding to conservative management.

Contraindications
1. Local infection in lumbar area.
2. Septicemia.
3. Blood dyscrasias or anticoagulant therapy.

Equipment. In addition to the items listed for lumbar puncture, a 10-ml syringe with a 22-gauge needle and a tourniquet are needed.
Positioning and Landmarks. Positioning and landmarks are as for lumbar puncture.

Procedure
1. Perform venipuncture in patient's arm and withdraw 5 to 10 ml of blood.
2. Perform lumbar puncture by "hanging drop" technique (see Lumbar Puncture) at the level the initial lumbar puncture was performed. Hold the needle in the epidural space.
3. Inject 2 to 4 ml of blood into the epidural space.
4. If the lumbar puncture is traumatic, discontinue the EBP, since the subsequent epidural clot may seal the hole. Furthermore, additional injection of blood may compress the nerve root.

Interpretation and Results. The patient will frequently report total relief of symptoms after getting up. Many clinical studies have confirmed the initial results of the procedure [74–77]. The EBP probably forms a gelatinous tamponade that prevents further leakage of spinal fluid, allowing the dura to heal [78]. It is interesting that prophylactic epidural injection of autologous blood has not been shown to prevent PLPH [79]. If the headache persists, the procedure can be repeated.

Complications. Most complications are minor. They include:

1. Transient paresthesia or radicular pain in lower extremities.
2. Nuchal stiffness during the injection.
3. Transient low-grade fever.
4. Abdominal cramping.
5. Tinnitus, dizziness, or vertigo [80,81].

Postprocedural Care. Keep the patient in bed for 0.5 to 1 hour. Provide liberal amounts of fluid.

Lateral C1–C2 Puncture

Lateral C1–C2 puncture is a spinoff of lateral cervical cordotomy [82, 83]. It is a handy alternative to lumbar puncture [84]. It may be performed with fluoroscopic control.

Indications
1. When lumbar puncture is technically difficult, e.g., in patients with morbid obesity, spinal deformities or midline fusion, arachnoiditis, and spinal stenosis.
2. To define the upper extent of a myelographic block demonstrated on a lumbar study.
3. In patients having cervical spine injury, in whom flexion is contraindicated.

Contraindications. Contraindications include intracranial mass and Arnold-Chiari malformation.

Positioning and Landmarks. The patient is positioned supine with the head and neck in alignment. The C1–C2 interlaminar space is capacious, since there is little overlap. The landmark for needle insertion is a point 1 cm caudad and 1 cm posterior (dorsal) to the tip of the mastoid process (Fig. 3-4).

Equipment. Equipment is the same as for lumbar puncture.

Procedure
1. Prepare skin with 70% alcohol or povidone-iodine solution.
2. Introduce an 18- to 20-gauge spinal needle at a point 1 cm caudad and 1 cm posterior to the mastoid tip. The tip of the needle is directed to the anterior third of the spinal canal to avoid injuring the cervical cord.
3. Advance the needle deliberately; confirm trajectory with fluoroscopy or x-ray film.
4. The familiar "give" is felt as the dura is traversed. Withdraw the stylet; collect CSF for analysis. Contrast agent may be instilled if myelography is to be performed.

Complications. Complications include cord or nerve root injury, which may cause pain, respiratory depression, or neurologic symptoms, and vertebral artery injury, evidenced as bleeding through the needle. Remove the needle promptly.

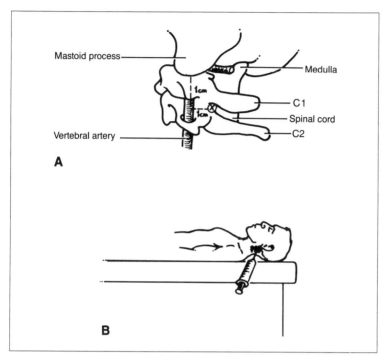

Fig. 3-4. Lateral C1–C2 puncture. A. Landmarks. B. Positioning.

Cisterna Magna Puncture

Indications and Contraindications. Indications and contraindications are the same as for the lateral C1–C2 puncture.

Positioning and Landmarks. Cisterna magna puncture may be performed with the patient in the sitting or recumbent position. The head should be well flexed. A horizontal line through the tips of the mastoid processes bisects the atlanto-occipital membrane. A vertical line from the inion through the spinous processes of the cervical vertebrae meets the horizontal at the needle entry point (Fig. 3-5). In the average adult, the cisterna magna is about 5 cm below the skin surface.

Equipment. Equipment is the same as for lumbar puncture.

Procedure. The step-by-step procedure is as follows:

1. Shave a small area of hair in the occipital-nuchal region; prepare the skin with 70% alcohol or povidone-iodine solution. No towels are necessary because landmarks may be occluded.
2. The head should be well flexed for maximum exposure of the space between the foramen magnum and C1.
3. Infiltrate the skin and soft tissues with 1% lidocaine.

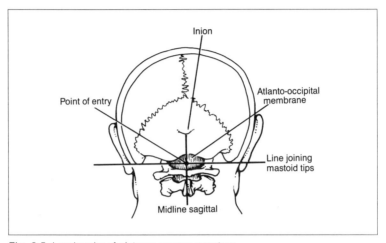

Fig. 3-5. Landmarks of cisterna magna puncture.

4. Two methods of cisterna magna puncture are described below, depending on entry site and direction of the needle.

DIRECT METHOD OF AYER [85]. Enter the skin in the midline just above the spinous process of C2 (with the head flexed, this is on a line joining both acoustic meati or the level of the glabella), and direct the needle rostrally to the space between the foramen magnum and C1. As the needle is advanced, one feels resistance as the atlanto-occipital ligament and the dura beneath it are encountered. When the needle perforates these two structures, its anterior end becomes fixed and difficult to move; on reaching the desired depth it becomes freely mobile, and CSF should flow at this stage. Do not insert the needle beyond 2 cm after puncturing the atlanto-occipital ligament to avoid injuring the medulla (Fig. 3-6).

INDIRECT METHOD OF ESKUHEN. Introduce the needle midway between the inion and the spinous process of C2 and direct it to the occipital squama. When bony resistance is appreciated, withdraw the needle slightly and reintroduce it more caudad, repeating this until the tip of the needle just passes under the free edge of the foramen magnum ("walking the needle"). Continue through the atlanto-occipital membrane and dura into the cisterna magna. Perforation of the dura is sometimes accompanied by sharp pain in the occipital region.

Complications. Complications include the following: hemorrhage from perforation of a vessel—lateral excursions may threaten the vertebral artery—and piercing of the medulla, which may cause vomiting, apnea, cardiac irregularity, or neurologic symptoms. Both lateral C1–C2 and cisterna magna puncture are useful procedures in specific circumstances. However, they must not be performed by the inexperienced in

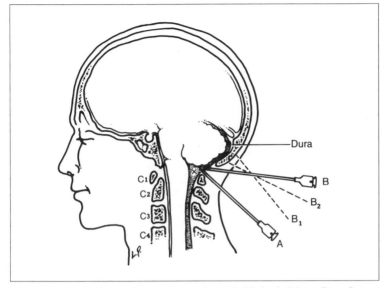

Fig. 3-6. Methods of cisterna magna puncture. A. Method of Ayer. B_1 to B_2 to B. Method of Eskuhen. x, Cisterna magna.

the absence of competent supervision. The lateral C1–C2 puncture is much safer and more widely used [86].

References

1. Katzman R., Pappius H. M. *Brain Electrolytes and Fluid Metabolism.* Baltimore: Williams & Wilkins, 1973.
2. Stern W. E., Coxon T. V. Osmolality of brain tissue and its relation to brain bulk. *Am. J. Physiol.* 206:1, 1964.
3. Yannet J. Changes in the brain resulting from depletion of extracellular electrolytes. *Am. J. Physiol.* 128:683, 1940.
4. Pollay M. Formation of cerebrospinal fluid. *J. Neurosurg.* 42:665, 1975.
5. Cushing H. Studies on the cerebrospinal fluid. I. Introduction. *J. Med. Res.* 26:1, 1914.
6. Dandy W. E. Experimental hydrocephalus. *Ann. Surg.* 70:129, 1919.
7. Epstein M. H., Feldman A. M., Brusilow S. W. Cerebrospinal fluid production: Stimulation by cholera toxin. *Science* 196:1012, 1977.
8. Milhorat T. H., Hammock M. K., Fenstermacher J. D., et al. Cerebrospinal fluid production by the choroid plexus and brain. *Science* 173:330, 1971.
9. Pollay M., Curl F. Secretion of cerebrospinal fluid by the ventricular ependyma of the rabbit. *Am. J. Physiol.* 213:1031, 1967.
10. McComb J. G. Recent research into the nature of cerebrospinal fluid formation and absorption. *J. Neurosurg.* 59:369, 1983.
11. Cutler R. W. P., Page L., Galicich J., et al. Formation and absorption of cerebrospinal fluid in man. *Brain* 91:707, 1968.

12. Weiss M. H., Wertman N. Modulation of CSF production by alterations in cerebral perfusion pressure. *Arch. Neurol.* 35:527, 1978.
13. Deane R., Segal M. B. The effect of vascular perfusion of the choroid plexus on the secretion of cerebrospinal fluid. *J. Physiol.* 293:18, 1979.
14. Carey M. E., Vela R. Effect of systemic arterial hypotension on the rate of cerebrospinal fluid formation in dogs. *J. Neurosurg.* 41:350, 1974.
15. Snodgrass S. R., Lorenzo A. V. Temperature and cerebrospinal fluid production rate. *Am. J. Physiol.* 222:1524, 1972.
16. Rosomoff H. L. Some aspects of hypothermia on the normal and abnormal physiology of the nervous system. *Proc. R. Soc. Br.* 149:358, 1956.
17. Holloway L. S., Cassin S. Cerebrospinal fluid dynamics in the newborn dog during normopoxia and hypoxia. *Am. J. Physiol.* 223:499, 1972.
18. Carey M. E., Davson H., Bradbury M. W. B. The effect of severe hypoglycemia upon cerebrospinal fluid formation, ventricular iodide clearance, and brain electrolytes in rabbits. *J. Neurosurg.* 54:370, 1981.
19. Edvinsson L., Hakanson R., Lindvall M., et al. Ultrastructural and biochemical evidence for a sympathetic neural influence on the choroid plexus. *Exp. Neurol.* 48:241, 1975.
20. Lindvall M., Edvinsson L., Ownman C. Sympathetic nervous control of cerebrospinal fluid production from the choroid plexus. *Science* 201:176, 1978.
21. Lindvall M., Edvinsson L., Ownman C. Effect of sympathomimetic drugs and corresponding receptor antagonists on the rate of cerebrospinal fluid production. *Exp. Neurol.* 64:132, 1979.
22. Edvinsson L., Nielsen K. C., Ownman C. Cholinergic innervation of choroid plexus in rabbits and cats. *Brain Res.* 63:500, 1973.
23. Haywood J. R., Vogh B. P. Some measurements of autonomic nervous system influence on production of cerebrospinal fluid in the cat. *J. Pharmacol. Exp. Ther.* 208:341, 1979.
24. Rubin R. C., Henderson E. S., Ommaya A. K., et al. The production of cerebrospinal fluid in man and its modification by acetazolamide. *J. Neurosurg.* 25:430, 1966.
25. McCarthy K. D., Reed D. J. The effect of acetazolamide and furosemide on cerebrospinal fluid production and choroid plexus carbonic anhydrase activity. *J. Pharmacol. Exp. Ther.* 189:194, 1974.
26. Key E. A. H., Retzius M. G. *Studien in der Anatomie des Nervensystems und des Bindegewebes.* Stockholm: Samson and Wallin, 1875.
27. Weed L. H. Studies on cerebrospinal fluid. III. The pathways of escape from the subarachnoid spaces with particular reference to the arachnoid villi. *J. Med. Res.* 31:51, 1914.
28. Arnold W., Ritter R., Wagner W. H. Quantitative studies on the drainage of the cerebrospinal fluid into the lymphatic system. *Acta Otolaryngol.* 76:156, 1973.
29. Cserr H. F., Osttach L. H. Bulk flow of interstitial fluid after intracranial injection of blue dextran 2000. *Exp. Neurol.* 45:50, 1974.
30. Milhorat T. H., Mosher M. B., Hammock M. K., et al. Evidence for choroid-plexus absorption in hydrocephalus. *N. Engl. J. Med.* 283:286, 1970.
31. Butler A. B., van Landingham K., McComb J. G. Pressure-facilitated CSF flow across the arachnoid membrane. In Ishii S., Nagai H., Brock M. (eds), *Intracranial Pressure V.* Berlin: Springer-Verlag, 1983.
32. Ehrlich C. 1902. Über die Beziehungen von Chemischer Constitution, Vertheliung, und pharmakologische Wirkung. In *Collected Studies in Immunity.* New York: John Wiley & Sons, 1906. Pp. 567–595.
33. Dobbing J. The blood-brain barrier. *Physiol. Rev.* 41:130, 1961.

34. Rapoport S. I. (ed.). *Blood-Brain Barrier in Physiology and Medicine.* New York: Raven Press, 1976.
35. Pollay M., Roberts P. A. Blood-brain barrier: A definition of normal and altered function. *Neurosurgery* 6:675, 1980.
36. Rapoport S. I. Pathological alterations of the blood-brain barrier. In Rapoport S. I. (ed.). Blood-Brain Barrier in Physiology and Medicine, New York: Raven Press, 1976. Pp. 129–152.
37. Chan P. H., Fishman R. A. The role of arachidonic acid in vasogenic cerebral edema. *Fed. Proc.* 43:210, 1984.
38. Fishman R. A., Chan P. H. Hypothesis: Membrane phospholipid degradation and polyunsaturated fatty acids play a key role in the pathogenesis of brain edema. *Trans. Am. Neurol. Assoc.* 106:58, 1981.
39. Unterberg A., Baethmann A. J. The kallikrein-kinin system as mediator in vasogenic brain edema. Part I: Cerebral exposure to bradykinin and plasma. *J. Neurosurg.* 61:87, 1984.
40. Groothuis D. R., Vick N. A. Brain tumors and the blood-brain barrier. *Trends in Neurosci.* 5:232, 1982.
41. Long D. M. Capillary ultrastructure and the blood-brain barrier in human malignant brain tumors. *J. Neurosurg.* 32:127, 1970.
42. Casanova M. F. Vasogenic edema with intraparenchymatous expanding lesions: A theory on its pathophysiology and mode of action of hyperventilation and corticosteroids. *Med. Hypotheses* 13:439, 1984.
43. Phillipon J., Foncin J. F., Grob R., et al. Cerebral edema associated with meningiomas: Possible role of a secretory-excretory phenomenon. *Neurosurgery* 14:295, 1984.
44. Bruce J. N., Criscuolo G. R., Merrill M. J., et al. Vascular permeability induced by protein product of malignant brain tumors: Inhibition by dexamethasone. *J. Neurosurg.* 67:880, 1987.
45. Bolwig T. G., Hertz M. M., Paulson O. B., et al. The permeability of the blood-brain barrier during electrically-induced seizures in man. *Eur. J. Clin. Invest.* 7:87, 1977.
46. Cutler R. W. P., Barlow C. F. The effect of hypercapnia on brain permeability to protein. *Arch. Neurol.* 14:54, 1966.
47. Neuwelt E. A., Frenkel E. P., Diehl J., et al. Reversible osmotic blood-brain disruption in humans: Implications for the chemotherapy of malignant brain tumors. *Neurosurgery* 7:44, 1980.
48. Neuwelt E. A., Balaban E., Diehl J., et al. Successful treatment of primary central nervous system lymphomas with chemotherapy after osmotic blood-brain barrier opening. *Neurosurgery* 12:662, 1983.
49. Neuwelt E. A., Barnett P. A., McCormick C. I., et al. Osmotic blood-brain barrier modification: Monoclonal antibody, albumin, and methotrexate delivery to cerebrospinal fluid and brain. *Neurosurgery* 17:419, 1985.
50. Rapoport S. I. Experimental modification of blood-brain barrier permeability by hypertonic solutions, convulsions, hypercapnia and acute hypertension. In Cserr H. F., Fenstermacher J. D., Fencl V. (eds.). *Fluid Environment of the Brain.* New York: Academic Press, 1975. Pp. 61–80.
51. Klatzo I. Neuropathological aspects of brain edema. *J. Neuropathol. Exp. Neurol.* 26:1, 1967.
52. Fishman R. A. Brain edema. *N. Engl. J. Med.* 293:706, 1975.
53. Miller J. D. The management of cerebral edema. *Br. J. Hosp. Med.* 21:152, 1979.
54. Langfitt T. W., Weinstein J. D., Kassel N. F., et al. Contributions of trauma, anoxia and arterial hypertension to experimental acute brain swelling. *Trans. Am. Neurol. Assoc.* 92:257, 1967.

55. Meinig G., Reulen H. J., Magawly C. Regional cerebral blood flow and cerebral perfusion pressure in global brain edema induced by water intoxication. *Acta Neurochir.* 29:1, 1973.
56. Corning J. L. Spinal anesthesia and local medication of the cord. *N.Y. State Med. J.* 42:483, 1885.
57. Laglia A. G., Eisenberg R. L., Weinstein P. R., et al. Spinal epidural hematoma after lumbar puncture in liver disease. *Ann. Intern. Med.* 88:515, 1978.
58. Tourtellotte W. W., Henderson W. G., Tucker R. P., et al. A randomized, double-blind clinical trial comparing the 22 versus 26 gauge needle in the production of the post-lumbar puncture syndrome in normal individuals. *Headache* 12:73, 1972.
59. Hollis P. H., Malis L. I., Zappulla R. A. Neurologic deterioration after lumbar puncture below complete spinal subarachnoid block. *J. Neurosurg.* 64:253, 1986.
60. Shaywitz B. D. Epidermoid spinal cord tumors and previous lumbar puncture. *J. Pediatr.* 80:638, 1972.
61. Vour'ch G. Continuous cerebrospinal fluid drainage by indwelling spinal catheter. *Br. J. Anaesth.* 35:118, 1963.
62. Aitken R. R., Drake C. G. Continuous spinal drainage in the treatment of postoperative cerebrospinal-fluid fistulae. *J. Neurosurg.* 21:275, 1964.
63. McCallum J., Maroon J. C., Janetta P. J. Treatment of postoperative cerebrospinal fluid fistulas by subarachnoid drainage. *J. Neurosurg.* 42:434, 1975.
64. Findler G., Sahar A., Beller A. J. Continuous lumbar drainage of cerebrospinal fluid in neurosurgical patients. *Surg. Neurol.* 8:455, 1977.
65. Post K. D., Stein B. M. Technique for spinal drainage. *Neurosurgery* 4:255, 1979.
66. Swanson S. E., Kocan M. J., Chandler W. F. Flow-regulated continuous spinal drainage: Technical note with case report. *Neurosurgery* 9:163, 1981.
67. Graf C. J. Comments. *Neurosurgery* 9:165, 1981.
68. Graf C. J., Gross C. E., Beck D. W. Complications of spinal drainage in the management of cerebrospinal fluid fistula. Report of 3 cases. *J. Neurosurg.* 54:392, 1981.
69. Nelson M. O. Postpuncture headaches—a clinical and experimental study of the cause and prevention. *Arch. Dermatol. Syph.* 21:615, 1930.
70. Jones R. J. The role of recumbency in the prevention and treatment of postspinal headache. *Anesth. Analg.* 53:788, 1974.
71. Krueger J. E., Stoetling V. K., Graf J. P. Etiology and treatment of post-spinal headaches. *Anesthesiology* 12:477, 1951.
72. Gormley J. B. Treatment of postspinal headache. *Anesthesiology* 21:565, 1960.
73. DiGiovanni A. J., Dunbar B. S. Epidural injection of autologous blood for post lumbar headache. *Anesth. Analg.* 49:268, 1970.
74. Glass P. M., Kennedy W. F. Jr. Headaches following subarachnoid puncture—treatment with epidural blood patch. *J.A.M.A.* 219:203, 1972.
75. Vandrell J. J., Bernards W. C. Epidural "blood patch" for the treatment of post spinal headaches. *Wisc. Med. J.* 72:132, 1973.
76. Ostheimer G. W., Palahniuk R. J., Schnider S. M. Epidural blood patch for post-lumbar-puncture headache. *Anesthesiology* 41:307, 1974.
77. Brodsky J. B. Epidural blood patch—a safe effective treatment for postlumbar-puncture headaches. *West. J. Med.* 129:85, 1978.
78. DiGiovanni A. J., Galbert M. W., Wahle W. M. Epidural injection of autologous

blood for postlumbar-puncture headache. II. Additional clinical experiences and laboratory investigation. *Anesth. Analg.* 51:226, 1972.

79. Balagot R. D., Lee T., Liu C., et al. The prophylactic epidural blood patch. *J.A.M.A.* 228:1369, 1974.
80. Cornwall R. D., Dolan W. N. Radicular back pain following lumbar epidural blood patch. *Anesthesiology* 43:692, 1975.
81. Shantha T. R., McWhirter W. R., Dunbar R. W. Case history: Complications following epidural "blood patch" for postlumbar-puncture headaches. *Anesth. Analg.* 52:67, 1973.
82. Mullan S., Harper P. V., Hekmatpanah J., et al. Percutaneous interruption of spinal-pain tracts by means of strontium 90 needle. *J. Neurosurg.* 20:931, 1963.
83. Rosomoff H. L., Brown C. J., Sheptak P. Percutaneous radiofrequency cervical cordotomy: Technique. *J. Neurosurg.* 23:639, 1965.
84. Zirvin J. A. Lateral cervical puncture: An alternative to lumbar puncture. *Neurology* 28:616, 1978.
85. Ayer J. B. Puncture of the cisterna magna. *J.A.M.A.* 81:358, 1923.
86. Ward E., Orrison W. W., Watridge C. B. Anatomic evaluation of cisternal puncture. *Neurosurgery* 25:412, 1989.

Suggested Readings

Davson H., Welch K, Segal M. B. *The Physiology and Pathophysiology of the Cerebrospinal Fluid.* London: Churchill Livingstone, 1987.
Wood J. H. (ed.). *Neurobiology of Cerebrospinal Fluid* (Vol. 1) New York: Plenum Press, 1980.
Wood J. H. (ed.). *Neurobiology of Cerebrospinal Fluid* (Vol. 2) New York: Plenum Press, 1983.

4. Electrophysiology

Cellular Electrophysiology

The lipid-protein cell membranes of neurons enclose high concentrations of potassium, negatively charged protein complexes, and lesser amounts of sodium and chloride. Extracellular fluid, in contrast, contains a high concentration of sodium and chloride.

Changes in the extracellular fluid concentration affect axons' resting and threshold potentials. The difference in concentration of potassium and chloride on either side of the membrane is maintained by the Na^+-K^+ adenosine triphosphatase (ATPase) pump, which actively pumps sodium out of, and potassium into, the cells. A resting membrane potential of -70 to -100 mV (inside negative with respect to outside) is thus maintained. An action potential occurs when the membrane is rapidly depolarized; the change in the membrane potential is sufficient to temporarily increase the membrane permeability for sodium, which rapidly enters the cell down its concentration gradient. Slightly later, a similar increase in membrane permeability for potassium repolarizes the membrane.

The action potential is propagated by saltatory conduction in myelinated nerve fibers or, in unmyelinated nerves, by local eddy currents. At the end of most neurons the action potential causes the release of a neurotransmitter (requires calcium influx) across a space known as the *synaptic cleft*. The neurotransmitter then acts at a receptor site, usually the postsynaptic neuron, where it in turn affects the membrane potential. Excitatory neurotransmitters (acetylcholine and glutamic acid) stimulate the receptor, which initiates a self-propagating action potential in the postsynaptic nerve. Inhibitory transmitters (glycine and gamma aminobutyric acid [GABA]) cause a reduction in excitability at the postsynaptic nerve, usually by facilitating the opening of chloride channels and the inflow of negatively charged chloride ions, resulting in hyperpolarization.

By altering the membrane's permeability to ions, (partial depolarization or repolarization), postsynaptic potentials inhibitory and excitatory (IPSP and EPSP), influence the ease with which an action potential may be elicited.

Electroencephalography

The electroencephalogram (EEG) is the brain's electrical activity as recorded from electrodes. The potential difference between pairs of electrodes or between an electrode and its reference point is amplified and then displayed on moving paper. Most often the electrodes are placed over the scalp. Specialized placement such as in the nasopharynx may be used to record activity of the anteromedial surface of the temporal lobe; sphenoidal electrodes record activity from the anteroinferior surface of the temporal lobe.

Certain activation procedures are used as part of the recording technique. Hyperventilation, which causes cerebral vasoconstriction, may accentuate EEG abnormalities. Recording during sleep or after a 24-hour period of sleep deprivation may provoke abnormalities that might otherwise be missed. The incidence of epileptiform discharge is increased when the EEG is recorded during sleep, especially in patients with partial complex seizures. Photic stimulation causes a rhythmic activity that is time-locked to the visual stimulus and has a frequency that is harmonically related to that of the flickering light. This is known as a "driving response," and may be detected over the posterior regions of the head.

EEG electrodes are connected in predetermined patterns, or *montages*, to permit the sequential recording of the electrical activity of various areas. The origin of the EEG is thought to be cortical, particularly from the postsynaptic potentials of the vertically oriented pyramidal cells. The cortical activity has a regular rhythm that seems to depend on the integrity of subcortical mechanisms.

The clinically relevant frequency range of the EEG includes the following bands:

Delta rhythm: less than 3.5 Hz
Theta rhythm: 4 to 7 Hz
Alpha rhythm: 8 to 13 Hz
Beta rhythm: greater than 13 Hz

The illogical sequence of the Greek letters can be understood in the context of a short historical review. Alpha and beta were the original ranges described by Berger, the pioneer of EEG, in 1929. Gamma rhythm, which is now a part of beta, originally referred to frequencies greater than 30 Hz. Delta rhythm was introduced by Walter in 1936 to describe all frequencies below alpha. He later designated theta for the band 4 to 7 Hz because he assumed it was of thalamic origin. The other Greek letters lambda and mu describe special EEG activities rather than bands.

Alpha rhythm (8–13 Hz) occurs during wakefulness, over the posterior regions, and is best seen with the patient resting and the eyes closed. Alpha is attenuated or abolished with eye opening. Not all activity in the alpha range is necessarily alpha rhythm; for instance, the mu rhythm (mu stands for motor) is within alpha range but differs from it in topography and physiologic significance, being strongly related to the motor cortex.

Beta rhythm (greater than 13 Hz) is found mainly over the frontal and central areas. It is especially prominent after the administration of barbiturates and benzodiazepines. Beta rhythm increases in amplitude over the area of a skull defect.

Theta activity (4–7Hz) is very prominent in children but becomes less so as they mature; it is also common in drowsiness and sleep.

Delta rhythm (less than 3.5 Hz) is the predominant activity in infants and is a normal finding during deep sleep in adults. When present in the awake, adult EEG, delta rhythm is pathologic.

Breach rhythm (6–11 Hz) is a mulike rhythm found in patients with skull defects after neurosurgical procedures.

Spike discharges are potentials with a sharp outline and a duration of less than 70 msec. A *sharp* wave has a duration of 70 to 200 msec. The presence of spike or sharp waves on the interictal EEG may be suggestive of the epileptiform activity of focal and generalized seizures. Three-per-second spike and wave complexes are seen in petit mal epilepsy. Delta slowing, occurring focally and consistently, is seen with mass lesions such as tumor or abscess. Focal theta and delta slowing is also seen in cerebral infarctions. Diffuse changes can be seen in hepatic failure or uremia or in postanoxic encephalopathies. These changes may range from mild disorganization and slowing of the background activity to diffuse high-voltage delta slowing. In the most severe cases, burst suppression, spindle coma, alpha coma, or an isoelectric (flat) tracing may be recorded. The EEG is often employed to gauge prognosis in coma and as a criterion for brain death. The EEG is most useful in the investigation of epilepsy.

A more recent application of electroencephalography in neurological critical care units is the continuous objective neurophysiological monitoring of comatose patients. EEG data is analyzed by a computer (processed EEGs). The technique involves the fast Fourier transformation of epochs of raw EEGs, usually 2 to 4 seconds long. The EEG is thereby characterized by power (amplitude squared) and frequency—power spectral analysis—and displayed in various ways. The principal advantage of power spectral analysis is that it offers data compression without sacrifice of too much information. When the EEG is used in this way continuously, the functional state of the brain can be known at all times, providing valuable information in the critical comatose patient [1].

Seizures and the Neurosurgical Patient

Seizures complicate many neurosurgical diseases. There is little doubt about their harmful effects. Apart from the physical danger posed to the patient by sudden, unprotected falls or inefficient respiratory effort, repetitive seizure activity may lead to structural changes, causing neuronal damage or the establishment of an epileptic focus. *Kindling* is the process whereby regular repetition of a stimulus in the brain leads to permanent augmentation of response locally or in a homologous area in the contralateral hemisphere [2]. Kindling may induce secondary dependent or independent foci; uncontrolled epilepsy is a progressive disease, clinically and anatomically. (The death rate among epileptics is higher than among controls, and it is especially higher during the first 10 years after diagnosis [3].)

An important cause of death and morbidity among epileptics is *status epilepticus*. Most authors accept any seizure lasting longer than 30 minutes, or a series of seizures without the person's regaining consciousness, as status epilepticus. Some 3.8 percent of epileptics have an episode of status at some point in their life, and this number is particularly high (9%) in patients with epilepsy secondary to a known underlying lesion. The risk of death from status has been estimated at between 1 and 20 percent in adults [4] and at 5 percent in children [5]. This mortality is in part due to cardiorespiratory arrest but more often is a result of the underlying disease (tumor, trauma, infection).

A risk of increased neurologic deficit is estimated at between 10 and 20 percent. Rapid control is the most important factor determining outcome. Initially, oxygen is given by mask or nasal catheter and an intravenous line is placed. Draw blood for analyses of glucose, electrolytes, and toxic agents. Since hypoglycemia is always a possibility, give 50 ml of 50 percent glucose. This is followed by 5 mg of diazepam intravenously. If the seizure continues or quickly returns (which often happens because of the rapid distribution of diazepam), additional doses of diazepam are given, not to exceed a total of 30 mg. The first injection of diazepam is followed by the intravenous administration of 1000 mg of phenytoin given slowly at a rate of no greater than 50 mg/minute, while monitoring the patient's vital signs. If the combination of diazepam and phenytoin does not abort the seizures, phenobarbital 10 mg/kg (100 mg in 1–2 minutes) may be given intravenously. If the seizures continue beyond 60 minutes, general anesthesia should be considered.

Seizures and Brain Tumors

The incidence of seizures in patients with supratentorial tumors is related to tumor type and location. Seizure frequency is inversely related to the degree of malignancy, varying from 50 to 81 percent with oligodendrogliomas to 40 to 66 percent among astrocytomas and to 19 to 26 percent in metastatic tumors. There is a relatively low incidence of seizures in patients with infratentorial tumors [6, 7].

The increased seizure frequency with the more histologically benign tumors is probably a function of lifespan. Seizure frequency also correlates well with tumor location. Cortex along the rolandic strips is highly susceptible to seizures; whereas the basicranial and occipital cortex is less vulnerable [8].

Subdural Empyema and Brain Abscess

Subdural empyema is a relatively uncommon condition that, until recently, has been associated with a very poor outcome. Seizures remain a frequent complication despite improved surgical therapy. Some 50 to 60 percent of patients with subdural empyema have seizures pre-operatively [9, 10]. Between 26 and 42 percent of patients continue to have seizures after surgery [10, 11].

The risk of occurrence of seizures in patients with brain abscess is between 36 and 79 percent [12–14]. Follow-up study indicates that 72% of patients develop seizures 1 to 15 years after operative therapy [15]. Intracranial suppuration seems to be associated with a sufficiently high risk of epilepsy to justify prophylaxis in virtually all cases [12].

Posttraumatic Seizures

Seizures are a known complication of head injury. Risk factors known to predispose to early seizures include linear skull fractures, depressed skull fractures, posttraumatic amnesia greater than 24 hours, focal neurologic deficit, and intracranial hematoma. One-fourth of seizures occur within 1 hour of injury, and an additional 25 percent occur within 24 hours. Delayed seizures are more likely to develop in those patients with acute hematoma, contusions, cortical lacerations or depressed skull fractures. Fifty percent of late seizures occur within the first year, with a progressive decrease in each subsequent year. The risk is no greater than in the general population after 5 years. Half of all late seizures are focal [16].

The risk of developing posttraumatic epilepsy can be assessed using Jennett's criteria [16]. Whether or not those patients whose risk is high (greater than 15%) should be given prophylaxis is a moot point. Although some authors advocate routine seizure prophylaxis for some patients (e.g., those with early seizures, depressed skull fractures, intracranial hematomas) [12, 16], the experience of Young et al. [17, 18] casts doubt upon the ability of phenytoin prophylaxis to prevent early or late posttraumatic seizures. Anticonvulsants are not benign drugs, and their use should be determined by solid criteria. In children, posttraumatic seizures occur in 7 percent of patients. Most such icti occur very early; repeat seizures are rare. In this cohort, early seizures carry no prognostic import for posttraumatic epilepsy [19].

Seizures and Aneurysmal Subarachnoid Hemorrhage

Early postaneurysmal subarachnoid hemorrhage (SAH) seizures can occur in up to 26 percent of patients with SAH; many occur at the time of the original hemorrhage, and repeat episodes may follow or herald rebleeding [20]. Late post-SAH seizure (more than 1 month after SAH or surgical treatment) has been observed in 10 percent of patients. There is an increased incidence in younger patients, in patients with middle cerebral and posterior communicating artery aneurysms, and in patients with intracerebral hematomas. Most seizures are generalized tonic-clonic and occur within 18 months of hemorrhage [21]. The risk of seizures and their consequences in the perioperative period of

SAH may justify anticonvulsant therapy during that period. Long-term therapy should be directed to those subgroups who show a propensity to seizure activity after definitive treatment of SAH.

Postoperative Seizures

Using the premise that trauma to the brain predisposes to seizure activity and that surgical manipulation is a traumatic event, many neurosurgeons administer prophylactic anticonvulsants to patients undergoing elective craniotomy. A few studies [22–25] have examined the efficacy of such practice, and generally the authors support it; supporting data is fragile however. In the early postoperative period, when cerebral edema is maximal, elevations of ICP from seizure activity are undesirable. Therefore it might be reasonable to recommend prophylaxis at least in the perioperative period. Whether all patients undergoing intracranial surgery should receive prophylaxis has not been resolved [12]. Obviously certain subgroups are at greater risk than others.

In general, the decision on what level of risk of seizure activity warrants prophylaxis must be individualized. There is little argument about using anticonvulsant medication once a seizure has occurred and recurring seizures are predictable. As a rule of thumb, since 10 to 15 percent of patients receiving anticonvulsant therapy may be expected to develop complications serious enough to warrant discontinuing or changing the drug, then a risk of epilepsy (or its consequences) of that magnitude or greater seems to be a reasonable point at which to consider prophylaxis [12].

Anticonvulsant Medications

Phenytoin (Dilantin). Phenytoin is useful for the treatment of many seizure types including generalized tonic-clonic, elementary and partial complex seizures. Its primary site of action is probably the motor cortex, where it inhibits the spread of seizure activity; possibly by promoting sodium efflux from neurons, phenytoin stabilizes the threshold against hyperexcitability and reduces post-tetanic potentiation at synapses. Loss of postetanic stimulation prevents the spread of epileptiform activity. Phenytoin is 90 percent protein-bound, with only 10 percent free to enter the CNS. This binding is responsible for several interactions with other substances.

Phenytoin exhibits dose-dependent pharmacokinetics, so that its apparent "half-life" changes with dose and serum level. However, many clinicians assume a half-life of approximately 24 hours and wait 5 to 7 days before assessing the patient's clinical response and measuring serum levels. Therapeutic blood levels are between 10 and 20 μg/ml. Therapeutic levels can be obtained in some patients by administering the drug once a day. Other patients may need more frequent doses. If therapeutic levels are required in a short time, a loading dose of 1 gm (or 10–15 mg/kg) is used. This loading dose can be given orally or intravenously (not to exceed 50 mg/min in adults or 1–3 mg/kg/min in neonates). Maintenance dosing may begin at 100 mg orally or intravenously three times daily and the dosage is then adjusted to suit individual requirements. Absorption is erratic after intramuscular injection and muscle necrosis may occur.

Toxic symptoms that are related to blood levels of the drug include nystagmus, ataxia, and blurred vision. Other side effects not related to blood levels of the drug include skin eruptions, teratogenesis, hepatitis, blood dyscrasias, and lupus. Hypertrichosis, gingival hyperplasia, and coarsening of facial features may trouble patients but rarely require withdrawal of medication.

Phenobarbital. Phenobarbital is effective in treating patients with generalized tonic-clonic seizures, and partial complex seizures. Its action as an anticonvulsant is the depression of repetitive electrical activity of multineuronal networks. It may be given intravenously, intramuscularly, or orally. Phenobarbital has a marked effect on the biotransformation of other medications. It has a long half-life and may be dosed once a day at bedtime. The dosage is generally 5 to 10 mg/kg. If levels must be achieved swiftly, a loading dose of 15 to 20 mg/kg can be given intravenously. Therapeutic blood levels are between 15 and 40 μg/ml. Toxic symptoms of the drug related to blood level include ataxia, sedation, and nystagmus; blood dyscrasias, hepatic changes, and skin rash may not be dose-related side effects.

Carbamazepine (*Tegretol*). Carbamazepine is used to treat generalized tonic-clonic seizures, elementary and partial complex seizures, and tic douloureux. It appears to act by reducing polysynaptic responses and blocking post-tetanic potentiation. Carbamazepine is usually a second line drug in seizure disorders. It is a relatively short-acting drug, reaching peak levels in 4 to 5 hours, with a half-life of about 12 hours. Carbamazepine undergoes autostimulation of its own metabolism with chronic therapy; therefore its half-life varies.

Therapeutic blood levels are between 5 and 12 μg/ml. Treatment is usually started at a low dose and gradually increased at weekly intervals until the best response is obtained. Dose-related toxicity includes vertigo, diplopia, dizziness, drowsiness, and unsteadiness. Other side effects, not necessarily dose-related ones, include blood dyscrasias and gastrointestinal disturbances. Periodic blood counts are advised after therapy is initiated.

Primidone (*Mysoline*). Primidone is chemically related to phenobarbital. It is converted to two metabolites—phenyethylmalonamide (PEMA) and phenobarbital—with antiepileptic activity. Primidone is used primarily for generalized tonic-clonic and complex partial seizures. The usual therapeutic dose is in the range of 20 mg/kg; a low dose (2–5 mg/kg) should be started and gradually increased to therapeutic levels. Therapeutic blood levels are between 8 and 12 μg/ml. Most of the toxic effects of chronic primidone therapy are similar to those of phenobarbital. Nystagmus and sedation are the most common toxic side effects.

Valproic Acid (*Depakene*). Valproic acid is used for many seizure types, including generalized tonic-clonic, complex partial, myoclonic, and absence seizures. It probably has the widest range of all the currently marketed antiepileptic drugs. Valproic acid is extensively protein-bound and may thus interact with other medications. It is usually given three or four times a day because of its relatively short half-life (7 to 9 hours); it peaks at 1 to 4 hours. It is relatively free of serious toxicity. Nausea, vomiting, and cramps are the most common untoward reactions. Hepatic toxicity has been noted, and if liver function tests become abnormal, the drug should probably be withdrawn.

Diazepam (*Valium*). Diazepam is used most frequently in the treatment of status epilepticus because it achieves a briefly high concentration in the blood. Brain and blood levels fall rapidly within 30 minutes of intravenous administration because of redistribution of the medication. Therefore, its administration must be followed by another medication in the treatment of status epilepticus. It and other benzodiazepams have little efficacy in chronic therapy. The drug is metabolized to a pharmacologically active metabolite. Diazepam has a half-life of 10 to 40 hours, and its metabolite may last for 3 or 4 days. The most prominent side effect is sedation.

Evoked Potentials

Sensory systems have been used most often for clinical evoked potential (EP) studies. Motor EPs can also be recorded and represent electrical activity of cortical neurons before a voluntary muscle movement is initiated. The sensory EP is a transient electrical response of the central nervous system (CNS) to a specific extrinsic stimulus. The CNS is constantly generating EPs in response to a battery of environmental stimuli. Diagnostic EPs require (1) a controlled, discrete stimulus; (2) recording from specific loci regions in the system pathway; and (3) elimination (usually by computerized signal averaging) of larger amplitude background electrical signals ("noise"), composed mostly of EEG but also of nonneural electrical activity that obscure the smaller amplitude EP ("signal"). The wave complexes of the EP are designated according to their electrical polarity (positive, P, or negative, N) and their location in the wave sequence (1,2,3, and so on) or their approximate poststimulus latency (in milliseconds).

Visual Evoked Potential

Although visual evoked potentials (VEPs) can be elicited by a variety of visual stimuli, the stimulus most frequently used is a reversible checkerboard pattern. The VEP is dominated by a large, V-shaped positivity with a peak latency of 100 ms (P100). There is some physiologic and technical variability in the latency and, to a lesser extent, the amplitude of P100. Ocular lesions produce abnormalities of the VEP by diminishing the effective stimulus reaching the retina. Diseases of the anterior visual pathway (optic nerve and chiasm) produce most of the clinical pathologic abnormalities of VEP. Demyelinating lesions (e.g., multiple sclerosis, optic neuritis) tend to prolong VEP latency, while preserving the configuration of P100 [26, 27].

Compressive, destructive (e.g., tumors of the orbit, sphenoid wing meningiomas, suprasellar meningiomas, pituitary tumors), or degenerative lesions that interrupt axons tend to diminish VEP amplitude and alter its configuration with or without prolongation of latency [28, 29]. Continuous intraoperative monitoring of visual function with VEP during parasellar surgery may alert the surgeon to excessive manipulation of the optic nerves [30, 31]. VEP abnormalities following head injury have been applied to the differential diagnosis of ocular injury and optic nerve trauma in altered states of consciousness [32, 33].

Brainstem Auditory Evoked Potential

Auditory EPs do not specifically localize to the auditory cortex as might be anticipated. Rather, they actually project over wide areas of the scalp. These nebulous hemispheric potentials (intermediate and late) have caused neurodiagnostic attention to focus on the more distinct potentials (early or short-latency) evoked from brainstem structures (brainstem AEP [BAEPs]).

The normal BAEP consists of a series five or more wave peaks appearing within the first 10 msec after the stimulus (broad-band clicks). These waves (positive polarity), numbered I through VII, appear to have the following origins [34, 35]: wave I, auditory nerve; wave II, cochlear nuclei (medulla)—although this is still controversial; wave III, superior olivary complex (pons); wave IV, lateral lemniscus (pons); wave V, inferior colliculus (midbrain); wave VI, medial geniculate; and wave VII, auditory radiations. Waves VI and VII are not present in conventionally recorded BAEPs in many normal individuals, which limits their clinical utility.

BAEPs are useful in evaluating the brainstem in patients with head injury and coma of unknown cause [36]. Demyelinating lesions of the brainstem (e.g., multiple sclerosis, central pontine myelinolysis) are detectable by BAEP [37, 38]. BAEPs have been used for the early diagnosis of posterior fossa tumors in patients with equivocal or negative neurologic and neuroradiologic findings [39, 40]. Intraoperative BAEPs are used to monitor the integrity of the neural pathways during tumor resection.

Somatosensory Evoked Potential

Somesthesis is made up of multiple modalities (e.g., touch, pin prick, vibration, joint position, and temperature), and it is possible to generate

EPs specific to one or another modality. However, most laboratories generate somatosensory evoked potentials (SEPs) from a percutaneous pulsed electrical stimulation (shock pulse) of a peripheral nerve, such as the median or ulnar in the arm or the peroneal or posterior tibial in the leg. This type of stimulus activates sensory axons without regard to their functional specificity. Nonetheless, SEPs are thought to arise in the posterior column–medial lemniscal system [41–43].

Because of the anatomic latitude spanned by the somatosensory system, it is frequently necessary to record from several sites along the pathway. This localizes the lesion by identifying the segment of the pathway in which the SEP is abnormal. With electrodes close to the spine, one may record "far-field" subcortical or spinal potentials in addition to "near-field" cortical potentials from scalp electrodes. Three to four early SEP wave peaks ("far-field" potentials) are recorded within the first 15 msec; their generators are not known with certainty, but they may arise from elements of peripheral nerve, spinal dorsal columns and nuclei, the medullary lemniscal pathway, and perhaps thalamic structures [44–46].

With upper limb stimulation the first cortical wave ("near-field" potential) of the SEP is a small negativity with a peak latency of about 20 msec (N1 or N20). When a lower leg nerve is stimulated, N1 is often not seen; instead, there is a large positivity at about 35 msec [47, 48].

Spinal cord function has been studied extensively by SEP [49]. Intraoperative recording of SEP has been used in a variety of procedures during which monitoring of cord function is critical, e.g., removal of intraspinal tumors and scoliosis surgery [50]. SEP analysis has been useful in the diagnosis of multiple sclerosis [51]. Tumors of the thalamus and the primary somatosensory area of the cortex spare P_{15} but abolish all other activity. In acoustic tumor surgery SEP can be used to monitor brainstem function when BAEP cannot be recorded because of eighth cranial nerve compromise. In head injury, measurements of central conduction time (CCT), i.e., the time delay occurring between an EP generated in a brainstem structure (P_3, medulla) and the first recordable cortical potential (N1, somatosensory cortex) at 10 and 35 days after injury, significantly correlate with patient outcome. Failure of transmission in the somatosensory system (e.g., prolonged CCT) is most likely due to shear injury from impact, or to ischemia [52–54].

Multimodality EPs (VEPs, BAEPs, SEPs) have been used to evaluate brain function and estimate prognosis following head injury [55–57], with variable results.

Motor Evoked Potential

The SEP is limited by the fact that it primarily monitors the dorsal columns. These have a different location and blood supply from those of the motor system. Accordingly, the SEP does not correlate adequately with motor function. The introduction of noninvasive transcranial stimulation of the brain has permitted a direct approach to the assessment of function of the central motor pathways. In cases where the SEP and the motor evoked potential (MEP) differ, the MEP has been the better predictor of motor function. MEPs are obtained by stimulating either the motor cortex of the brain or the motor pathways of the spinal cord and then recording nerve action potentials from motor nerves or mechanical activity in muscle.

MEPs recorded from the intermediolateral tract of the spinal column are faster than SEPs transmitted by the dorsal columns. They may be more readily affected by injury to the anterior cord than are SEPs traveling in the dorsal columns. Levy et al. recorded MEPs elicited by stimulation of the spinal cord and by transcranial stimulation of the motor cortex in humans [58–61]. More work is needed before these techniques can be universally applied.

Electromyography

Electromyography (EMG) is the clinical study of the electrical activity of muscle. EMG is helpful when the clinical examination is equivocal or difficult. EMG findings are not pathognomonic of a specific disease but can be used as corroborative data when other evidence (e.g., clinical) supports the diagnosis. EMG is frequently used in conjunction with nerve conduction studies (see below). The muscles examined are selected on the basis of the clinical presentation. The study is performed by inserting a recording electrode into the muscle, initially at rest and then with graded contraction. The muscle potentials are displayed on an oscilloscope and fed through a loudspeaker for simultaneous visual and acoustic analysis. Electrical activity recorded at rest arises from insertion or movement (*insertion activity*) of the needle and is due to mechanical stimulation or injury of the muscle fibers. It usually stops within 2 to 3 seconds of the movement. Spontaneous activity at rest may be found at the end plate region but not elsewhere (*end plate potentials*).

During activity, excitation of a single motor neuron activates the muscle fibers that it serves (*motor unit*). This generates a compound potential (usually biphasic or triphasic). The configuration and dimensions (amplitude, duration) of individual motor units are usually constant provided the electrode is undisturbed. With graded contraction the firing rate of the various motor units increases until it reaches a certain frequency, when additional units are recruited, resulting in a continuous burst of activity on the screen (*interference pattern*).

Pathologic Activity

When the muscle is at rest, insertion activity is seen only when some viable muscle fiber is left. It is prolonged in denervated muscle, polymyositis, and myotonic disorders.

Fibrillation potentials are small-amplitude, short-duration action potentials that arise spontaneously from single muscle fibers. They are found in denervated muscle provided some viable tissue remains, and they usually persist until the muscle is reinnervated or degenerates. They are also found in primary muscle disorders. *Positive sharp waves* are usually found in association with fibrillation potentials and are thought to arise from single fibers that have been injured. *Fasciculation potentials* are due to spontaneous activation of muscle fibers in individual motor units. They are of similar dimension to motor unit potentials, and may be found in normal patients or in those with chronic partial denervation. *Myotonic discharges* are high-frequency action potentials evoked by electrode movement or by tapping or contraction of the muscle. Their frequency and amplitude wax and wane; consequently the activity sounds like a dive bomber. They are found in patients with myotonic disease. *Myokymic discharges* are spontaneously occurring grouped action potentials, each group being followed by a brief period of silence. They occur in patients with radiation myelopathy, multiple sclerosis, chronic radiculopathy, or entrapment neuropathy [62].

During Activity

Motor unit potentials may be altered by a change in the number of functional fibers in the motor unit—*myopathic disorders*, or in the number of functional units—*neuropathic disorders*. In the former the mean duration and amplitude of the motor unit potentials are shortened, and there is an increased tendency for polyphasic potentials. In the latter, the motor unit potentials are longer, have a larger amplitude than normal, and may be polyphasic.

Nerve Conduction Studies

Nerve conduction studies (NCSs) assess peripheral motor and sensory nerve function by evaluating the EP following nerve stimulation. There are three kinds of NCSs: sensory, mixed nerve, and motor nerve conduction studies. Sensory NCSs are performed by stimulating orthodromically or antidromically. With the orthodromic method the sensory *nerve conduction velocity (NCV)* is determined by stimulating the distal part of the nerve and recording the *compound nerve action potential (CNAP)* proximally. For antidromic stimulation, the stimulating and recording electrodes are switched. The averaged CNAP is a triphasic wave; its latency, amplitude and conduction velocity are measured. Unlike motor nerve conduction, the sensory conduction time is equal to the latency. Therefore, sensory NCV is calculated by dividing the distance by the latency. The mixed NCV can be studied by stimulating the distal part of the mixed nerve (sensory and motor fibers) and recording the CNAP proximally. The mixed NCV is calculated as for the orthodromic sensory NCV. The clinical significance of the mixed NCV is essentially the same as that of the sensory NCV. Motor nerve conduction studies require the stimulation of a peripheral nerve with a supramaximal stimulus at each of two proximal points along the course of the nerve and simultaneously recording the *compound muscle action potential (CMAP)* from the muscle innervated by the nerve. The time required for this response with distal stimulation is the *terminal latency*. To obtain the conduction time, the terminal latency is subtracted from the latency at the proximal point of stimulation—*proximal latency*. The distance from the proximal to the distal point of stimulation is measured. The NCV is determined by dividing this distance by the conduction time. The directly (orthodromic) evoked compound muscle action potential recorded after stimulation of a peripheral nerve is called an *M wave*. It is described in terms of its latency, amplitude, and configuration. Antidromic activation of the anterior horn cells causes the discharge of an action potential, which is conducted orthodromically along the axon resulting in a small muscle potential. This late response is known as the *F wave* or *F response*. Its stimulus threshold is usually higher than that required for the H reflex and M response. The major application of F waves is in the assessment of central conduction. The H reflex (Hoffmann), another late response, is a monosynaptic reflex. The afferent limb consists of group Ia afferent fibers, from muscle spindles, and the efferent limb consists of alpha motor axons. The reflex arc is within the particular spinal cord segment. The stimulus threshold is lower than that required to evoke an M response. Late response studies are useful in a number of peripheral nerve disorders. Significant prolongation of H reflex and F response latency may be seen at a time when conventional methods do not show an abnormality.

NCSs can be used to identify the location of peripheral nerve disease and to differentiate this from disorders of muscle or neuromuscular conduction. NCSs can also help to separate axonal degeneration from segmental demyelination. Sensory CNAPs are of much lower amplitude than CMAPs and are more sensitive than motor conduction studies in detecting early or mild neuropathy.

Electrophysiologic alterations apparent on NCSs may include conduction block or slowing, as seen with segmental demyelination or with narrowing of the axons. Demyelinating neuropathies are typically associated with prolonged latencies and a pronounced slowing of conduction. A conduction block causes a reduction in amplitude with stimulation proximal to the block— in amplitude with relatively normal distal stimulation. Conduction slowing results in prolonged latency. A block is more common in rapidly developing disorders, and slowing is more representative of chronic disease. In traumatic nerve injuries there is either a conduction block with an amplitude change or axonal disruption with fibrillation potentials.

In addition, *reduced or absent responses* from wallerian degeneration after axonal disruption or axonal degeneration, may be seen, as in the "dying-back" neuropathies. Axonal neuropathies are particularly common in toxic and metabolic disorders. The major change on NCS is the reduced amplitude of the potentials.

One of the most common focal mononeuropathies is carpal tunnel syndrome. The sensory latency through the carpal tunnel is the most sensitive measurement in identifying the earliest abnormality. More severe compression reduces the amplitude of the sensory nerve action potential and prolongs the latency to a greater extent and over a longer distance. Severe median neuropathy at the wrist increases the distal motor latency to the thenar muscles and reduces the compound motor action potential.

References

1. Bickford R. G. Computer analysis of background activity. In Remond A. (ed.). *EEG Informatics. A Didactic Review of Methods and Applications of EEG Data Processing.* Amsterdam: Elsevier, 1977.
2. Goddard G. V., McIntyre D. C., Leech C. K., et al. A permanent change in brain function resulting from daily electrical stimulation. *Exp. Neurol.* 25:295, 1969.
3. Hauser W. A., Annegers J. F., Elveback C. R. Mortality in patients with epilepsy. *Epilepsia* 21:399, 1980.
4. Oxbury J. M., Whitty C. W. M. Causes and consequences of status epilepticus in adults: A study of 66 cases. *Brain* 94:733, 1971.
5. Aicardi J., Chevrie J. J. Convulsive status epilepticus in infants and children: A study of 239 cases. *Epilepsia* 11:187, 1970.
6. Lund M. Epilepsy in association with intracranial tumors. *Acta Psychiatr. Neurol. Scand.* 8(Suppl.):1, 1952.
7. Youmans J. R., Cobb C. A. Glial and neuronal tumors of the brain in adults. In Youmans J. R. (ed.). *Neurological Surgery.* Philadelphia: W. B. Saunders Co., 1982. Pp. 2759–2835.
8. Rasmussen T., Blundell J. Epilepsy and brain tumors. *Clin. Neurosurg.* 7:138, 1959.
9. Anagnostopoulos D. I., Gortvai P. Intracranial subdural abscess. *Br. J. Surg.* 60:50, 1973.
10. Cowie R., Williams B. Late seizures and morbidity after subdural empyema. *J. Neurosurg.* 58:569, 1983.
11. Hitchcock E., Andreadis A. Subdural empyema: a review of 29 cases. *J. Neurol. Neurosurg. Psychiatr.* 27:422, 1964.
12. Deutschman C. S., Haines S. J. Anticonvulsant prophylaxis in neurological surgery. *Neurosurgery* 17:510, 1985.
13. Gupta P. L., Legg N. J., Scott D. F. Epilepsy following surgical treatment of intracranial abscess. *Electroencephalogr. Clin. Neurophysiol.* 30:470, 1971.
14. Northcroft O. B., Wyke B. D. Seizures following surgical treatment of intracranial abscess. *J. Neurosurg.* 14:249, 1957.
15. Legg N. F., Gupta P. C., Scott D. F. Epilepsy following cerebral abscess: A clinical and EEG study of 70 patients. *Brain* 96:259, 1973.
16. Jennett B. *Epilepsy after Non-missile Head Injuries.* (ed. 2) London: Heinemann, 1975.
17. Young B., Rapp R. P., Norton J. A., et al. Failure of prophylactically administered phenytoin to prevent early posttraumatic seizures. *J. Neurosurg.* 58:231, 1983.
18. Young B., Rapp R. P., Norton J. A., et al. Failure of prophylactically admin-

istered phenytoin to prevent late posttraumatic seizures. *J. Neurosurg.* 58:236, 1983.
19. Amacher A. L. *Pediatric Head Injury. A Handbook.* St Louis; W.H. Green, 1988. P. 229.
20. Hart R. G., Byer J. A., Slaughter J. R., et al. Occurrence and implication of seizures in subarachnoid hemorrhage due to ruptured intracranial aneurysms. *Neurosurgery* 8:417, 1981.
21. Rose F. L., Sarner M. Epilepsy after ruptured intracranial aneurysm. *Br. Med. J.* 1:18, 1965.
22. Kvam D. A., Loftus C. M., Copeland B., et al. Seizures during the immediate post-operative period. *Neurosurgery* 12:14, 1983.
23. Mathew E., Sherwin A. L., Welner S. A., et al. Seizures following intracranial surgery: Incidence in the first post-operative week. *Can. J. Neurol. Sci.* 7:285, 1980.
24. North J. B., Hanieh A., Challen R. G., et al. Post-operative epilepsy: A double-blind trial of phenytoin after craniotomy. *Lancet* 1:384, 1980.
25. North J. B., Penhall R., Hanieh A., et al. Phenytoin and postoperative epilepsy: A randomized double-blind trial. *J. Neurosurg.* 58:272, 1982.
26. Halliday A. M., McDonald W. F., Mushin J. Visual evoked response in the diagnosis of multiple sclerosis. *Br. Med. J.* 4:661, 1973.
27. Shahroki F., Chiappa K. H., Young R. R. Pattern shift visual evoked responses: Two hundred patients with optic neuritis and/or multiple sclerosis. *Arch. Neurol.* 35:65, 1978.
28. Halliday A. M., Halliday E., Kriss A. The pattern-evoked potential in compression of the anterior visual pathways. *Brain* 99:357, 1976.
29. Holder G. E. The effects of chiasmal compression on the pattern visual evoked potential. *Electroencephalogr. Clin. Neurophysiol.* 45:278, 1978.
30. Wilson W. B., Kirsch W. M., Neville H., et al. Monitoring of visual function during parasellar surgery. *Surg. Neurol.* 5:323, 1976.
31. Feinsod M., Selhorst J. B., Hoyt W. F., et al. Monitoring optic nerve function during craniotomy. *J. Neurosurg.* 44:29, 1976.
32. Feinsod M., Auerbach E. Electrophysiological examination of the visual system in the acute phase after head injury. *Eur. Neurol.* 9:56, 1973.
33. Vaughan H. G. Jr., Katzman R. Evoked response in visual disorders. *Ann. N.Y. Acad. Sci.* 112:305, 1964.
34. Jewett D. L., Williston J. S. Auditory-evoked far fields averaged from the scalp of humans. *Brain* 94:681, 1971.
35. Picton T. W., Hillyard S. A., Krausz H. I., et al. Human auditory evoked potentials. I. Evaluation of components. *Electroencephalogr. Clin. Neurophysiol.* 36:179, 1974.
36. Uziel A., Benezech J. Auditory brain-stem responses in comatose patients: Relationship with brain-stem reflexes and levels of coma. *Electroencephalogr. Clin. Neurophysiol.* 45:515, 1978.
37. Stockard J. J., Rossiter V. S., Wiederholt W. C., et al. Brainstem auditory-evoked responses in suspected central pontine myelinolysis. *Arch. Neurol.* 33:726, 1976.
38. Stockard J. J., Stockard J. E., Sharborough F. W. Brain stem auditory evoked potentials in neurology: Methodology, interpretation, clinical application. In Aminoff M. J. (ed.). *Electrophysiologic Approaches to Neurologic Diagnosis.* New York: Churchill Livingstone, 1986. Pp. 467–534.
39. Selters W. A., Brackmann D. E. Acoustic tumor detection with brain stem electric response audiometry. *Arch. Otolaryngol.* 103:181, 1977.
40. Daly D. M., Roeser R. J., Aung M. H., et al. Early evoked potentials in patients

with acoustic neuroma. *Electroencephalogr. Clin. Neurophysiol.* 43:151, 1977.

41. Cracco R. Q. Spinal evoked response in normal adults and in patients with complete spinal cord lesions. *Electroencephalogr. Clin. Neurophysiol.* 34:816, 1973. (Abstr.)

42. Ertekin C. Studies on the human evoked electrospinogram. II. The conduction velocity along the dorsal funiculus. *Acta Neurol. Scand.* 53:21, 1976.

43. Giblin D. R. Somatosensory evoked potentials in healthy subjects and in patients with lesions of the nervous system. *Ann. N.Y. Acad. Sci.* 112:93, 1964.

44. Allison T., Goff W. R., Williamson P. D., et al. On the neural origin of early components of the human somatosensory evoked potential. In Desmedt J. E. (ed.). *Clinical Uses of Cerebral, Brainstem and Spinal Somatosensory Evoked Potentials. Progress in Clinical Neurophysiology* (vol. 7). Basel: S. Karger, 1980. Pp. 51–68.

45. Cracco R. Q., Cracco J. B. Somatosensory evoked potential in man: Far field potentials. *Electroencephalogr. Clin. Neurophysiol.* 41:460, 1976.

46. Wood C. C., Allison T., Goff W. R., et al. Neural origins of short-latency somatosensory evoked potentials: A review. In Nash C. L., Brown R. H. (eds.). *Proceedings of the Spinal Cord Monitoring Workshop: Data Acquisition and Analysis.* Cleveland: Case Western Reserve University, 1980. Pp. 129–156.

47. Desmedt J. E., Ceron G. Somatosensory evoked potentials to finger stimulation in healthy octogenarians and young adults: Wave forms, scalp topography and transit times of parietal and frontal components. *Clin. Neurophysiol.* 50:404, 425, 1980.

48. Dorfman L. J. Indirect estimation of spinal cord conduction velocity in man. *Electroencephalogr. Clin. Neurophysiol.* 42:26, 1977.

49. Ganes T. Somatosensory conduction times and peripheral, cervical and cortical evoked potentials in patients with cervical spondylosis. *J. Neurol. Neurosurg. Psychiatr.* 43:683, 1980.

50. McCallum J. E., Bennett M. H. Electrophysiological monitoring of spinal cord functions during intraspinal surgery. *Surg. Forum* 26:469, 1975.

51. Eisen A., Odusote K. Central and peripheral conduction times in multiple sclerosis. *Electroencephalogr. Clin. Neurophysiol.* 48:253, 1980.

52. Nakanishi T., Shimada Y., Sakuta M., et al. The initial positive component of the scalp-recorded somatosensory evoked potential in normal subjects and in patients with neurological disorders. *Electroencephalogr. Clin. Neurophysiol.* 45:26, 1978.

53. Hume A. L., Cant B. R. Conduction time in central somatosensory pathways in man. *Electroencephalogr. Clin. Neurophysiol.* 45:361, 1978.

54. Hume A. L., Cant B. R. Central somatosensory conduction time in comatose patients. *Ann. Neurol.* 5:379, 1979.

55. Greenberg R. P., Becker D. P., Miller J. D., et al. Evaluation of brain function in severe human head trauma with multimodality evoked potentials. I. Evoked brain-injury potentials, methods, and analysis. *J. Neurosurg.* 47:150, 1977.

56. Greenberg R. P., Becker D. P., Miller J. D., et al. Evaluation of brain function in severe human head trauma with multimodality evoked potentials. II. Localization of brain dysfunction and correlation with postraumatic neurological conditions. *J. Neurosurg.* 47:163, 1977.

57. Greenberg R. P., Newlon P. G., Hyatt M. S., et al. Prognostic implications of early multimodality evoked potentials in severely head-injured patients. A prospective study. *J. Neurosurg.* 55:227, 1981.

58. Levy W. J. Spinal evoked potentials from the motor tracts. *J. Neurosurg.* 58:38, 1983.

59. Levy W. J., York D. H. Evoked potentials from the motor tracts in humans. *Neurosurgery* 12:422, 1983.
60. Levy W. J., McCaffrey M., York D. H., et al. Motor evoked potentials from transcranial stimulation of the motor cortex in cats. *Neurosurgery* 15:214, 1984.
61. Levy W. J., McCaffrey M., York D. H., et al. Motor evoked potentials from transcranial stimulation of the motor cortex in humans. *Neurosurgery* 15:287, 1984.
62. Albers J. W., Allen A. A., Bastron J. A., et al. Limb myokymia. *Muscle Nerve* 4:494, 1981.

Suggested Readings

Aminoff M. J. (ed.). *Electrodiagnosis in Clinical Neurology* (*2nd ed.*). New York: Churchill Livingstone, 1986.
Oh S. J. *Clinical Electromyography. Nerve Conduction Studies.* Baltimore: University Park Press, 1984.
Niedermeyer E., Lopes da Silva F. (eds.). *Electroencephalography* (2nd ed.). Baltimore: Urban & Schwarzenberg, 1987.

II. Clinical Neurosurgery

5. Preoperative Assessment of the Neurosurgical Patient

The goal of preoperative assessment is to reduce operative risk and perioperative problems by anticipating and correcting potential difficulties before surgery. Consultation between the neurosurgeon and neuroanesthesiologist provides the information exchange necessary for smooth execution of the operation. Medical conditions may influence the course of neurologic disease; correspondingly, neurologic disease or treatment of it may confound an existing medical condition. The following section will describe preoperative considerations in the patient undergoing major cranial or spinal operation.

General Medical Status

A thorough history and physical examination are the first steps in evaluating a patient. Pertinent areas to consider include the patient's cardiovascular, pulmonary, metabolic and renal, and hematologic status.

Cardiovascular Status

Inquire about dypsnea, exercise tolerance, arrhythmias, angina, peripheral edema, hypertension, cardiac failure, and cardiac medications. *Hypertensive* patients function with a *right-shifted cerebral blood flow* (CBF) *autoregulatory curve.* Hypertension influences intraoperative hemodynamics. Hypovolemia related to chronic hypertension prediposes to hypotension from anesthetic agents. Of particular importance is a recent myocardial infarction (MI) (excess cardiac mortality of major surgery is 25% within 3 weeks of MI, 10% within 3 months, and 5% within 6 months).

The urgency of the procedure should thus be weighed against the cardiac risk. Generally, most patients will require a preoperative 12-lead electrocardiogram (ECG). If significant cardiac disease is suspected, a cardiologist should be consulted. Patients with significant cardiac risk may require a Swan-Ganz catheter for optimal perioperative management. Generally, cardiac medications should be continued until surgery, with the exception of aspirin, which should be discontinued 1 to 2 weeks before.

Pulmonary Status

Factors predisposing to perioperative pulmonary morbidity include long-term cigarette smoking, chronic obstructive or restrictive pulmonary disease, acute respiratory infection, and morbid obesity. Smoking is best discouraged perioperatively (smokers have 3 times as many postoperative pulmonary complications as nonsmokers). If feasible, provide preoperative instruction in use of an incentive spirometer. For patients likely to require respiratory support postoperatively, obtain preoperative arterial blood gases (ABGs) on room air to establish a baseline. Virtually all adult patients will need a chest x-ray film. Patients who cannot be expected to be ambulant after surgery—due to paraplegia, altered consciousness, or prolonged intensive care—require a program of chest physiotherapy and respiratory therapy that may be instituted before surgery. Patients receiving bronchodilator therapy should continue with their regimen to reduce the risk of bronchospasm.

Metabolic and Renal Status

A history of polyuria, polydypsia, edema, recent change in weight, and diuretic use should be sought. Chronic diuretic therapy may decrease total body potassium. Intraoperative volume expansion may further lower the serum potassium level, which predisposes to cardiac arrhythmias and increased sensitivity to muscle relaxants.

Hyperventilation, which is often used to reduce intracranial pressure (ICP), causes alkalosis, provoking an intracellular shift of potassium in place of hydrogen, which shifts extracellularly in an effort to correct alkalosis, making serum potassium level an important determination in this situation.

Laboratory investigations play an important role in assessing metabolic and renal status. Examination of serum electrolytes, blood urea nitrogen (BUN), creatinine, glucose, serum proteins, liver function tests, and urinalysis will uncover potential problems. Note significant recent trends as well as absolute values.

Patients with known diabetes mellitus need optimal stabilization, especially since high-dose steroids and surgical stress often exacerbate hyperglycemia. In addition, diabetic patients tend to heal poorly. Patients with acromegaly (growth hormone [GH]-secreting pituitary adenoma) may be diabetic or have abnormal glucose tolerance. Following the successful removal of a GH-secreting pituitary adenoma, these patients require less insulin in the postoperative period; the reduced requirement is probably related to a decrease in levels of circulating GH levels.

Patients with poor kidney function are less tolerant of fluid loading. The use of hypervolemic hemodilutional therapy for cerebral vasospasm in aneurysmal subarachnoid hemorrhage presents a significant challenge in such patients. Medications in patients with poor kidney function may have to be adjusted in line with creatinine clearance.

Renal dysfunction may cause coagulopathies from altered platelet function. Obtain a bleeding time if this is suspected.

Liver disease may confound anesthetic management because many drugs are detoxified in the liver. Coagulopathies from factor deficiences and thrombocytopenia are common in patients with severe hepatic dysfunction.

Suboptimal nutritional status (low serum proteins and transferrin) is associated with poor wound healing. Conversely, morbid obesity may predipose to thromboembolic or pulmonary complications in the postoperative period. Positioning obese patients on the operating table is difficult. A large panniculus restricts respiratory excursion. In the prone position, intraabdominal venous return is compromised and may result in intraoperative hypotension and hemorrhage from epidural veins during lumbar spine surgery.

Nausea and vomiting may accompany increased ICP, particularly in children, and may result in electrolyte imbalance or even weight loss.

Patients with status douloureux tic may be so frightened of opening their mouths that they neither eat nor drink. They may become dehydrated or malnourished. Children with hypothalamic tumor may show failure to thrive and poor nutritional status.

Intracranial disease may give rise to the syndrome of inappropriate secretion of antidiuretic hormone (SIADH). The syndrome is characterized by hyponatremia with a normal intravascular volume. It is exacerbated by fluid overload (common in the perioperative period) and may worsen cerebral edema or precipitate seizures.

Hematologic Status

A careful history, physical examination, and screening laboratory tests will identify most hemostatic defects. Spontaneous bleeding (hematomas, epistaxis, ecchymosis, or hematuria) suggests a congenital or acquired bleeding defect. A drug history of aspirin or warfarin should be sought. Useful screening tests include platelet count, bleeding time, protime (PT), and partial thromboplastin time (PTT).

Preoperative Rounds

The house staff should review the operative list. Be sure that cases have been scheduled as planned. If combined procedures are being done with other specialities (e.g., plastic surgery, orthopedics), they should be informed about any changes. The preoperative checklist should include the following:

1. *Informed operative consent.* The patient should be fully informed about the indications for surgery and its limitations, alternatives, risks, and expected outcome. Preferably, a responsible relative should be included in the preoperative discussion. The papers should be signed and witnessed. Separate forms may be required for blood products or heterologous tissue (e.g., bone grafts, dural substitutes).
2. Confirm the availability of banked blood. Directed donor blood is

becoming increasingly popular and can be arranged for elective cases.

3. Finalize arrangements with the patient's family about how they will be notified of the outcome of surgery. In major referral centers where many patients are out-of-town residents, give due consideration to family members who may not accompany them.

4. *Laboratory assessment.* Ensure that any significant abnormalities have been addressed. Request follow-up values after treatment. Communicate with the anesthesiologist about any concerns.

5. *Medications.* Patients taking cardiac or diabetic medications, anticonvulsants, and steroids should generally continue taking these until surgery. Check with the medical consultant or anesthesiologist for guidance. Prophylactic antibiotics (if used) should be ordered for the patient in the operating room. Sedatives, narcotics, and hypnotics, especially if long-acting, should be prescribed cautiously in patients with intracranial disease because they may confound neurologic assessment. Steroids (typically, dexamethasone 10 mg orally or intravenously) are useful before elective craniotomy for intracranial lesions (e.g., tumors) where cerebral edema may be a problem postoperatively. This helps to limit the insult from mechanical trauma to the brain during exposure, retraction, and other direct brain manipulation. Steroids are continued for a short period postoperatively and then tapered off gradually. Prophylactic anticonvulsants may be indicated if the procedure involves a corticectomy or an epileptogenic area of the brain.

6. *Surgical preparation.* Patients undergoing a craniotomy require a povidone-iodine or hexachlorophene shampoo the night before surgery. Most surgeons defer the shaving of hair until just before surgery. For spine or peripheral nerve operations, the area(s) of interest should be prepared accordingly.

7. *Premedication.* This will be ordered by the anesthesiologist.

8. Ensure that all pertinent plain x-ray films (spine or skull), computed tomography (CT) scans, and magnetic resonance images (MRI), angiograms, and myelograms will be available in the operating suite. *Confirm that the labels on the images are consistent and match clinical expectations. Errors of lateralization are unacceptable in neurosurgery.*

Neurosurgical Diagnostic Procedures

Angiography

Conventional Cerebral Angiography

Angiography plays a significant role in the diagnosis and surgical management of aneurysms, arteriovenous malformations (AVMs), atherosclerotic vascular disease, and some tumors. A knowledge of angiographic anatomy is necessary for interpretation of cerebral angiograms. *Intraoperative angiography,* in selected cases, facilitates the surgical management of AVMs and aneurysms. *Postoperative angiography* may be used to assess the completeness of resection of an AVM or confirm satisfactory placement of an aneurysm clip.

The technique of subtraction removes bony structures from the radiograph, allowing for better visualization of vessels; subtraction angiography is particularly useful for studying vessels of the neck, skull base, and posterior fossa. Dehydration and poor renal function are potentially hazardous in patients receiving radiopaque diagnostic agents. A BUN and serum creatinine should be obtained before proceeding.

Postangiogram orders are written by the neuroradiologist; generally, the patient is placed on bed rest for 6 to 8 hours with frequent clinical monitoring. Pressure packs may be placed over the puncture site. Neurologic complications of cerebral angiography include seizures, embolic stroke, drowsiness, or mild disturbances in vision. Local complications include hematoma, arterial laceration, and pseudoaneurysm formation. Systemic complications range in severity from a sensation of flushing, cutaneous hives, and laryngeal stridor to cardiovascular collapse and renal failure. Fortunately, severe complications are rare.

Digital Subtraction Angiography

Digital subtraction angiography (DSA) is a method for electronic processing of fluoroscopic images. A computer subtracts the mask image from the vascular images, removing soft tissue and bone densities that might obscure vascular anatomy. DSA requires a lower concentration of contrast than conventional angiography. DSA has improved the speed of angiographic examinations since subtracted images are obtained almost immediately. Although DSA was originally developed for intravenous injection, intravenous DSA (IV-DSA) is being supplanted by intraarterial DSA (IA-DSA). IV-DSA requires a higher contrast load and has less resolution than IA-DSA. One advantage of IV-DSA is that it eliminates the risk of intraarterial injection and possible cerebrovascular accident from intraarterial embolization. Both IV-DSA and IA-DSA offer less resolution than conventional angiography. DSA can be done on an outpatient basis [1–4].

Nuclear Medicine

Brain Scanning

Radionuclide brain scanning has been replaced to a large extent by CT and MRI. The study is generally performed in two phases: *dynamic* and *static.* Dynamic images are obtained by performing rapid sequential images following intravenous injection of a radionuclide (e.g., technetium 99m pertechnetate). Potassium perchlorate is given orally to block the normal uptake by choroid plexus prior to injecting technetium. Static images are acquired following the dynamic study.

The *dynamic brain scan* demonstrates rapid symmetric perfusion in both hemispheres. Asymmetry may be noted in the venous phase due to normal variations in venous anatomy. Radionuclide flow studies may be employed adjunctively in the determination of brain death. The study may be performed at the bedside. Flow through the carotid arteries to the base of the skull without intracerebral filling and lack of visualization of major venous sinuses on immediate static imaging is corroborative evidence of brain death [304].

The normal *static brain scan* shows activity in the suprasellar and sylvian regions. The venous sinuses (sagittal and transverse) also show activity. There is minimal activity within the brain on the static study if the blood-brain barrier is intact. Areas of disruptions in the blood-brain barrier (infarctions, cerebritis, and tumors) appear as "hot-spots" or focal increased activity.

Radionuclide Cerebrospinal Fluid Imaging

Radionuclide cerebrospinal fluid (CSF) imaging has been used in the investigation of hydrocephalus and CSF fistula. CSF circulation in adult-onset communicating hydrocephalus (AOCH) or normal pressure hydrocephalus (NPH) has been a particular area of investigation. The agent (indium 111 DPTA) is injected intrathecally by lumbar puncture. Thoracolumbar spine images are obtained at 2 and 4 hours, followed by cranial images at 6, 24, and 48 hours. A normal study demonstrates progressive radioactivity in a caudo-craniad direction. Serial images show movement through the subarachnoid spaces (basal cisterns, interhemispheric and sylvian fissures, and convexities). In normal pressure hydrocephalus there is early ventricular entry, persisting for 24 to 48 hours.

Isotope Cisternography

Radioisotope cisternography is useful in the evaluation of *skull base CSF fistula*. The test is performed by instilling human serum albumin tagged with technetium 99 or indium 111 into the subarachnoid space by lumbar puncture. To diagnose and localize the source of a CSF rhinorrhea, cotton pledgets are placed in the nasal passages to trap the escaping CSF. Nasal secretions ordinarily contain some unbound isotope; CSF rhinorrhea is indicated if there is a significant difference in radioactivity between the nasal pack on one side compared to that on the other and between the nasal pledgets and serum. **Shunt patency** has been evaluated using technetium-99-labeled isotope. The radioisotope is injected into the shunt reservoir or tubing; imaging within 30 to 60 minutes shows activity in the peritoneal cavity. Reflux into the ventricular system and clearance of radioactivity from the ventricles after a few hours completes the examination. Distal shunt obstruction may be inferred by a lack of diffuse activity in the abdomen; likewise, proximal shunt obstruction may show up as lack of clearance of isotope from the ventricle.

Computed Tomography

Since its introduction, CT has continued to undergo technologic evolution. Currently, fourth-generation scanners are in use. CT scanning is not a direct x-ray film of the brain, but rather a mathematical image reconstruction of its tissue densities. CT is noninvasive and rapid. Intravascular contrast CT is used to demonstrate a break in the integrity of the blood-brain barrier as occurs with tumors, abscesses, and fresh infarcts. The enhancement of AVMs and aneurysms is probably due to the iodine content of the circulating blood pool.

CT of the spine is important in the evaluation of lumbar disk disease, lumbar spinal stenosis, and spine trauma [5, 6]. Intrathecal contrast CT (myelography, cisternography) is helpful in the investigation of spinal lesions and CSF fistula. CT is indicated for such a wide range of intracranial and spinal pathologic states that it is difficult to imagine any diagnostic situation to which it could not contribute in some way. Specific CT findings in various lesions are discussed separately.

Magnetic Resonance Imaging

Although the use of MRI in medicine was first suggested in 1971, it has only been since the mid-1980s that the use of MRI has become widespread in the United States. Some of the unique features of MRI include the ability to image in any plane (axial, sagittal, and coronal), to visualize flowing blood, and to acquire chemical data.

A very simplified summary of the technique follows. The patient is placed within a powerful magnetic field that causes the protons in the tissues to align themselves in the orientation of the magnetic field. Introducing a specific radiofrequency (RF) pulse into the field perturbs the protons causing them to resonate and change their axis of alignment. When the RF pulse is removed, the protons "relax" and return to their original alignment. In so doing, the RF energy that was absorbed is emitted and subjected to computer analysis, from which a magnetic resonance image is constructed. The MRI essentially produces a map of hydrogen ion (proton) concentration. Hydrogen lends itself to examination by MRI because of its natural abundance in the body and the strong signal it emits.

After the RF pulse, the magnetization returns to equilibrium by a dynamic process described by two time constants T1 (spine-lattice relaxation) and T2 (spin-spin relaxation), both determined by the tissues being examined.

The appearance of the final image is modified by the RF pulse sequences set by the operator and the tissue parameters. Tissue parameters that affect MRI include *proton density T1 and T2 relaxation times.*

Proton density (PD) images are water density images; increases in the local concentration of water cause an increased intensity in the PD image. PD images are useful in imaging white matter disease (e.g., demyelinating lesions) where there is an increase in water content that is recognizable as an increased brightness. In general, the *longer the T1* and the *shorter the T2,* the *less intense (darker) the signal;* the *shorter the T1* and the *longer the T2,* the *more intense (brighter) the signal.* Solids (bone, calcium) and bulk water (e.g., CSF), rapidly flowing blood, and edema have much longer T1 and appear dark on T1-weighted images. Bound water (i.e., highly proteinaceous fluids), fat, and subacute blood have a short T1 and appear bright on T1-weighted images. T1-weighted images are best for evaluating anatomy because of the excellent resolution with this sequence. T2-weighted images are very sensitive in detecting pathologic conditions since these usually increase parenchymal edema, which appears bright on a T2-weighted study. Other things that appear bright on a T2-weighted image (long T2 signal) include fat, subacute blood, and CSF. Dark areas (short T2) on T2-weighted studies include bone or calcium, rapidly flowing blood, and acute blood.

The operator can alter two variables, repetition time (TR) and echo time (TE), to alter the contributions of any of the three tissue-specific characteristics to the intensity of the MRI; this is known as image weighting.

MRI has better resolution than CT and provides greater anatomic detail; it has a distinct advantage in the posterior fossa and cervicomedullary junction because of the lack of bone artifact. It also has an increased sensitivity to white matter lesions, especially demyelinating disease [7, 8].

Both CT and MRI scanners may cause claustrophobic patients a great deal of anxiety; sedation may be necessary to obtain good quality images. It is cumbersome to obtain an MRI on a critically ill patient because the strong magnetic field and radiofrequency transmission involved are liable to interfere with monitoring equipment. Recently, support and monitoring equipment (e.g., ventilators, transducers, ICP monitors, arterial lines, cardiac monitors, medication delivery pumps) have been adapted by eliminating ferromagnetic materials and using extension cables and telemetric monitoring to allow critically monitored patients to undergo MRI scanning [120].

Myelography

Myelography is the radiographic visualization of the spinal cord and nerve roots after a radiopaque substance is injected into the spinal subarachnoid space. Currently, two nonionic water-soluble contrast agents, iohexol (Omnipaque) and iopamidol (Isovue), are used for cervical, thoracic, and lumbar myelography. Myelography is generally performed under fluoroscopic guidance. The contrast agent is introduced through a lumbar or C1–C2 puncture. Contrast agent should not be allowed to enter the cranial vault since seizures may result. The patient is given clear liquids before the study; after the myelogram, the patient is kept in bed with the head slightly elevated, and fluids are encouraged. Postmyelogram low pressure headaches, nausea, and vomiting may confine some patients to bed for one to several days.

Spinal lesions demonstrable on myelography may be divided into (1) extradural lesions (e.g., herniated intervertebral disks, nerve sheath tumors, epidural abscess or hematoma, and metastatic lesions), (2) intradural-extramedullary lesions (e.g., meningioma, neurofibroma, drop metastases from a medulloblastoma, lipoma, and dermoid), and (3) intradural-intramedullary lesions (e.g., ependymoma, astrocytoma, and syringomyelia). Postmyelogram CT scanning is useful, especially in the cervical region. This defines the relationship of structural lesions to the cord and nerve roots [10].

Ultrasonography

Cranial Ultrasonography

Cranial ultrasound examinations are performed in infants with patent anterior fontanels. Sedation is rarely required. The study can be performed at the bedside. Indications include suspected hydrocephalus; it is also used as a screening test for infants with myelomeningocele or those at risk for intraventricular hemorrhage.

Coronal, axial, and sagittal views are usually obtained. Spontaneous intracranial hemorrhage is common in premature infants and may be seen in up to 70 percent of cases [305]; this may be germinal matrix hemorrhage or intraventricular hemorrhage. The germinal matrix is a highly vascular structure most prominent in the region between the head of the caudate nucleus and the thalamus. It is here that subependymal hemorrhage often originates. It may be confined to that area or extend into the cerebrum or ventricles. These hemorrhages may be diagnosed and followed by serial cranial ultrasound.

Germinal matrix hemorrhage is classified according to progressive severity from grades I through IV. Intraventricular hemorrhage is frequently complicated by posthemorrhagic hydrocephalus; generally, the degree of hydrocephalus is proportional to the amount of hemorrhage. Another important use of cranial ultrasound is in the diagnosis of hydrocephalus and abnormal CSF collections such as the Dandy-Walker malformation, arachnoid cysts, and holoprosencephaly. *Intraoperative* ultrasound is discussed in Chapter 6; *carotid ultrasound* is discussed under carotid endarterectomy.

Positron Emission Tomography

Positron emission tomography (PET) is an imaging technique that measures the location and concentration of physiologically active compounds labeled with positron emitters. The technique is based on the physics of positron annihilation and detection and the mathematical formulations developed for x-ray CT. PET provides insight into the brain's biologic functioning. A radiolabeled compound or isotope that decays by positron emission is chosen for its ability to trace specific biologic processes. Positron-emitting nuclides of biologic importance include oxygen 15, carbon 11, and nitrogen 13. These nuclides have a relatively short half-life and a low radiation dose. Because of their short half-life, positron-emitting radionuclides generally must be produced on site and rapidly synthesized into compounds of biologic interest. This requires a cyclotron for radionuclide production and is a capital-intensive project requiring a skilled team of specialists, putting it out of the reach of all but a few facilities. Physiologic measurements that are feasible with PET include CBF, cerebral glucose metabolism, and cerebral oxygen metabolism [11, 12].

Preoperative Care In Specific Neurosurgical Conditions

Intracranial Aneurysm

Almost 75 percent of nontraumatic subarachnoid hemorrhage (SAH) is the result of a ruptured aneurysm. About 20 percent of patients with SAH have associated intracerebral hemorrhage (ICH). The typical presentation of an SAH includes headache (usually described as the "*worst I have ever had*"), meningism, altered consciousness, and focal deficits such as paresis, anisocoria, aphasia, or visual field defect [13].

Most warning leaks are missed by first-contact physicians; this is tragic, for the subsequent hemorrhage is catastrophic in more than half of patients. The incidence of aneurysmal SAH is about 10.3 per 100,000 people per year [15]. Patients are usually in their fourth to sixth decades and females predominate. Not infrequently, patients present with an unruptured aneurysm, manifested by third nerve palsy or other local compressive effects.

Diagnosis

Every patient will require a complete history and physical examination, with emphasis on the central nervous system (CNS) and cardiorespiratory systems. It is particularly important to assess the patient's state of hydration, electrolyte balance, and hematocrit.

It is common practice to classify patients with SAH according to their clinical condition. The clinical grading scale most widely used is that of Hunt and Hess (Table 5-1) [16]. Standard grading of patients allows

Table 5-1. Clinical Grading of Subarachnoid Hemorrhage

Grade 0	Unruptured aneurysm
Grade 1	Asymptomatic; minimal headache or slight nuchal rigidity
Grade 2	a. Moderately severe headache, nuchal stiffness, no neurologic deficit b. Cranial nerve palsy
Grade 3	Drowsiness, confusion, mild focal deficit
Grade 4	Stupor, moderate to severe hemiparesis, possibly early decerebrate rigidity and vegetative disturbances
Grade 5	Deep coma, decerebrate rigidity, moribund

Note: Any serious systemic disease (hypertension, diabetes, chronic pulmonary disease, severe arteriosclerosis) or severe cerebral vasospasm places the patient in the next less favorable category.
Source: Hunt, W. E., Hess, R. M. Surgical risk as related to time of intervention in the repair of intracranial aneurysms. *J. Neurosurg.* 28:14, 1968.

for statistical comparisons between groups of patients when results of various treatment regimens are compared (Table 5-1).

Recently, a new grading scale has been proposed by the World Federation of Neurological Surgeons (WFNS) Committee on Universal Subarachnoid Hemorrhage Grading Scale. This has grades I through V and uses the Glasgow Coma Scale (GCS) for evaluating the level of consciousness (Tables 5-2, 5-4) [306, 312]. The WFNS committee also resolved that the Glasgow Outcome Scale (GOS) be used for the classification of outcome in SAH patients [307].

The diagnosis of SAH is confirmed by demonstration of blood or blood products in the subarachnoid space. Next, the source of bleeding is identified.

Computed Tomography. The initial diagnostic test in a patient suspected of having an SAH is an unenhanced CT scan. The reliability of CT scanning in SAH has been well documented [17–20]. A negative

Table 5-2. World Federation of Neurological Surgeons (WFNS) Committee on Universal Subarachnoid Hemorrhage (SAH) Grading Scale

WFNS grade	GCS score	Motor deficit
I	15	Absent
II	14–13	Absent
III	14–13	Present
IV	12–7	Present or absent
V	6–3	Present or absent

Source: Drake, C. G. Report of World Federation of Neurological Surgeons Committee on Universal Subarachnoid Hemorrhage Grading Scale. *J. Neurosurg.* 68:985, 1988.

Table 5-3. Computed Tomography Scan Grading of Subarachnoid
Hemorrhage

Grade 1	No blood detected
Grade 2	Diffuse deposition or thin layer with all vertical layers of blood; interhemispheric, insular cistern, ambient cistern, <1 mm thick
Grade 3	Localized clots or vertical layers of blood >1 mm thick
Grade 4	Diffuse or no subarachnoid blood but with intracerebral or intraventricular clots

Source: Fisher C. M., Kistler J. P., Davis, J. M. Relation of cerebral vasospasm to subarachnoid hemorrhage visualized by computed tomographic scanning. *J. Neurosurg.* 6:1, 1980.

CT scan does not exclude the diagnosis of a recent SAH. If clinical suspicion is high, a lumbar puncture is warranted. CT scan characteristics of SAH are due to the density of the extravasated blood. The density depends on the volume of the hemorrhage, the hematocrit of the blood, and the time elapsed since the bleed. The greater the volume of blood and the less dilution with CSF, the higher the density on CT.

The longer the blood lies in the subarachnoid space, the more dilution and resorption occur, so that after 5 or 6 days, CT no longer reliably detects SAH [20]. CT identifies blood in the subarachnoid space in approximately 90 percent of patients in the first 24 hours and over 50 percent of patients within the first week after the hemorrhage.

Fisher, Kistler, and Davis established a grading scale to assess SAH visualized on CT scan (Table 5-3) [21]. The location of the aneurysm may be suggested by the distribution of blood in the cisterns or the location of an associated ICH. With contrast-enhanced CT, the aneurysmal sac itself may enhance. If the aneurysm is completely thrombosed, the central portion fails to enhance and may have an attenuation coefficient similar to that of brain tissue. Occasionally, the shadow of a sac may be visible because it is surrounded by blood. Giant aneurysms (exceeding 2.5 cm) may calcify following thrombosis and become apparent on nonenhanced CT. Acute hydrocephalus following SAH is readily apparent on CT [22].

Arterial narrowing (vasospasm) frequently occurs following SAH. There is a strong positive correlation between the location and quantity of SAH and the distribution and intensity of vasospasm [23]. Vasospasm may lead to infarction, recognizable as low-density areas on CT scan.

Alterations in neurologic status following SAH may be due to rebleeding, delayed cerebral ischemia (DCI) due to vasospasm, or acute hydrocephalus; CT can differentiate between them.

Lumbar Puncture. If the CT is negative and clinical suspicion warrants it, a lumbar puncture is performed. A rule of thumb is as follows: patients suspected of having SAH whose neurologic examinations are normal and who would not be hospitalized if their CSF were clear should have a lumbar puncture. The tap should be atraumatic. The CSF should be immediately centrifuged and examined for xanthochromia.

Angiography. Once the diagnosis of SAH has been confirmed by CT or lumbar puncture, cerebral angiography is indicated. This determines the source of hemorrhage. Close consultation between the neurosurgeon and neuroradiologist is necessary to ensure that the study answers all relevant questions.

Complete cerebral angiography includes visualization of the anterior (internal carotid) and posterior (vertebrobasilar) circulations. Magnification and subtraction techniques as well as oblique and special (surgical) views are necessary to define the neck and configuration of the aneurysm and display surrounding vessels. These images assist the surgeon in deciding on the best surgical approach. Saccular aneurysms most commonly occur at arterial bifurcations. About 85 percent of all aneurysms are located on the anterior circulation; 15 percent are located on the posterior circulation. Twelve to thirty percent of patients harbor multiple aneurysms, and 9 to 19 percent of patients have bilateral aneurysms [25]. Nehls, Flom, and Carter have proposed an algorithm to identify the site of rupture in patients with multiple intracranial aneurysms [26]. Pointers include the presence of local vasospasm and an irregular contour of the aneurysm sac (Murphy's tit).

An AVM will be present in about 1 percent of patients with an intracranial aneurysm [24]; such aneurysms may be multiple and are often located on the major feeding artery of the AVM.

Occasionally, the initial angiogram will fail to reveal the source of the hemorrhage. If the initial study reveals any abnormality such as focal cerebral vasospasm, repeat the study in about a week. If the initial study is entirely normal, i.e., without any vasospasm and all vessels adequately visualized with magnified subtracted views, a repeat study is unlikely to be fruitful. These patients generally have a good prognosis [27, 28].

In the cooperative study, repeat carotid angiography revealed aneurysm in 16.5 percent of patients in whom the first angiogram was normal [29]. The angiogram may be repeated during the perioperative period if the patient deteriorates and vasospasm is suspected. If spasm has been present, a repeat study just before elective surgery may be necessary. Significant reduction in arterial caliber may indicate a need to delay surgery.

Digital occlusion of the contralateral common carotid artery during injection (cross-compression) provides a useful view of the arteries supplying both hemispheres. In addition to diagnosis, cross-compression may be invaluable in surgical management (e.g., in evaluating the patient's suitability for carotid ligation).

An aneurysm may be missed for several reasons: (1) inadequate technique, (2) arterial spasm, which may seal off the aneurysm neck and prevent contrast filling of the sac, and (3) observer error, usually in the setting of multiple lesions (i.e., the most obvious finding is identified but others lurk in the background). The most frequent associated intracranial lesion is a second aneurysm. Aneurysms of the middle cerebral artery (MCA) and posterior cerebral artery (PCA) tend to be symmetric on both sides—so-called mirror aneurysms. Multiple aneurysms are more common in women than in men, in patients with chronic hypertension, and in patients with sickle cell disease [25, 308, 309].

Certain atypical features, e.g., a patient under 18 years of age or an aneurysm located on the distal tree (especially if multiple), should raise the question of bacterial endocarditis or other infective sources (mycotic aneurysms) and certain diseases (coarctation of the aorta, fibromuscular hyperplasia, polycystic kidney disease).

Magnetic Resonance Imaging. Acute SAH is not readily detectable on MRI. However, in the subacute phase SAH becomes bright (high signal intensity) on both T1- and T2-weighted images. Old SAH may be seen on MRI as superficial siderosis (linear areas of marked T2 shortening and low signal intensity) [30, 31]. The aneurysm sac may be visible as a flow void. MRI is therefore useful in patients who may have sustained an earlier SAH and in whom the CT scan was negative.

Common Associated Problems

Rebleeding. Aneurysmal rebleeding following SAH carries a high morbidity and mortality. The peak incidence of rebleeding is within the first 24 to 48 hours following SAH. The rate of rebleeding decreases rapidly in the 4 weeks after the initial hemorrhage. After 6 months the risk of rebleeding continues at the rate of about 3 percent per year [32].

The worse the clinical grade on admission, the greater the likelihood of rebleeding. Hypertension increases the likelihood of rebleeding. The best method for avoiding rebleeding is treatment of the aneurysm by clip ligation as soon as possible. However, not all patients are candidates for early operation; these patients pose a significant management problem.

While awaiting surgery, the risk of rebleeding can be decreased by several methods, including reducing the transmural pressure across the wall of the aneurysm. *Transmural pressure* is the difference between arterial pressure (within the aneurysm sac) and the ICP (outside the sac). By lowering blood pressure and avoiding sudden or uncontrolled decreases in ICP, transmural pressure is reduced. Blood pressure is closely monitored, preferably by arterial line, and therapy is designed to keep pressure within the upper range of normal to maintain an adequate cerebral perfusion pressure (CPP). Wide fluctuations are best avoided; prolonged hypotension or hypovolemia during the period of peak incidence of vasospasm (approximately 5–10 days following SAH) are especially undesirable [33, 34]. Hydralazine (Apresoline) or labetalol (Normodyne) are reasonable choices for managing blood pressure in these patients. Other measures such as avoiding straining, anxiety, or pain (see the section on preoperative orders) are also important in preventing sudden elevations of transmural pressure that may result in rebleeding.

Another factor promoting increased transmural pressure is a sudden reduction in ICP. The typical situation predisposing to this is ventriculostomy and CSF drainage for treatment of hydrocephalus following SAH. Sudden loss of large quantities of CSF may drastically reduce ICP and increase transmural pressure. Intermittent lumbar punctures in this setting are apt to produce similar net effects.

Administration of the antifibrinolytic agent *epsilon-aminocaproic acid (EACA or Amicar)* reduces rebleeding. It acts by reducing the fibrinolytic reaction that is part of the overall meningeal reaction to blood in the subarachnoid space [35, 310, 311]. Antifibrinolytic agents reduce the overall risk of rebleeding in the first 2 weeks after SAH while a patient is awaiting surgery. An initial loading dose of 5 gm intravenously (or orally) followed by continuous infusion of 1.0 to 1.25 gm doses at hourly intervals will usually achieve a rapid therapeutic plasma level of 0.130 mg/ml of drug. This is the concentration apparently necessary for the inhibition of fibrinolysis. Administration of more than 30 gm/24 hours is not recommended. If satisfactory levels are not rapidly attained, Amicar may not prevent rebleeding during the first 2 days after SAH; unfortunately, this lag corresponds to the period of highest risk for rebleeding. Although antifibrinolytic therapy reduces the risk of rebleeding, it does not reduce overall mortality since there is a proportional increase in thrombotic and ischemic sequelae. These side effects of pulmonary emboli, venous thrombosis, cerebral infarcts, and hydrocephalus have limited its popularity. However, a recent Canadian study of the use of the calcium channel blocker nimodipine in subarachnoid hemorrhage suggests that some patients on antifibrinolytic therapy and nimodipine may have a lesser incidence of delayed ischemic side effects [43].

Cerebral Vasospasm. Intracranial arterial narrowing (cerebral vasospasm) may occur following SAH. The etiology, pathogenesis, and treatment of vasospasm remain a subject of intense research [36]. Perioperative vasospasm increases morbidity and mortality after aneurysm surgery. A distinction should be made between *angiographic spasm* on the one hand and ischemic neurologic deficit secondary to cerebral arterial spasm on the other (*clinical vasospasm*). Not all patients with angiographic spasm will be symptomatic. Overall, angiographically apparent spasm is seen in 30 to 65 percent of all patients with SAH, and about 30 percent of all patients with angiographically apparent spasm will develop ischemic neurologic deficits. Clinical features include a change in the level of consciousness and new or worsening focal deficit. These deficits are the most common cause of morbidity in these patients. CT is necessary to rule out hydrocephalus or bleeding, two conditions that must be considered in the differential diagnosis.

The risk of cerebral infarction from vasospasm can be reduced by avoiding hypovolemia, hypotension, and hyponatremia [37, 38].

Current concepts in management of cerebral vasospasm include the following:

1. *Volume expansion and hemodilution* (with colloid and crystalloid) and *induced hypertension* (with dopamine or dobutamine) to increase CPP [38] and augment CBF. This therapy has been successful in reversing the effects of vasospasm, but can be complicated by rerupture of an untreated aneurysm.
2. *Calcium channel blocking drugs* such as *nimodipine* and *nicardipine,* which may act by cerebral protection and vasodilatation of small cerebral arteries, may reduce ischemic neurologic deficits from aneurysmal SAH and vasospasm [39–42]. In a recent Canadian nimodipine study, treatment with oral nimodipine was associated with a significant number of patients with good neurologic outcome. Compared with untreated patients, fewer patients treated with nimodipine developed ischemic deficits from vasospasm. These results were primarily in grade 3 and 4 patients; grade 5 patients had an almost uniformly poor outcome regardless of treatment. The drug is quite safe, the most serious side effect being hypotension in a small number of patients [43].
3. *Interventional radiologic techniques* with balloon angioplasty is used to directly dilate constricted cerebral arteries in spasm in patients with ischemic neurologic deficit [44]. Only a small number of cases have been performed and there are few qualified practitioners of this technique. Although reports have been promising, further results are awaited before wider application.

Intracranial Hypertension. Rupture of an intracranial aneurysm may severely disrupt intracranial vascular dynamics (see Chap. 1). ICP rises significantly as blood is liberated into the subarachnoid space [45]. Intracranial hypertension following aneurysmal rupture may be compounded by an intracranial hematoma or cerebral edema. Significant mass effect from a hematoma may require urgent craniotomy for clot evacuation and treatment of the aneurysm. In some cases, ICP monitoring is necessary for optimal management of intracranial hypertension. Such intervention is more often required in poorer-grade patients in whom sustained elevations of ICP and lower levels of CBF are likely.

Hydrocephalus. Acute hydrocephalus after aneurysmal SAH is not uncommon. In one recent series, hydrocephalus (defined as ventricular size above the age-corrected 95th percentile) was found in 34 (20%) of 174 patients with SAH who survived the first 24 hours and underwent CT scanning within 72 hours [22]. Hydrocephalus may be secondary to intraventricular hemorrhage and obstruction of CSF pathways (noncommunicating); more commonly, SAH interferes with CSF reabsorption (communicating hydrocephalus).

Clinically, there may be progressive deterioration in the level of consciousness, slow pupillary reaction, and hyponatremia that develops insidiously. If the patient is symptomatic, one may place an external ventriculostomy for temporary CSF drainage. Eventually, some patients will require an internal CSF shunt.

Seizures. Seizures develop in approximately 10 to 15 percent of patients following SAH. Aneurysms of the middle cerebral artery are associated with the highest incidence of seizures in patients with ruptured aneurysm. The younger the patient, the greater the risk; in addition, the presence of an intraparenchymal hemorrhage makes seizures more likely. Seizures are associated with increased CBF and ICP, and may precipitate rebleeding. Patients at significant risk should be given prophylactic anticonvulsant therapy [313].

Cardiovascular Events. Hypertension following aneurysmal rupture may be a response to increased ICP and ischemia. Hypertension is an important negative prognostic factor [46]. Significant sustained elevations of blood pressure may result in rebleeding.

In planning antihypertensive therapy, one must consider the dual and often conflicting goals of preventing rebleeding and preserving an adequate cerebral perfusion. Sudden reductions in blood pressure may precipitate or worsen a neurologic deficit [33].

Cardiac complications following SAH include MI and arrhythmias. ECG abnormalities are seen in up to 50 percent of patients with aneurysmal SAH. Serious arrhythmias (e.g., supraventricular tachyarrhythmias, ventricular flutter or fibrillation, ventricular premature complexes, and torsade de pointe) may occur in 40 percent of patients. These are more common in the first 24 hours after SAH. Other abnormalities include sinus tachycardia or bradycardia, prolonged QT intervals, ST segment elevation or depression, broad or inverted T waves, and prominent U waves. These changes reflect subendocardial damage secondary to hypothalamic stimulation and an increase in sympathetic tone. ECG monitoring and cardiologic assessment are recommended for virtually all patients with SAH. Catecholamine blockade is effective in treating ventricular arrhythmias and in preventing subendocardial lesions associated with SAH. Beta blockers such as propranolol, labetalol, or esmolol are the most appropriate antihypertensive agents to use in these patients [47–49].

Pulmonary Edema. Pulmonary edema sometimes occurs following SAH; the patient may present with breathing difficulties, irregular respirations, and frothy sputum [50]. Intubation and ventilatory support with positive end-expiratory pressure (PEEP) and large doses of a diuretic, such as furosemide (Lasix), may be required [51].

Fluid and Electrolyte Problems. These include *hyponatremia, hypernatremia, SIADH,* and *diabetes insipidus.* These are more likely with aneurysms of the anterior communicating artery than all other sites combined, presumably because they are close to the hypothalamus. Most commonly they occur between the third and seventh days following SAH [52] and may be precipitated or aggravated following surgery.

SIADH. Diagnostic criteria are serum sodium under 135 mEq/liter, serum osmolality under 280 mOsm/kg, urinary sodium over 25 mEq/liter, and a urine osmolality greater than the plasma osmolality. In mild cases the treatment is water restriction (800–1000 ml/24 hours). However, this may decrease intravascular volume and cerebral perfusion, which is undesirable in these patients. More serious cases require the judicious use of hypertonic saline infusion (3% NaCl) and perhaps furosemide. If such therapy is embarked on, fluid and electrolyte levels must be monitored diligently.

DIABETES INSIPIDUS. The diagnosis should be entertained if the urine output is more than 500 ml/2 hours or 300 ml/hour. The urine specific gravity is less than 1.005, urine osmolality is between 50 and 150 mOsm/kg, and serum sodium levels are over 150 mEq/liter. Accurate monitoring and correction of fluid balance are necessary. Impaired mental status may preclude appropriate responses to thirst. Desmopressin acetate (DDAVP), a synthetic analog of the neurohypophyseal nonapeptide arginine vasopressin, is the treatment of choice for central diabetes insipidus. It may be given intravenously, subcutaneously, or intranasally; the typical dose is 0.5 ml (2.0 μg) to 1.0 ml (4.0 μg) intravenously or subcutaneously daily, usually in two divided doses. It has less pressor activity and a longer duration of action compared with aqueous vasopressin [53].

Total blood volume may be reduced following SAH from bed rest, supine diuresis, or pooling in peripheral vascular beds. Such volume contraction may predispose to or exacerbate ischemic infarction [34].

Pyrexia. Blood within the subarachnoid space may cause a temperature elevation of 1° to 2°F. The deleterious effects of temperature elevation on cerebral metabolism and blood flow have been discussed in Chap. 1. Fever should be controlled by antipyretics, cooling blanket, or tepid sponging.

The goals of management in the preoperative period for patients with ruptured intracranial aneurysm are as follows: (1) avoid rebleeding, (2) maintain adequate cerebral perfusion despite intracranial hypertension and cerebral vasospasm, and (3) reduce morbidity from associated medical complications.

Typical Preoperative Orders for Ruptured Intracranial Aneurysm

1. Provide bed rest in a tranquil environment; minimize stimulation from visitors, television, telephone, and radio.
2. Prevent Valsalva's maneuvers. Take temperatures orally. Provide a high fiber diet and stool softeners, e.g., Colace, 100 mg orally twice daily.
3. Exclude caffeine and tobacco.
4. If the patient's level of consciousness is impaired, institute nasogastric tube feeding or intravenous hyperalimentation to preserve nutritional status.

5. Elevate head of bed 15 to 30 degrees to facilitate venous drainage and CSF outflow. Note that increased ICP and communicating hydrocephalus occur in a significant number of patients with SAH.
6. Pneumatic compression stockings may prevent deep venous thrombosis in comatose patients.
7. Restless patients may require restraint with loose mittens, although a mild sedative is often sufficient.
8. Prescribe a sedative such as phenobarbital 60 to 120 mg daily either orally or intravenously. This agent may also be used as an anticonvulsant.
9. Prescribe a mild analgesic for headache and neck pain such as acetaminophen 650 mg with codeine 60 mg orally every 3 to 4 hours.
10. Prescribe anticonvulsants prophylactically, e.g., diphenylhydantoin (Dilantin) in a loading dose of 1 gm followed by 300 mg orally or intravenously daily in divided doses every 8 hours or a single dose at night. Doses should be adjusted to achieve a blood level of 10 to 20 μm/ml.
11. Prescribe the antifibrinolytic agent epsilon-aminocaproic acid to prevent rebleeding [46, 54]. It may be given intravenously as a continuous infusion or orally. A loading dose of 5 gm is followed by 1.0 to 1.25 gm doses at hourly intervals thereafter. A total dose of more than 30 gm within 24 hours is not recommended.
12. Prescribe the calcium channel blocker nimodipine in a dose of 60 mg by mouth or nasogastric tube every 4 hours begining within 96 hours of the event through 21 consecutive days in Hunt and Hess grades I–III patients. The major side effect is hypotension (4% of patients). Currently, an intravenous preparation is available for investigational use only.

Monitoring

With few exceptions, patients are managed in a neurosurgical or equivalent intensive care unit. Frequent neurologic checks are performed in a standard fashion and are clearly recorded. Level of consciousness and clinical grade of SAH are charted according to the Glasgow coma scale (Table 5-4) and on the Hunt and Hess scale (see Table 5-1).

1. Monitor central venous pressure. A Swan-Ganz catheter is preferable in patients with underlying cardiopulmonary disease.
2. Use an arterial line for continuous blood pressure monitoring.
3. Use a Foley catheter (if necessary). Chart intake and output. Check urine specific gravity or osmolality as necessary. Weigh the patient daily.
4. If indicated, perform ICP monitoring in poorer-grade patients with severe SAH, intraparenchymal hemorrhage, or cerebral edema.

Timing of Aneurysm Surgery

There is little question that surgical treatment of cerebral aneurysm prevents early and long-term rerupture. The more vexatious question is

Table 5-4. Glasgow Coma Scale

Eyes	Open	Spontaneously	4
		To verbal command	3
		To pain	2
		No response	1
Best motor response	To verbal command	Obeys	6
		Localizes	5
	To pain	Flexion—withdrawal	4
		Flexion—abnormal (decorticate)	3
		Extension (decerebrate)	2
		No response	1
Best verbal response		Oriented and converses	5
		Disoriented and converses	4
		Inappropriate words	3
		Incomprehensible sounds	2
		No response	1
Total			3–15

Source: Teasdale G., Jennett B. Assessment and impaired consciousness. A practical scale. *Lancet* 2:81, 1974.

when to embark on it (*early versus late operation*). Years ago, early operation was marred by prohibitive statistics relating to outcome, and delayed surgery became the modus operandi. However, many patients succumbed while awaiting surgery. Advances in operative technique and perioperative care have encouraged a move toward early operation. *Early* surgery is justifiable [41, 42] on the grounds that surgery is the definitive method for preventing rebleeding, the risk of which is greatest immediately following SAH. Further, symptomatic vasospasm reaches its peak in the second week after SAH. This interval is unfavorable for surgical intervention.

Also favoring early surgery is the fact that aggressive treatment of vasospasm can be more safely undertaken when the aneurysm has been excluded from the circulation. A less compelling argument is the advantage of subarachnoid toilet (lavage) during early surgery as a means of reducing the incidence of vasospasm [55]. Early surgery is reasonable in good-risk patients.

Delaying surgery for about 2 weeks after SAH tends to avoid the element of vasospasm and de facto selects the best surgical candidates for surgery. The brain is less "tight" and subarachnoid dissection is easier. Moreover, intrinsic cerebrovascular autoregulatory mechanisms are returning to normal, reducing the likelihood of postoperative ischemic vascular complications. Opponents cite the threat of rebleeding during the waiting period, although the use of antifibrinolytic agents helps to reduce this risk. [56, 57]. The special circumstance of emergency surgery presents little argument, i.e., when patients arrive critically ill from a life-threatening intracerebral clot, shift of intracranial contents, and escalating ICP. Such patients may benefit from urgent craniotomy for clot evacuation and clip ligation of the aneurysm if it is readily accessible. Still, operation upon patients graded 4 or worse carries significant morbidity and mortality, with few exceptions [56, 57].

Intracerebral Hematomas

The incidence of spontaneous ICH varies among series of acute stroke [58]. The incidence increases with age, peaking between 65 and 80 years. Females appear to be more prone to develop ICH. ICH may be primary (most are associated with systemic hypertension) or secondary, i.e., from other causes such as aneurysms, arteriovenous malformations, tumors, and blood dyscrasias (leukemias, hemophilia). Approximately 50 percent of primary ICHs occur in the corpus striatum, 15 percent in the thalamus, 10 to 15 percent in the pons, 10 percent in the cerebellum, and 10 to 20 percent in the cerebral white matter.

Clinical presentation depends on location of the hemorrhage. There is usually a sudden deterioration in the level of consciousness and vital functions and the development of a focal deficit. The site of the hemorrhage has a direct bearing on prognosis.

Diagnosis

Laboratory investigation for coagulopathy (PT, PTT, Platelet count, bleeding time) and blood should be typed and cross matched.
Computed Tomography. CT scan is the first choice in suspected ICH. This should be a nonenhanced study. Acute hemorrhage appears as a well-demarcated area of homogeneous high density. There may be mass effect, shift, or surrounding edema. The lesion becomes less dense as clot resolution progresses. An intraventricular hemorrhage is reabsorbed more quickly than is an intraparenchymal clot. An underlying vascular lesion (especially an AVM) may be apparent on contrast-enhanced CT.
Angiography. If the location of the ICH is atypical for a hypertensive hemorrhage, an angiogram may reveal the source of hemorrhage. Certain sites of ICH suggest aneurysm, e.g., within the sylvian fissure (middle cerebral aneurysm) or between the anterior frontal lobes (anterior communicating artery aneurysm). In dire circumstances it seems unwarranted to delay surgical management to perform angiography.

Treatment

Medical Treatment. Many patients arrive in an altered state of consciousness and can deteriorate quickly. The first priority is to ensure an adequate airway and proper gas exchange. Close monitoring of vital signs and neurologic status in an intensive care setting is necessary.

Systemic hypertension and cardiac dysrhythmias frequently occur with ICH from compensatory brainstem mechanisms to maintain CBF. Overzealous antihypertensive treatment of this initial cardiovascular response may drastically reduce CPP and have an adverse effect on neuronal function. If the neurologic condition improves or remains stable and arterial hypertension persists, a hitherto undiagnosed hypertensive state may exist that requires appropriate therapy. There may be a history of poor compliance with antihypertensive therapy.

Parenteral medications are more effective in this setting, with hydralazine or labetalol being reasonable choices. If the situation is more desperate, sodium nitroprusside (Nipride) is a more potent agent.

Intracranial hypertension should be treated according to the outline in Chap. 2.

Prophylactic anticonvulsant therapy may be initiated with diphenylhydantoin sodium, especially when the ICH resides in the more epileptogenic zones (temporal, parietal, frontal).

Coagulopathies are treated with appropriate component transfusions.

Surgical Treatment. The advisability of surgery is based on several factors: location and size of ICH, the patient's clinical condition, and potential for useful recovery. There is no uniformity of opinion. Some surgeons propose a more aggressive approach [60]; others sound a cautionary note, advocating medical or delayed surgical management [61, 62].

Surgical treatment is usually by craniotomy to evacuate the hematoma. One must be fastidious about hemostasis to reduce the likelihood of a delayed hemorrhage. Stereotaxis evacuation of ICH has also been reported [63].

Cerebellar Hemorrhage and Infarction

These conditions are considered together because of their similarities and potentially treacherous clinical course. The cerebellum is the site of hemorrhage in about 10 percent of ICH, mostly in hypertensive patients. Cerebellar infarcts are usually due to emboli of cardiac origin to the territory of the posterior inferior cerebellar artery (PICA), and 40 percent of these patients are hypertensive. Cerebellar infarcts may be grossly hemorrhagic in about 25 percent of cases. *Clinical presentation* includes headache, nausea, vomiting, and cerebellar signs. With increasing mass effect there may be hydrocephalus with progressive alteration in mental status and sixth cranial nerve palsy or gaze paresis. Further compression may compromise the brainstem, and the patient may slip rapidly into coma. At this stage few patients are salvageable.

Diagnosis

CT provides the diagnosis. Acute hemorrhage appears as a well-demarcated area of homogeneous high density. There may be mass effect, shift, or surrounding edema. With an infarct, there is a zone of hypodensity and significant mass effect. If an AVM or aneurysm is suspected, angiography will be necessary.

Treatment

Suboccipital craniectomy with evacuation of the hematoma or necrotic tissue (infarct) is the surgical treatment of choice [64]. Stable, alert patients with small lesions, without brainstem findings or hydrocephalus, and in whom basal cisterns are normal or only minimally compressed may not require surgical therapy.

Arteriovenous Malformations

AVMs are congenital vascular anomalies in which an abnormal communication exists between an artery and a vein. The malformations are found throughout the CNS, most often in the cerebral hemispheres. *Clinical manifestations* include hemorrhage (subarachnoid, intraparenchymal, or intraventricular), seizures, focal neurologic deficit, and headache. The average annual risk of first hemorrhage from an AVM is about 3 percent. After a single hemorrhage the risk of rebleeding is 6 percent in the first year and 2 to 3 percent per year thereafter [65, 314, 315].

Seizures are a more likely presentation of large AVMs with superficial components in the cerebral hemisphere. The younger the patient at diagnosis, the more likely it is that epilepsy will develop. Focal neurologic deficit may be due to cerebral ischemia from vascular shunting by a high-flow AVM (intracerebral steal).

Diagnosis

Cerebral angiography is an important tool for diagnosis and surgical planning. Angiography demonstrates enlarged feeding arteries, the nidus of the malformation (appears as a tangle of vessels), and early draining veins. The mass is typically a non-space-occupying one, except when associated with an ICH. CT scans may reveal a hemorrhage, usually intraparenchymal [66]. *MRI* provides an excellent image of AVMs in a three-dimensional perspective and its relationship to regional structures. Because of the signal void of flowing blood, there is a serpiginous area of negative signal representing enlarged feeding arteries and draining veins [67]. AVMs may be graded according to degree of complexity for the purposes of determining resectability and surgical risk [316].

Treatment

Medical Treatment. Preoperatively the patient is prescribed anticonvulsants prophylactically or, if seizures are the presentation, continued on the existing regimen. Dexamethasone is started about 24 hours pre-operatively to reduce postoperative cerebral swelling.

Surgical Treatment. The ideal treatment for most AVMs is complete excision by craniotomy [68]. There is some controversy regarding the indications for surgery in unruptured AVMs [308]. If the AVM resides in or is juxtaposed to eloquent cortex, craniotomy may be performed under local anesthesia with cortical mapping of important areas [69].

Embolization. Embolization may be used preoperatively to devascularize a malformation as an adjunct to surgical excision. It may be the sole treatment for some AVMs. Preoperative embolization is done at least a week before surgery because of the possibility of ischemia or edema in the surrounding brain following embolization. Surgery should follow embolization as soon as feasible to obviate the formation of collaterals. Intravascular thrombosis is induced by injecting thrombogenic particles (silicone pellets, cyanoacrylate glues) into a feeding artery from where they are drawn into the malformation by blood flow. Emboli may stray into the adjacent normal circulation, resulting in a deficit [70, 319].

Radiotherapy. Stereotactic radiosurgery is the use of focused, high-dose radiation to obliterate an AVM. This may be done with the Leksell gamma knife (cobalt), proton beam therapy using the Bragg peak phenomenon (which is of limited availability), or stereotactic linear accelerators. This modality is suited to small, deep AVMs or patients with inoperable AVMs [71, 320, 321].

Epilepsy

Partial epilepsies are the most common form of seizure disorder, occuring in two-thirds of adult patients with epilepsy and about 40 percent of children with epilepsy. Patients with partial complex epilepsy, especially with secondary generalization, are more likely to have medically intractable epilepsy (MIE) [72].

Partial epilepsies (also known as focal epilepsies) are seizures in which the first clinical and electroencephalographic (EEG) changes indicate activation of an anatomic or functional system limited to a part of one or both cerebral hemispheres. When consciousness is not impaired, the seizure is classified as an elementary partial attack; with impaired consciousness, the seizure is classified as a complex partial attack (psychomotor epilepsy). Partial seizures may generalize to tonic-clonic (grand mal) seizures [73].

Selection Criteria for Surgery

Patient selection for resective surgery rests on the following tenets: identifying a focus of origin of the seizures and ensuring that such a focus resides in a region where surgical treatment is not fraught with unacceptable operative risk. Since the major impact of epilepsy surgery is on seizure frequency, it should be determined beforehand whether such outcome will have a substantial impact on the patient's life.

Employment following epilepsy surgery is far more contingent on preoperative employment prospects and neuropsychological status than on seizure control per se [74]. Patients without other serious neurologic or psychiatric problems are better candidates. The patient and family should be resolved to endure the seemingly lengthy selection process for surgery and aftercare.

There are currently two major neurosurgical approaches to the treatment of MIE:

1. Resection of seizure focus. About 80 percent of demonstrable focal epileptic zones in patients with MIE are within the anterior temporal lobe, making anterior temporal lobectomy (and its variations) the commonest procedure for epilepsy. Usually the focus is in the hippocampus; neuropathologic correlates include gliosis from postnatal trauma, hamartomas, occult tumors, and small AVMs [75].
2. Corpus callosotomy (partial or complete division of the corpus callosum).

Preoperative Testing

Electroencephalogram. The goal of preoperative testing is to identify an epileptogenic zone. Protocols vary among different institutions. Methods include the following:

1. Scalp EEG recording of interictal events.
2. EEG and video monitoring, which allows simultaneous recording of clinical and EEG data.
3. Chronically implanted electrodes (subdural, epidural, or depth electrodes) for ictal and interictal recording. Plates or grids for subdural or epidural monitoring are placed at craniotomy. Long-term monitoring and functional mapping are possible with this technique. Prophylactic antibiotics are given for the duration of electrode implantation because of the risk of infection. To increase the likelihood of precipitating seizure activity during monitoring, seizure medications are decreased, and the patient is denied sleep [76].
4. Intraoperative recording from the surface of the brain (electrocorticography [ECoG]). EcOG may be performed under local or general anesthesia [77, 78]. Some neurosurgeons use EcoG data to modify temporal lobe resections, as opposed to performing a standard temporal lobe resection.

Satisfactory EEG criteria for predicting the success of surgery remain controversial [79–81]. EEG findings at variance with the clinical presentation or that are equivocal suggest the need for further investigation [82]. More invasive and selective electrode placement may be required [83–85].

In a comparison of the reliability of EEG techniques in identifying the best area of resection to abolish seizures, the site of ictal onset on depth electrode recording was most accurate, followed by the location of interictal activity with scalp EEG recording, and finally the locus of hypometabolism on PET scanning [86].

Neuroimaging. Neuroimaging tests include the following:

1. CT scan. In addition to the lesions mentioned, another finding on CT is subtle enhancement ipsilateral to the epileptogenic focus compared with the contralateral side [87].
2. MRI scan.
3. PET—The most reliable finding has been on interictal PET scans following the injection of 18_F-fluorodeoxyglucose (FDG), showing hypometabolism ipsilateral to the temporal lobe focus [88].

Neuropsychological. The patient's functional neurologic status may be further evaluated by a battery of tests, e.g., the Wechsler adult intelligence and memory scales and Wisconsin card-sorting test (these tests mainly assess temporal lobe function) [322]. The Wada test is for lateralization of speech dominance and the ability of each hemisphere to support short-term memory. Sodium amytal is injected into the carotid, and tests for speech and memory are conducted [323, 324].

Pituitary and Suprasellar Tumors

The classification of pituitary tumors has been modified based on recent histopathologic studies, rendering the old tinctorial classification of chromophobe, basophilic, and eosinophilic adenomas obsolete. Pituitary adenomas may be *functional* or *nonfunctional* (undifferentiated) [89–91].

Functional tumors are those that secrete excessive quantities of a hormone and cause symptoms due to that hormone. Nonfunctional tumors do not secrete physiologically active hormones and usually cause symptoms by compressing neighboring structures.

The functional group includes (1) growth hormone (GH) cell adenoma, (2) prolactin (PRL) cell (lactotropic cell) adenoma, (3) mixed (Gh and PRL) cell adenoma, (4) corticotroph (ACTH) cell adenoma, (5) thyrotroph (TRH) cell adenoma, (6) gonadotroph (LSH and FSH) cell adenoma, and (7) acidophil stem cell adenoma, a single cell type with composite features of GH- and PRL-secreting cells.

Functional tumors comprise 75 percent of all pituitary adenomas. Of these, *prolactinomas* represent 40 to 50 percent; *somatotropin (GH) adenomas,* 15 to 25 percent; and *corticotropin-secreting adenomas* account for 5 percent. *Thyrotropin* and *gonadotropin-secreting adenomas* number less than 1 percent of all pituitary adenomas. The TRH cell adenoma causes thyrotoxicosis due to secretion of thyrotropin [329]. These tumors have been discovered chiefly in patients with long-standing primary hypothyroidism.

Tumors of the neurohypophysis are rare. Other lesions encountered in the sella and suprasellar region include meningiomas, craniopharyngiomas, mucocele of the sphenoid sinus, abscesses, and granulomas.

Regardless of secretory activity, *prolactinomas* constitute the largest group of pituitary adenomas—about 25 percent. In females, prolactinomas produce menstrual dysfunction (primary or secondary amenorrhea and oligomenorrhea) and galactorrhea. Prolactinomas are a common and important cause of infertility, accounting for 20 to 30 percent of cases [325]. In men, they are associated with impotence or subtle loss of libido and hypogonadism; more often they become clinically apparent only when the tumor enlarges to cause symptoms from mass effect and hypopituitarism. In general, prolactinomas in males are larger at presentation than in females. Hyperprolactinemia per se is not associated with any particularly serious cause of morbidity; bone demineralization has been associated with long-term hyperprolactinemia [326].

Growth hormone (GH) adenomas result in acromegaly, characterized by acral enlargement of the hands and feet, prognathism, macroglossia, thickened skin, galactorrhea, abnormal carbohydrate metabolism, cardiac disease, and peripheral nerve entrapment. Because acromegaly decreases life expectancy and is esthetically displeasing, early diagnosis and prompt treatment are important.

Biochemical features include an *elevated basal GH* and *somatomedin-C*; GH fails to suppress with glucose loading. *Corticotroph cell adenomas* fall into two categories—those that secrete ACTH and result in Cushing's disease or Nelson's syndrome and the silent tumors that contain ACTH and other fragments of the pro-opiocortin molecule, but are not associated with clinical or biochemical evidence of ACTH excess. Functioning corticotroph cell adenomas in Cushing's disease are most often microadenomas, whereas those in Nelson's syndrome are usually large and invade neighboring tissue. Both Cushing's disease and Nelson's syndrome have a definite female preponderance.

Clinical features of Cushing's disease include centripetal obesity ("moon facies," buffalo hump, supraclavicular fat pad), purple striae, ecchymoses, emotional disturbances or frank psychosis, amenorrhea and hirsutism in women, glucose intolerance, and hypertension. Cushing's disease poses a significant threat to health and life expectancy. Cushing's disease in children is a rare condition, initially manifested by impaired skeletal growth and obesity. Early treatment is necessary since resumption of normal growth can be achieved in patients treated before epiphyseal fusion occurs [327, 328].

Gonadotrophin (LH-FSH) secreting tumors are uncommon, and because of a relative lack of symptoms they frequently go undetected. *Nonfunctional tumors* cause symptoms from *mass effect*. With growth and extension into the suprasellar region, these large pituitary adenomas may cause visual symptoms from compression of the afferent visual pathways; initially there is a *bitemporal upper quadrantanopsia* that may evolve into a *bitemporal hemianopsia*. Other symptoms from compression include headaches due to stretching of the dura and pituitary insufficiency. Lateral invasion into the cavernous sinus may compromise the third through sixth cranial nerves. Prolactin may be mildly elevated from compression of the stalk, interfering with release of prolactin inhibiting factor (PIF)—the so-called *stalk effect*. In some instances, a particularly severe sudden headache with obtundation is a result of *pituitary apoplexy*. Pituitary apoplexy is a relatively rare manifestation of pituitary tumors that results from hemorrhage into or acute infarction of a pituitary tumor. The classic picture is one of sudden visual loss, severe headache, meningism, oculomotor palsies, and a declining level of consciousness [95].

Varying degrees of *panhypopituitarism* from compression of the normal gland are also the result of mass effect. Further extension of a suprasellar tumor anteriorly or laterally may produce various neurologic symptoms. With anterior (frontal) extension, personality changes, anosmia, dementia, or generalized seizures may occur. Lateral extension into the middle fossae may result in partial complex seizures (uncinate fits), homonymous hemianopsia from optic tract involvement, and hemiparesis from impingement on the cerebral peduncle.

Empty sella syndrome (ESS, Intrasellar arachnoid diverticulum) is the result of intrasellar herniation of the suprasellar cistern with or without an incompetent diaphragma sella. ESS may be primary or secondary (i.e., following pituitary adenomectomy or hypophysectomy). The CSF pulsation within the herniated arachnoid diverticulum flattens the pituitary gland and gradually enlarges the sella. The syndrome is often encountered in obese middle-aged, hypertensive females. Symptoms include vague headaches, CSF rhinorrhea, hypopituitarism, and visual symptoms; in most cases, ESS is not associated with significant symptoms [92, 93]. Treatment may be required for CSF rhinorrhea or visual problems.

Nelson's syndrome is the result of pituitary adenoma that develops (or was already present) in a patient who has undergone adrenalectomy for Cushing's disease.

Nelson and Meakin first reported hyperpigmentation associated with an enlarging adrenocorticotropin (ACTH)-secreting adenoma 3 years following bilateral adrenalectomy in a patient with a normal sella and Cushing's disease [330]. There is a 5 to 10 percent incidence of sella enlargement and hyperpigmentation following bilateral adrenalectomy for Cushing's disease. The tumors associated with Nelson's syndrome are invasive in 10 to 25 percent of cases.

Diagnosis

Endocrine Evaluation. There are a number of tests available for studying pituitary endocrine function, and one may adopt various combinations in arriving at an "endocrine profile."

Most include:

Pituitary-adrenal axis: AM serum cortisol, 24-hour urinary 17-ketoste-
roids, and 17-hydroxycorticosteroids.
Pituitary-gonadal axis: serum luteinizing hormone (LH), follicle-stimu-
lating hormone (FSH), estradiol, and testosterone.
Pituitary-thyroid axis: free and total thyroxine (T_4), triiodothyronine (T_3)
levels, and TSH.

In addition, one should obtain baseline PRL and GH levels if a secretory
tumor is suspected. Further tests of stimulation and suppression are
usually required depending on the clinical presentation and the results
of the initial battery.

PRL. There are numerous causes of hyperprolactinemia encountered
in clinical practice other than pituitary tumors. A drug history is important in the assessment of any patient with hyperprolactinemia. Serum
prolactin is elevated in about three-fourths of patients with pituitary tumors either from PRL secretion by the tumor or because the tumor compresses the pituitary stalk and prevents dopaminergic suppression of
PRL release (stalk effect). PRL levels over 20 ng/ml are abnormal. Between 20 and 150 ng/ml may be due to stalk or drug effect (e.g., phe-
nothiazines, antidepressants, intravenous but not oral cimetidine, oral
contraceptives). PRL levels above 200 ng/ml should be considered to
be due to a prolactinoma until proved otherwise.

Dynamic tests of prolactin secretion have provided useful information
about the mechanism of control of prolactin secretion in normal and
hyperprolactinemic patients but are of limited value in the differential
diagnosis of hyperprolactinemia.

GH. In normal individuals, basal GH levels are usually less than 5 ng/
ml. In patients with acromegaly, GH levels are usually greater than 10
ng/ml. This relationship is not invariable, and acromegalic patients may
have normal GH levels.

Further confirmation by an abnormal GH-glucose suppression test, i.e.,
failure of GH to fall below 2 ng/ml after an oral glucose load, may be
necessary. Increased secretion of GH following the administration of
thyrotropin-releasing hormone (TRH) occurs in some patients with acromegaly but does not affect GH levels in healthy patients.

Somatomedin-C (SMC). This is a peptide released from the liver and
other sources. It is an indirect measure of GH activity. Normal values
are from 0.34 to 2.0 U/ml in men and 0.45 to 2.2 U/ml in women.

Cushing's Disease

The term Cushing's *syndrome* refers to hypercortisolism per se, while
Cushing's *disease* is reserved for those patients with hypercortisolism
from a pituitary tumor. Cushing's disease is the commonest cause of
endogenous adrenocortical hyperfunction (Cushing's syndrome)—
about 75 percent of cases.

Defining the etiology of Cushing's syndrome by endocrinologic testing is extremely important because many pituitary tumors that cause hypercortisolism are small and may not be demonstrated even on high-quality CT scans or MRI. About 70 to 90 percent of patients with Cushing's disease harbor a pituitary adenoma at the time of diagnosis, while the remainder may have hyperplasia of the pituitary corticotropes [331].

One of the most basic endocrinologic features of Cushing's syndrome is the absence of a normal diurnal cortisol rhythm. The rationale behind the endocrinologic diagnosis of Cushing's disease is that the CRF-ACTH axis retains some of its normal homeostatic responses to circulating levels of cortisol (but is "reset" to respond to higher glucocorticoid levels) unlike Cushing's syndrome from an adrenal tumor or ectopic ACTH-producing tumor, which exhibit autonomous cortisol secretion and therefore fail tests of feedback inhibition. CRF may differentiate Cushing's disease from ectopic ACTH secretion. In Cushing's disease, there is a significant rise in ACTH following CRF administration, whereas, in patients with ectopic ACTH secretion and adrenal tumors, ACTH fails to respond to CRF.

Plasma cortisol levels (normally 5–25 ng/ml) are elevated, as are its urinary excretion products—urinary free cortisol (UFC, normal 20–90 µg) and 17-hydroxysteroids (normally under 12 mg/day). ACTH assay shows increased or high-normal levels in Cushing's disease; a high plasma ACTH is also seen in ectopic ACTH-producing tumor. A low plasma ACTH is obtained in adrenal tumor or primary adrenal hyperplasia.

With the overnight low-dose dexamethasone suppression test (DST), an oral dose of 0.5 mg (low dose) of dexamethasone in normal individuals will suppress the ACTH-adrenal axis. This will be reflected in serum cortisol levels below 5 µg/dl, urinary ketogenic steroids less than 5 mg/24 hr, and UFC less than 20 µg/24 hours. Patients with Cushing's syndrome fail to show such suppression. In response to a 2-mg (high-dose) dexamethasone suppression test, the majority of patients with Cushing's disease should suppress their parameters greater than 50 percent of baseline. An ectopic source of ACTH or adrenal tumor will not be significantly suppressed by either the 0.5-mg or 2.0-mg dose. Almost all patients with Cushing's disease will show a positive response to the metapyrone stimulation test, whereas patients with Cushing's syndrome from an adrenal tumor or ectopic ACTH-producing tumor will either show no change or a decrease in the parameters of cortisol secretion (metapyrone unresponsive). Petrosal sinus sampling may establish a differential in ACTH levels between the left and right sinuses draining the pituitary gland and may distinguish between Cushing's disease and adrenal or ectopic Cushing's syndrome [94].

Neuroophthalmologic Assessment. Suprasellar extension of a pituitary tumor and compression of the overlying optic chiasm produces a progressive decrease in visual acuity and visual field defects. The classic deficit is a bitemporal hemianopsia. Visual field examination may be done by confrontation, tangent screen, Goldmann perimeter, or computerized automated perimetry (Octopus). Confrontation fields are simple and can be done by the nonophthalmologist at the bedside. Fundoscopy may show early signs of primary atrophy. Papilledema is an unusual finding with pituitary adenomas but may be seen with subfrontal extension. Extraocular palsies, the result of cavernous sinus involvement, occur in fewer than 10 percent of patients. Significant visual symptoms are less often seen in patients with pituitary adenomas than previously because of earlier diagnosis.

Radiologic Evaluation. There has been a progressive evolution in the diagnostic modalities for pituitary tumor; skull x-rays and sella polytomography have given way to high resolution CT and MRI.

CT SCAN (MICROADENOMAS). These are tumors smaller than 10 mm in diameter. Thin-section (1.5–2.0 mm) CT scans (enhanced and nonenhanced) in the direct coronal plane give the best results. The height of the gland (normal maximum 7–8 mm), contour of the diaphragma sellae (usually flat or concave), appearance of the suprasellar cistern, and pituitary stalk can be assessed in this study. Bone windows are obtained to visualize the sella floor and the sphenoid sinus septa.

The normal pituitary gland and infundibulum are outside the blood-brain barrier. Therefore, they appear heterogenous on contrast-enhanced CT and thus could be misinterpreted as containing a microadenoma [96, 97]. Most pituitary lesions do not enhance or show less enhancement than the normal pituitary. CT scan criteria of a microadenoma include (a) focal hypodense or hyperdense lesions, (b) elevated diaphragma sella, (c) abnormal gland height, (d) displaced infundibulum, and (e) erosion of the sella floor. None of these per se is diagnostic; furthermore, many patients with microadenoma show no radiographic abnormalities [98].

CT SCAN (MACROADENOMAS). These are large tumors (>10 mm in diameter). They may be isodense or hyperdense on unenhanced scans and have variable patterns of enhancement. Their most reliable feature is that they originate within the sella. They may extend superiorly into the suprasellar region or inferiorly into the sphenoid sinus with erosion of the sellar floor.

MRI. MRI is currently the preferred imaging technique for the diagnosis of pituitary lesions [99, 100]. It yields a more precise anatomic image and no radiation is involved. Multiplanar imaging (sagittal, coronal, and axial) provides a three-dimensional view of the lesion. Vascular lesions (aneurysms) that may mimic tumors in this region can be differentiated by MRI, obviating the need for angiography. MRI is more sensitive for detecting tissue abnormality, although specificity is not as accurate. On T1- and T2-weighted images, the normal gland is isointense with normal brain. Most adenomas are isointense to hypointense to normal gland on T1-weighted sequences and show variable intensity on T2-weighted images.

SKULL FILMS. Enlargement of the sella usually without bone destruction is seen with pituitary adenomas and the empty sella syndrome [101].

The commonest tumor to enlarge the sella is a nonsecreting adenoma; they are frequently discovered incidentally on skull radiographs obtained for other purposes. Hormone-secreting tumors usually present clinically when smaller than 10 mm (microadenoma) and are usually associated with a normal-sized sella. Pneumatization of the sphenoid sinus begins anteriorly and proceeds posteriorly and laterally. Various degrees of pneumatization of the sphenoid may be seen in adults. Appreciation of sella and sphenoid anatomy is important in planning transsphenoidal surgery.

Angiography. Currently, angiography has limited use in the evaluation of patients with pituitary tumors. Its main role was to exclude aneurysms or other vascular anomalies and to determine the position of the carotid siphons. The availability of MRI has curtailed the need for arteriography.

Treatment

Perhaps as important as knowledge of existing therapeutic options is a grasp of how they are most successfully applied. Pituitary adenomas may be treated surgically, medically, or with radiation. In many instances, the therapeutic endpoint is "control" rather than "cure" of the endocrinopathy. To further muddy the waters, the definition of successful treatment of some syndromes varies from one series to another.

Acromegaly. Successful treatment results in clinical improvement, reduction in basal GH levels to less than 5 ng/ml, normal somatomedin-C levels, and normal GH dynamics (e.g., suppression by glucose).

Cushing's Disease. Successful treatment results in clinical improvement, return of cortisol and ACTH levels to normal, and the return of normal cortisol suppression after the administration of low-dose dexamethasone. The small size of most corticotrope adenomas and their frequent location deep within the central wedge of the pituitary make discovery at the time of surgery difficult. In the most experienced hands, the cure rates of adult noninvasive adenomas are 83 to 95 percent [115].

Prolactinoma. Unlike Cushing's disease and acromegaly, the argument for treatment (medical or surgical) of a prolactinoma is more complicated. Generally, the criteria for surgical removal include (1) desire for pregnancy in women, (2) primary amenorrhea, (3) intolerance to medication, (4) personal choice, and (5) acute progressive visual loss. Criteria for control include normalization of prolactin, relief of clinical symptoms, and no evidence of recurrence. It is possible to remove all of the tumor and still have persistent hyperprolactinemia from pituitary stalk damage [111, 112].

Nonfunctional Tumors. Here success is measured in relief of symptoms (e.g., visual) and completeness of tumor removal.

Medical Treatment. Bromocriptine (Parlodel) has been used in the treatment of a number of pituitary tumors. Bromocriptine is an ergot derivative structurally related to dopamine and is a dopamine receptor agonist. Dopamine appears to be the hypothalamic factor (prolactin-inhibiting factor [PIF]) that inhibits PRL secretion. Prolactinomas have been particularly successfully managed with bromocriptine. It is effective in reducing tumor size and PRL levels in prolactinomas [102, 103]. The reduction in tumor volume seems to be due to a decrease in cell size (the major change being in the cytoplasm) rather than cell number.

Bromocriptine is usually given orally in doses of 2.5 to 10.0 mg 3 to 4 times a day. It must be taken continuously; if discontinued, the tumor may rapidly reexpand [104, 105].

Bromocriptine is also effective in the treatment of acromegaly. Comparatively higher doses (5–20 mg 3 times daily by mouth) are required. Unlike PRL, GH rarely falls to normal levels, although most patients show clinical improvement and reduction in tumor size. Again, clinical regression occurs if the medication is discontinued [106, 107].

Results of bromocriptine therapy in the management of Nelson's syndrome and Cushing's disease are less convincing. Nonetheless, bromocriptine produces some suppression of both pituitary adrenocorticotropin (ACTH) levels and circulating steroids. Side effects of bromocriptine therapy include nausea, vomiting, and postural hypotension [108].

The normal pituitary almost doubles in size during pregnancy; in the presence of a PRL-secreting adenoma there is some risk of compression of the optic pathways [109]. Careful monitoring of patients with prolactinomas during pregnancy is important. *Somatostatin analog (SMS 201-995, Sandostatin)* is a derivative of somatostatin, a naturally occurring peptide in humans. It is effective in inhibiting GH release in most acromegalic patients and has been used as an effective adjunct to surgery for large GH-secreting adenomas [333, 334].

Surgical Treatment. Surgical extirpation is the preferred treatment of most pituitary tumors. The transsphenoidal approach is favored by most neurosurgeons since it is safer and more effective than craniotomy.

The goals of surgical management include (1) decompression of neural structures, particularly the optic pathways, (2) correction of endocrine dysfunction, (3) histologic diagnosis, and (4) complete removal of the tumor.

The *Hardy Classification* (based on radiographic anatomy and operative findings) of adenomas according to grade I to V (degree of sella destruction) and stage O, A to E (extrasellar extension) is of value in estimating prognosis and comparing results [110]. Treatment modalities include the following:

1. *Transsphenoidal microsurgical adenomectomy.* This is the procedure of choice for tumors occupying the sella whether or not there is sphenoid extension and for tumors with vertical suprasellar expansion without significant lateral extension [111].

   Preoperative cortisone supplementation is important in patients undergoing pituitary surgery. Hydrocortisone 100 mg is given intravenously before surgery and continued postoperatively to forestall collapse of the pituitary-adrenal axis. The procedure has low morbidity and mortality in experienced hands. The neurosurgeon is able to visually differentiate pituitary gland from tumor. Although the approach is through a nonsterile field (sinuses), meningitis is rare.

Control rates of functional adenomas with transsphenoidal adenomectomy are between 75 and 80 percent in most surgical series.

In *prolactinomas,* the highest surgical cure rates are obtained in patients with tumors smaller than 10 mm (microadenomas), PRL levels under 200 ng/ml (75–80% cure rate), and short duration of symptoms. Postoperative PRL values are an index of the likelihood of cure [112–114].

Patients with *pituitary apoplexy* and compression of the optic pathways require urgent surgical decompression.

Cushing's disease can be life-threatening, and even when a microadenoma is not found many neurosurgeons recommend a total hypophysectomy and replacement hormonal therapy. This may not be appropriate in children or in women of child-bearing age; medical therapy, bilateral adrenalectomy, or radiotherapy should be considered.

Some patients with Cushing's disease in whom a discrete tumor is not identified have diffuse hyperplasia or histologically normal glands. This raises the possibility of a hypothalamic disorder in at least some cases.

Nelson's syndrome poses a more tenacious surgical problem; usually transsphenoidal adenomectomy is combined with radiation therapy.

Control rates in *nonfunctional* tumors are less than those obtained with functional tumors. This is most likely related to the fact that most nonfunctional adenomas have attained an enormous size before the patient comes to surgery.

Before surgery the patient's nose, gums, and teeth should be examined. Some surgeons use prophylactic antibiotics.

2. *Craniotomy.* Although the transsphenoidal approach is used in most cases, the *transcranial approach (subfrontal or pterional)* is preferable for tumors with significant intracranial extension into the subfrontal (anterior fossa) or parasellar regions (middle fossa).

Morbidity exceeds that for transsphenoidal adenomectomy with the possible exception of CSF leak. Further, there is a risk of damage to the optic apparatus and pituitary stalk.

3. *Radiotherapy.* The role of radiotherapy has become less prominent in recent years with the evolution of more effective neurosurgical and medical therapy. Radiation is reserved for adjunctive therapy. Main modes of delivery include conventional radiation by cobalt or linear accelerator generators and heavy particle radiation (protons), which is currently available in only a few centers worldwide. These gen-

erators, working on the principle of the Bragg peak, deliver radiation to a discrete targeted locus. The effect of radiotherapy may be delayed for months. In general, radiation is employed when medical and surgical therapy have failed to control symptomatic recurrent disease.

Neurosurgical Infections

Subdural Empyema

Subdural empyema is a serious intracranial infection. It is frequently a complication of paranasal sinusitis, trauma, or meningitis (in infants). Because of the origin in the sinuses, anaerobic organisms are commonly isolated. In infantile meningitis, *Haemophilus influenzae* and *Streptococcus pneumoniae* are important causative organisms. Patients are usually very ill, febrile, and may have focal neurologic deficits or seizures.

CT scan may show a minimal collection with little mass effect and contrast enhancement over the convexities. Associated findings of sinusitis or mastoiditis may be present [335].

Systemic antibiotics are directed to the organisms isolated. Surgical drainage is usually necessary since the pus lies in the relatively avascular plane between the subarachnoid space and the dura. Multiple burr holes with copious irrigation may be sufficient in some cases; other patients will require craniotomy for adequate drainage. The pus is frequently tenacious and may extend over a large area, making removal difficult. Venous sinus or cortical vein thrombosis may complicate subdural empyema [336].

Cerebral Abscess

Brain abscess is usually due to contiguous spread from a paranasal sinus, mastoid, or middle ear, or metastatic spread from a distant infection. About 80 percent of patients with brain abscess have a known predisposing factor.

Frontal or ethmoidal sinusitis may lead to a frontal lobe abscess; maxillary or sphenoid sinusitis may spread to the frontal or temporal lobes; and mastoid sinusitis may result in cerebellar or temporal lobe abscess.

Metastatic brain abscesses usually develop in the distribution of the middle cerebral artery by hematogenous spread from the lung, tooth, or heart (bacterial endocarditis). These abscesses are often multiple and are located at the junction of the grey and white matter.

Frequently, brain abscess complicates an open head injury, especially in penetrating wounds with retained indriven fragments. Brain abscesses are caused by a number of organisms including anaerobic and aerobic bacteria. Common anaerobes are the *Bacteroides* species and anaerobic streptococci. Aerobic streptococci are frequent in many series; gram-negative aerobes (haemophilus species, enterobacteriaceae) are prominent in isolates from patients with chronic sinusitis. *Staphylococcus aureus* is commonly isolated from posttraumatic abscesses.

In the immunocompromised host, more exotic pathogens such as *Nocardia asteroides, Listeria monocytogenes,* and mycobacterium species must be considered.

Clinical presentation may include headache, fever, seizure, altered mental status, and focal deficits corresponding to the location of the abscess. There may be a history of a predisposing condition such as bronchiectasis, bacterial endocarditis, penetrating head injuries (gunshot wounds or stab wounds), tooth infections, or intravenous drug abuse.

Diagnosis. The erythrocyte sedimentation rate (ESR) is elevated in the majority of cases. The peripheral white count is elevated in a minority of cases. Lumbar puncture is unlikely to yield significant bacteriologic information and may be contraindicated in the face of a mass lesion because of the risk of herniation.

CT has played a critical role in the contemporary management of cerebral abscesses by providing early diagnosis and thereby reducing mortality [337]. *CT findings* depend on the maturity of the abscess. In *mature lesions,* the abscess is well-encapsulated and the contrast-enhanced CT scan shows a low-density lesion with ring enhancement and surrounding edema. Usually the ring is thin. The ring of enhancement does not necessarily represent the actual capsule but rather an area of blood-brain–barrier breakdown that can be seen with cerebritis.

Ring enhancement is not pathognomonic of cerebral abscesses and the differential diagnosis should include cystic gliomas, resolving infarcts, or metastatic tumors.

In the *early (cerebritis)* stage, patchy contrast enhancement may occur within an area of low density. There may also be ventricular or meningeal enhancement, indicating ventriculitis or meningitis.

Treatment MEDICAL TREATMENT. Selected patients may be managed successfully without surgical intervention. When the condition is diagnosed early, appropriate antibiotic therapy and serial CT scanning to follow progression of the abscess has been successful in some cases.

Selection of *antibiotic therapy* depends on the results of culture and sensitivity; however, antibiotic therapy may be empirical when the abscess is not aspirated or while awaiting culture results.

The duration of antibiotic therapy varies from 4 to 6 weeks depending on the particular circumstances. Medical therapy alone is usually insufficient in a patient who shows progressive neurologic deficit or alteration in level of consciousness from mass effect. Similarly, abscesses enlarging on serial CT scanning despite medical treatment should be aspirated or excised, if feasible [338].

The role of *corticosteroids* in the management of brain abscess is controversial. Steroids are of benefit in reducing cerebral edema, but this may be outweighed by their negative effect on host immune mechanisms. Steroids retard encapsulation, decrease leukocyte migration, and inhibit gliosis, which may favor abscess progression. However, when there is significant mass effect from cerebral edema, a short course of steroids may improve the neurologic status. Corticosteroids should be withdrawn as soon as the patient's condition permits.

SURGICAL TREATMENT. Surgical options include CT-guided stereotactic (closed) or ultrasound-guided (open) needle aspiration and craniotomy for abscess excision.

Stereotactic aspiration is accomplished through a burr hole under local anesthesia. Repeat aspirations may be done, if necessary. There is a greater likelihood of abscess recurrence with aspiration than complete excision. Aspiration is particularly suitable for deep lesions in patients with medical contraindications to craniotomy or multiple abscesses. If the abscess is accessible and CT suggests evacuable pus with a formed capsule, the abscess may be removed by craniotomy. Total excision is most feasible with lobar or cerebellar abscesses. Patients with abscesses that are refractory to repeat aspirations and antibiotic therapy may also require complete excision [339].

Neurocysticercosis

Neurocysticercosis is a CNS infection with the larval form of *Taenia solium,* the pork tapeworm. Recent migration patterns from endemic areas have made neurocysticercosis more common in North America.

Clinical Presentation. Clinical presentation includes seizures, symptoms of intracranial hypertension, and focal neurologic abnormalities. Four forms of cerebral cysticercosis are described: meningeal, parenchymal, ventricular, and mixed lesions. Cysts may be single or racemose. Hydrocephalus is a common complication.

Diagnosis. The typical CT findings are single or multiple low-density cystic lesions with ring enhancement. MRI demonstrates a cystic lesion with a well-defined mural nodule or a large racemose cyst lacking a mural nodule.

CSF shows a pleocytosis (especially eosinophils), elevated protein, and hypoglycorrhachia.

Serological tests on the CSF and serum (Cysticercosis enzyme-linked immunosorbent assay (ELISA) and indirect hemagglutinin [IHA]) are commonly used.

Treatment. Praziquantel, in a dose of 50 mg/kg/day in three divided doses over 14-days, is effective. Surgical treatment may be required for decompression and evacuation of a cyst [340].

Toxoplasmosis

Toxoplasmosis is due to infection with the protozoan *Toxoplasma gondii,* whose definitive host is the cat. CNS infection is common in immunocompromised hosts. Infection may be meningoencephalitis or single or multiple mass lesions.

There has been a rise in CNS toxoplasmosis with the increasing incidence of acquired immunodeficiency syndrome (AIDS); it is currently the most common CNS infection in these patients.
Diagnosis. The organism has rarely been isolated from the CSF, which shows a mild lymphocytic pleocystosis and slightly elevated protein.

Serological diagnosis by indirect hemagglutinating antibody (IHA), indirect fluorescent antibody (IFA), or the Sabin-Feldman dye test are confirmatory.

CT findings of multiple ring enhancing lesions or homogeneously enhancing lesions in a patient with AIDS is highly suggestive of toxoplasmosis.

Lesions may be biopsied if accessible; histologic sections show trophozoites and cysts.
Treatment. Treatment is with a combination of pyrimethamine and sulfadiazine. Pyrimethamine is given in a dose of 100 mg orally on day 1 followed by 25 mg once a day thereafter; sulfadiazine is given 4 to 6gm daily by mouth. Both are continued for 4 to 5 weeks.

CNS Mycoses

Cryptococcus is the commonest mycotic infection of the CNS. It is associated with debilitating disease in most instances, and the primary site is usually the lung or skin. Spread to the CNS is hematogenous. The infection may be a meningitis (especially basilar), meningoencephalitis, or focal mass lesion. Patients present with headache, cranial nerve palsies, and nuchal rigidity.
Diagnosis. CSF is positive with the India ink preparation for cryptococcal infection. Positive cultures in most fungal infections require many weeks. Serologic testing is helpful in cryptococcal, candida, and coccidioides infections.

Fungal mass lesions may appear on contrast CT as ring enhancing nodules.

Amphotericin B is an effective therapeutic agent. It is given intravenously in a dose of 0.3 mg/kg/day for 6 weeks after a 1-mg test dose. CSF penetration is poor [341, 342].

Herpes Simplex Encephalitis (HSE)

Herpes Simplex Virus Type 1 (HSV-1) is the most common cause of nonepidemic acute viral encephalitis in the United States. Herpes simplex encephalitis usually occurs in an immunocompromised host. The infection is due to HSV-1 or, rarely HSV-2. The virus has a predilection for the temporal lobes, perhaps because of its proximity to the trigeminal ganglion, where latent HSV infection has been shown to occur in a significant number of autopsy specimens.

Clinical Features. Initially, there is a febrile illness with headaches and malaise that soon progresses to seizures, alteration in level of consciousness, personality changes, and focal deficits. Untreated, the patient rapidly slides into coma. Progressive intracranial hypertension and herniation may result without prompt diagnosis and therapy.

Diagnosis. CSF shows pleocytosis and raised immunoglobulin (Ig) levels.

CT scan reveals low-density enhancing lesions in the temporal lobe. Acute and convalescent sera and CSF should be obtained for HSV antibody levels.

The EEG shows slowing or periodic discharge over the temporal lobes.

Brain tissue is required for definitive diagnosis. The biopsy is taken from the most suggestive site based on clinical and diagnostic evidence. Biopsy material is examined by routine histology, electron microscopy, and HSV isolation by tissue culture.

Mortality is high when diagnosis is delayed. Outcome is critically dependent on the patient's level of consciousness at the inception of treatment.

Treatment. Acyclovir (Zovirax) is the drug of choice and is quite effective; it is superior to vidarabine (which was previously the drug of choice). Generally, treatment is begun at or soon after the brain biopsy. Acyclovir is administered intravenously in a dose of 10 mg/kg every 8 hours.

ICP monitoring and treatment with mannitol or barbiturates may be required for intracranial hypertension in critical patients [343].

Head Injury

Head injuries account for about 50 percent of all trauma fatalities and extract a huge economic and social toll from society. The yearly incidence of significant head injury is about 200 cases per 100,000 population for all regions of the United States. Prevention will always remain our best defense against this challenge. Primary mechanical brain injury that occurs at the moment of impact cannot be addressed by any currently available therapy. The main thrust in the management of craniocerebral trauma is preventing secondary insults to the already traumatized brain.

Most patients are initially seen in the emergency room. With the recent evolution of emergency medical care in many parts of the country, some estimate of the approaching patient's condition is available to the waiting trauma team. Trauma management is a team effort, and many interventions need to proceed quickly and simultaneously.

Priorities in management include airway and ventilation followed by circulation. No matter the urgency of neurologic trauma, no priority exceeds that of securing the airway and ensuring that patient is breathing adequately. Unconscious patients should be intubated immediately to protect the airway, since aspiration can cause sudden pulmonary compromise leading to hypoxia and hypercapnia, which worsens the brain injury. Even without aspiration, between 30 and 50 percent of patients in traumatic coma are hypoxic when first treated. ABGs should be obtained as soon as possible to establish a baseline and guide further treatment.

Head injury very rarely produces shock, except in the terminal phases of brain death, where medullary failure causes intractable hypotension, or when extensive scalp injuries are left unattended for prolonged periods with profuse blood loss. Hypotension must be assumed to be due to chest, abdominal, or extremity injury until proved otherwise. The significance of hypotension cannot be overemphasized; the excess mortality from hypotension in patients with equivalent degrees of head injury is at least 40 percent. Bradycardia associated with hypotension often means cervical spine injury.

To reverse possible hypoglycemia or narcotic overdose that may contribute to neurologic depression, we advise administering 50 ml of 50% dextrose and 0.4 mg of naloxone intravenously to comatose patients after obtaining blood and urine specimens for routine chemistries and toxicologic studies.

Diagnosis

History and Physical Examination. Most often the history comes from paramedics, police officers, or bystanders. If family members are available, obtain some information regarding previous health status, medications, and allergies. The neurosurgeon must synthesize the often truncated historical data with the clinical presentation.

Vital signs are of course an immediate priority. Associated injuries must be immediately identified to establish management priorities. A *cervical injury must be presumed to exist;* keep the head and neck in neutral alignment, and obtain a cross-table lateral cervical spine (C-spine) x-ray film. A normal lateral C-spine, including the C7–T1 junction, without prevertebral swelling is a good screening study in the majority of cases. To complete the evaluation, however, other views must be obtained. It is important to leave a well-fitting cervical collar in place until the C-spine series has been completed and cleared of injury. *Inspect* the *scalp carefully* for lacerations, avulsions, and penetrating wounds. These are commonly missed if located in the dependent occipital area. If an open wound is identified, no further probing is necessary, since it must be debrided and closed. The practice, sometimes advocated, of probing lacerations with a gloved finger has little to commend it. Dislodgment of a bone fragment from a lacerated cerebral artery or a torn venous sinus may create problems of a magnitude to discomfit the perpetrator for some time. Bleeding from scalp lacerations must be controlled, whether by pressure, hemostat, or scalp suture.

Basilar skull fractures can be diagnosed by indirect clinical evidence. Circumscribed unilateral or bilateral periorbital ecchymosis (*raccoon eyes*) indicate fracture of the floor of the anterior fossa. Direct orbital trauma may result in a similar finding. Blood in the external canal indicates a basilar fracture through the lateral portion of the temporal bone. If the fracture is medial to the tympanic membrane, a hemotympanum may be seen.

Ecchymosis overlying the mastoid (*Battle's sign*) is usually delayed for 12 to 24 hours after initial injury; it represents blood dissecting to the skin from a mastoid fracture. Leakage of CSF from the nose (*rhinorrhea*) or ear (*otorrhea*) is due to a meningeal tear at the site of a basilar fracture and carries a risk of infection (meningitis, cerebral abscess).

The *initial neurologic examination must be rapid and thorough;* immediate diagnostic and therapeutic decisions hinge on these findings. The examiner should determine the level of CNS function by the GCS [312] (see Table 5-4). The scale records the patient's responses (eye opening, best motor response, and best verbal response) to verbal and painful stimuli. A numerical scale assigns a discrete value (from 3 to 15) to the examination. The scale has gained international acceptance. It is highly reliable with little interobserver variation. It has been used to compare the results of various treatment modalites among different groups of patients.

The integrity of midbrain, pontine, and medullary function is determined by cranial nerve examination. The pupillary light reflex involves the optic (second) and oculomotor (third) cranial nerves. The oculocephalic reflex (doll's eyes maneuver), which evaluates connections between the vestibular apparatus, pontine gaze centers, and the sixth and third nerve nuclei in the pons and midbrain, requires vigorous rapid head turning and can *only* be done if cervical spine injury has been excluded by appropriate investigation. If a cervical injury does exist, the pathway can still be evaluated by the oculovestibular reflex (caloric testing).

Supraorbital pressure can be used to elicit a facial grimace to test seventh cranial nerve (facial) function in a comatose patient. Respiratory pattern, cough, and gag reflexes reflect lower cranial (ninth and tenth) nerve and medullary function.

Skull X-Ray Films. Traditionally, skull x-ray films have been obtained in the evaluation of head injury, but the introduction of CT scanning has greatly diminished their use [116]. However, CT bone windows often fail to disclose the true extent of fractures of the vault; anteroposterior, lateral, and Towne's views of the skull would be useful in those situations. Skull x-ray films should be obtained for penetrating injuries or depressed fractures. The films should be "bright lighted" so that any areas of soft tissue swelling may be more easily seen.

Skull fractures may be *linear* (most common), *depressed, comminuted, diastatic, compound, closed,* or a combination. The presence of a skull fracture does not imply that there is a severe or even any intracranial injury. In the absence of complications or intracranial injury, skull fractures per se usually are not clinically significant; in fact, energy used to fracture the skull is not available to injure the brain. Severe neural injury can and does occur in the absence of a skull fracture. Although a linear fracture in early childhood nearly always heals without incident, occasionally the fracture does not heal and the diastatsis between the fracture edges increases. This is referred to as a "*growing*" skull fracture. It reflects the development of a leptomeningeal cyst at the site of a skull fracture where a dural laceration allowed the arachnoid to pout out into the fracture site. CSF pulsation causes thinning of the dura, enlargement of the cyst, and erosion of the bone edges. Growing fractures are usually seen in children under 3 years of age, occur most frequently in the parietal bone, and develop within the first 2 to 6 months after a linear skull fracture.

The scalp is swollen, there may be a history of seizures, and skull x-ray films show a diastatic fracture that has increased in size from the prior film.

Depressed fractures refer to skull fractures in which a bony segment is sunken below the outer table of the skull. They are the result of a large amount of kinetic energy dissipated over a small area of the skull. Examples include being struck on the head with a baseball bat, golf club, or the butt of a gun. There is a spectrum of severity from inconsequential to surgical emergency. They are clinically significant if (1) the fragments are depressed below the inner table of the adjacent calvarium, (2) they are open, (3) they lie over a dural sinus, or (4) they are associated with underlying cortical injury.

A *tangential* view is helpful in determining the amount of depression of the bony fragments. A depression of 1.0 cm or more is liable to cause damage to the underlying brain. Depressed bone fragments may tear the dura and allow air, bacteria, or foreign bodies into the cranial cavity. *External compound fractures* result from a communication with the scalp. *Internal compound fractures* communicate with the paranasal sinuses. Infection may complicate a compound fracture. Basilar skull fractures are particularly difficult to detect. Clinical signs include CSF rhinorrhea or otorrhea, Battle's sign or raccoon's eyes, and hemotympanum. If the fracture involves the facial canal, there may be a facial nerve palsy. Presumptive radiologic signs include air-fluid levels from blood or CSF within the sinus and air within the cranial cavity (pneumocephalus).

Linear fractures of the calvaria are radiolucent with a very well-defined border. It is possible to mistake a normal suture or vascular groove for a linear fracture. Simple linear skull fractures extend through both tables of the skull and therefore are more lucent than vascular grooves. They do not have the sclerotic borders seen with vascular grooves, and they rarely bifurcate—another finding with vascular grooves. Suture lines on the outer table of the skull have a serrated appearance, whereas the suture on the inner table of the skull is a straight line and may be mistaken for a fracture. The pediatric skull presents unique problems because of the presence of normal sutures and synchondroses in the early years of life. In particular, the mendosal suture of the occipital bone may be mistaken for a fracture.

Computed Tomography. CT is currently the most efficient tool in the triage of head injury. The initial trauma CT scan should always be nonenhanced (i.e., without contrast). It should be noted that IV-dye given for renal visualization (IVP) before the cranial CT may make it impossible to assess the presence of intracranial blood. It may be necessary to sedate or even paralyze a very agitated patient to obtain good-quality images free of motion artifact. If there are unexplained alterations in neurologic status after an initial CT, the scan may be repeated to look for delayed hemorrhages or cerebral edema.

A full discussion of the subtleties of CT in cranial trauma is beyond the scope of this book; what follows are common and useful features.

MIDLINE. Starting with the basal cut, look for the midline structures: the third and fourth ventricles, pineal gland calcification, and falx cerebri. Are any of these structures shifted from their usual midline position?

BLOOD. Is there any blood in the intracranial space? Fresh blood appears hyperdense (white).

SUBARACHNOID HEMORRHAGE. *Trauma is the commonest cause of a SAH.* SAH may appear as a bright line along the margin of the falx or a hazy density over the tentorium cerebelli. SAH may also fill the basal cisterns, sylvian fissure, and cerebral sulci. Intraventricular hemorrhage (IVH) may be visualized as a blood-fluid level in the lateral ventricle. Although IVH usually clears, it may cause CSF obstruction and hydrocephalus.

EPIDURAL HEMATOMA. Epidural hematoma (EDH) appears on nonenhanced CT scans as a peripherally located, lentiform (convexity medial), hyperdense area. The ipsilateral hemisphere is often compressed by the hematoma, with intracranial contents shifting to the opposite side. Clasically, an EDH is associated with a fracture across the course of the middle meningeal artery that lacerates the vessel, resulting in arterial bleeding. Venous hemorrhage is also a known cause of EDH. An associated fracture may not be apparent on CT if it is not in the plane of the CT cuts; a plain skull x-ray film, however, will usually demonstrate it.

SUBDURAL HEMATOMA. *Subdural hematomas develop between the inner layer of dura and the arachnoid.* They are crescentic extracerebral collections of blood seen over one or both hemispheres. The inner margin is concave while the outer margin is convex, following the contour of the cranial vault.

Subdural hematomas may have three evolutionary stages: acute, subacute, and chronic.

1. *Acute subdural hematoma* is hyperdense. It may vary from very small to a large collection with significant shift. The adjacent calvarium

may obscure a small collection; adjusting the window level may segregate the bony density from blood. The hematoma is often associated with significant underlying brain injury, swelling, and shift, well out of proportion to the mass effect from the clot itself. This picture reflects the intrinsic brain injury at the time of impact.

2. *Subacute subdural hematoma.* There is a time lapse of up to 2 weeks for a subdural collection to acquire the characteristics of a subacute hematoma (depending on its original size). Because of a gradual decrease in density of the blood with time, the area is isodense; therefore it is difficult to distinguish between it and normal brain on CT. With contrast-enhanced CT there may be a rim of enhancement due to injured brain and organizing membrane.

3. *Chronic subdural hematoma* appears as a hypodense extraaxial collection on nonenhanced CT. It usually takes 3 to 4 weeks to evolve a hypodense subdural hematoma. There may be a blood-fluid level within the collection. A membrane (which may calcify) is frequently evident. Clinical presentation includes seizures, headaches, altered level of consciousness, or focal deficit. Patients with chronic subdural hematoma are generally old, alcoholic, or demented and may give a history of multiple instances of head trauma. More commonly there is no recollection of head injury. The hematoma may be bilateral without shift of the midline ("balanced subdurals") or unilateral and still no shift because there is significant cerebral atrophy. In children, these collections may be associated with dilatation of the lateral ventricles. The ventriculomegaly is thought to result from impaired absorption of CSF by the arachnoid villi.

CONTUSIONS. Contusions are small specks of blood usually interspersed with hypo- or isodense injured brain tissue ("salt and pepper" appearance), sometimes surrounded by edema. They are frequently found in the anterior temporal and frontal lobes because the contour of the anterior fossa is rough and the sphenoid ridge limits the forward motion of the temporal lobe during deceleration injury. Contusions may be single or multiple, large or small. The distinction between contusion and ICH may occasionally present difficulty. Generally, ICH is a homogenous density with well-defined margins.

EDEMA. *Diffuse cerebral swelling* may be inferred by the small size of the ventricles or effacement of the basal cisterns. Early on there may be no detectable change in brain density. SAH is a frequently associated finding [118].

Cerebral edema is common in patients with diffuse axonal shearing injury. Diffuse swelling of both hemispheres as an acute cerebral reaction to injury is common in children, probably from hyperemia [119]. Localized areas of edema appear on nonenhanced CT scans as low-density areas with mass effect.

CISTERNS. Totally obliterated cisterns (i.e., no CSF density visible) on good-quality scans imply significant cerebral swelling and poor intracranial compliance.

BONE. This is best examined on the bone windows setting. While doing so, note any intracranial air (black dots or globules); any fluid levels in the frontal, ethmoid, sphenoid, or mastoid air sinuses; the degree and site of scalp swellings; and the orbits and globes. The only significant depressed skull fractures that may escape this survey are those situated rostrally on the calvarium.

Magnetic Resonance Imaging. The use of MRI has been limited in the patient with multisystem trauma, since most of the monitoring and support equipment contain ferromagnetic material and cannot be brought into the suite. Furthermore, the RF pulses generated in the scanner interfere with most equipment. Recently, support and monitoring equipment have been adapted (ventilators, transducers, ICP monitors, arterial lines, cardiac monitors, medication delivery pumps) by eliminating ferromagnetic materials, the use of extension cables, and telemetric monitoring to allow critically monitored patients to undergo MRI scanning [120]. Although some monitoring artifact is encountered, it is not a significant problem.

Edema appears as a decreased signal intensity on T1-weighted images and increased signal intensity (or white) on T2-weighted images. The role of MRI in trauma remains to be defined.

Treatment: Severe Head Injury

Medical Treatment. Medical treatment for severe head injury is discussed below.

ICP. A great deal of the medical management of the head-injured patient centers on control of ICP. ICP monitoring is a guide to the treatment of raised ICP. (Methods for monitoring and treating patients with elevated ICP have been discussed in Chap. 2 and will not be discussed here.)

STEROIDS. There is no acceptable evidence that steroids are of any value in the treatment of brain injury; indeed, given the deleterious effects of steroids on the immune and other systems, the risk-benefit ratio is probably unfavorable [121].

ANTICONVULSANTS. If there is good reason for the use of an anticonvulsant (prophylactic or therapeutic), phenytoin sodium is usually the first choice. A loading dose of 1 gm intravenously or by mouth is given followed by 300 to 400 mg daily, in divided doses. Serum phenytoin levels are checked after starting therapy; the maintenance dose may then be altered accordingly to maintain therapeutic blood levels.

FLUID AND ELECTROLYTES. A Foley catheter should be placed for monitoring of urine output. Much has been made about running the patient "dry." In adults, urinary output should be at least 30 ml/hour, and hypovolemia should be avoided. A reasonable choice for intravenous therapy is 5% dextrose in water with one-half normal saline and 20 mEq of potassium chloride per liter at 80 to 125 ml/hour depending on needs. Electrolytes are checked frequently. Hyponatremia can worsen cerebral edema. SIADH may complicate head injury. The diagnostic criteria and treatment have been considered in the section on SAH.

NUTRITIONAL SUPPORT. Elevated energy expenditures and increased protein catabolism can occur in patients with severe head injury. Although these effects of trauma have long been recognized in nonneurosurgical patients, only recently has specific attention been directed toward the metabolic changes in severe neurosurgical trauma [122–124]. Nasogastric feeding is the usual method of nutritional support in the patient who is unable to eat by mouth. The economic and physiologic benefits of this route are well known. In patients requiring long-term enteral nutrition, gastrostomy or jejunostomy can prevent problems such as nasal and esophageal erosion, feeding tube dislodgment, and aspiration pneumonia. The percutaneous insertion of a gastrostomy tube is a good alternative. Ileus often prevents successful early enteral nutritional support. Enteral feeding is poorly tolerated during the first 14 days following severe head injury. Tolerance of enteral feedings is inversely related to increased ICP and the severity of brain injury. Aspiration pneumonitis may occur in almost 22 percent of patients with intracranial hypertension from regurgitation of tube feedings [125]. In one recent study the mean duration from injury to initiation of full-strength, full-rate tube feedings was 11.5 days. Total parenteral nutrition (TPN) should preferably be started within 3 days after injury in the severely brain-injured and be continued until enteral feedings can be safely administered [125, 126]. The drawbacks of TPN in the neurosurgical patient are the large volumes of fluid required; hyperglycemia, which may exacerbate ischemic neuronal injury; and sepsis.

Surgical Treatment. Surgical treatment for severe head injury is discussed below.

SCALP INJURIES. Abrasions and contusions require routine wound care. Subgaleal and superiosteal hematomas usually resorb spontaneously and practically never require needle aspiration, which may predispose to infection. In closing contaminated scalp lacerations, place interrupted monofilament sutures through all layers of the scalp after thorough cleansing and debridement. Give due attention to tetanus prophylaxis.

SKULL FRACTURES. *Nondepressed skull fractures* seldom require surgical treatment other than repair of an associated scalp laceration.

Growing skull fractures in children frequently require dural repair and cranioplasty.

With clinically significant *closed depressed fractures,* the reasons for surgical treatment (elevation of bone fragments and wound closure) are to correct a cosmetic defect and reduce the incidence of posttraumatic seizures.

Compound depressed fractures require exploration, debridement of devitalized soft tissues, elevation of the indriven bone fragments, debridement of injured brain, repair of dural lacerations, and wound closure. Prompt treatment is recommended as delay is associated with a significant increase in the risk of infection. Replacement of bone fragments at the time of surgery may preclude the need for a second operation to perform a cranioplasty. If closure was delayed (which could increase the risk of infection), deferred cranioplasty would be preferable.

Basilar skull fractures without CSF leak generally do not require operative treatment. Basilar skull fracture with CSF fistula (rhinorrhea or otorrhea) is managed expectantly since the overwhelming majority will cease spontaneously. The diagnosis is suspected when there is a clear or serosanguineous, nonmucoid nasal, or aural discharge. With CSF rhinorrhea, or strong suspicion of it (upper facial fractures), nasotracheal intubation and nasogastric tube placement should be avoided if possible, lest additional damage to or penetration of the skull base occur.

The patient should be placed in a head up 15- to 30-degree position to minimize the leak and cautioned to avoid blowing the nose. Coexistent hydrocephalus may prolong a CSF leak; obtain a CT scan to establish this if suspected. The use of prophylactic antibiotics in CSF fistula is controversial, since there is a risk of selecting drug-resistant bacteria [127]. Should unexplained fever or meningeal signs develop, perform a lumbar puncture. Examine the CSF (including culture and sensitivity) and begin appropriate antibiotic therapy as indicated. If CSF leak persists for more than 72 hours, lumbar spinal drainage for 3 to 5 days should be considered (see Chap. 3). If the leak ceases within a week, no further therapy is necessary beyond observation. If the leak persists despite conservative management, further workup to localize the leak—metrizamide CT scan or radioisotope cisternography—is indicated [128]. Surgical repair of the fistula is then tailored accordingly [129].

ACUTE TRAUMATIC HEMATOMAS. When indicated, surgical treatment must be pursued with dispatch. The decision for surgical intervention in the case of traumatic intracerebral hematoma depends on size of the hematoma and its location, the degree of mass effect, and the patient's clinical condition. In general, all significant acute epidural and most subdural hematomas will require surgical evacuation. Currently, surgical treatment is guided by CT scan; before the CT era, burr-hole exploration was very common. Acute traumatic intracranial hematomas are generally evacuated through large craniotomy flaps ("trauma flap"). Decompression and meticulous hemostasis are the goals of surgical treatment.

GUNSHOT WOUNDS TO THE HEAD. Civilian gunshot wounds to the head are usually due to small-caliber, low-velocity missiles. All patients should receive tetanus prophylaxis and those with obvious cortical injury should receive anticonvulsant prophylaxis. Surgical priorities include removal of debris and bone fragments (if readily accessible), evacuation of an associated hematoma, hemostasis, and dural closure. ICP monitoring is usually required for patients with 8 or worse on the GCS. Intracranial hypertension may result from cerebral edema and should be treated in general as it is in elevated ICP. Cerebrospinal fluid fistulas, posttraumatic epilepsy, meningitis, and cerebral abscess are common complications encountered with gunshot wounds to the head.

GUNSHOT WOUNDS TO THE SPINE. The commonest location is the thoracic spine. These injuries may result in a flaccid paraplegia with complete sensory loss to the cord below the level of injury from trauma. When the trajectory is through the gastrointestinal tract into the spinal canal, there is significant risk of infection (meningitis, epidural abscess). Spinal stability is almost never compromised to any significant extent with gunshot wounds to the spine. Spinal shock is managed by volume support, central venous pressure monitoring, and pressors if needed. Plain x-ray films of the spine may assist in the evaluation of the bullet trajectory and defining associated bony injury. CT scanning through the involved segments (with contrast) can evaluate a CSF leak or assess the integrity of the thecal sac and its relationships. Operative intervention may be required in the patient who is worsening neurologically due to a definable mass lesion (hematoma, missle or bone impingement, epidural abscess) or to close a persistent CSF leak. Delayed complications include posttraumatic syringomyelia, pain syndromes, and problems of immobility in the spinal cord–injured patient.

Treatment: Minor Head Injury

Defined as patients with a GCS score between 13 and 15, minor head injuries constitute almost 50 percent of all head injuries [130]. Patients with minor head injury tend to be young (11–20 years). The group with the highest risk of minor injuries are students; falls and sporting accidents are common causes [130]. There is controversy regarding admission policies and management of minor head injury [131]. In a recent retrospective review of 373 adult patients admitted for minor closed head injury (GCS 13–15), the neurologic examination in the emergency room was the best predictor of subsequent deterioration or the presence of an operative hematoma [132]. The only patients with a GCS score of 15 who required surgical evacuation of extraaxial hematoma had a relevant focal neurologic deficit with or without abnormal mental status. A GCS of 13 or 14 was associated with a 2 percent risk of an operative hematoma or of subsequent clinical deterioration. Based on their data, these authors recommended that CT scan of the head be obtained on all patients with a GCS score less than 15, abnormal mental status, or hemispheric neurologic deficit [132].

If no operative lesion is found, the patient should be admitted for observation. Those patients with a GCS score of 15, normal mental status, and no hemispheric neurologic deficit may be discharged home to be observed by a competent observer despite basilar or calvarial skull fracture, loss of consciousness, or cranial nerve deficit. No benefit was gained from skull radiography in any group [132].

Complications of Head Injury

CSF Fistula. The most common cause of a CSF leak is trauma. The floor of the frontal fossa is susceptible to fracture because it is thin.

The defect is usually located in the cribriform plate. Posttraumatic CSF fistulas occur in approximately 2 to 3 percent of all patients with head injuries. Most CSF fistulas seal spontaneously. CSF rhinorrhea ceases in over 85 percent of patients within the first week following injury, and otorrhea ceases spontaneously in virtually all cases. Meningitis may occur with persistent CSF leak, especially after 7 days. *Streptococcus pneumoniae* is the most common infecting organism. The prognosis for children with meningitis secondary to a CSF fistula appears to be worse, and a more aggressive surgical approach is warranted in pediatric cases [136].

Carotid-Cavernous Sinus Fistula. Carotid-cavernous sinus fistula may be due to laceration of the carotid artery in the cavernous sinus from a basilar fracture or a penetrating orbitocranial injury.

Extracranial Vascular Injury. Injury to major neck vessels and carotid or vertebral arteries from rotational vectors may result in intimal dissection, thrombosis, and vessel occlusion. This results in cerebral ischemia, which may present with hemiplegia or other focal deficit [133]. A high index of suspicion is necessary for early diagnosis, since there is frequently very slight or no sign of external injury and the symptoms of ischemia may be delayed or masked by the comatose state [134]. Vascular injury should be suspected if a hemispheric focal deficit develops or exists in the setting of an initially negative CT scan. Important signs include an ipsilateral Horner's syndrome from injury to the cervical sympathetic chain, a carotid bruit, and associated mandibular fracture [135]. Angiography is the definitive diagnostic study. A delayed CT scan may show hypodensity within a vascular distribution representing infarction.

Infection. Infection may complicate open fractures of the cranial vault and base and lead to meningitis, cerebral abscess, or subdural empyema. Meningitis that appears within 3 days of a skull fracture is most likely due to *Streptococcus pneumoniae.* If meningitis develops 5 days or more after a head injury, a wide variety of organisms should be considered, including staphylococci, gram-negative rods, and anaerobes. The staphylococci are best treated with a penicillinase-stable penicillin, such as nafcillin, intravenously. If methicillin-resistant *Staphylococcus aureus* (MRSA) are isolated or encountered frequently, vancomycin in doses of 2 gm/day in divided doses should be used instead. The addition of rifampin 600 mg orally every 12 to 24 hours enhances the treatment of MRSA meningitis. Gram-negative rods (*E. coli, Klebsiella,* and *Pseudomonas*) may be successfully treated by the third-generation cephalosporins (e.g., ceftazidime [Fortaz] and ceftizoxime [Cefizox]). Metronidazole (Flagyl) has excellent CSF penetration and is effective against anaerobic organisms. It is given in a dose of 500 mg every 6 hours.

Cerebral abscess and subdural empyema are common complications of cranial missle injuries.

Posttraumatic Epilepsy. *Early* posttraumatic epilepsy is defined as at least one recurrent seizure occuring within 1 week of head injury without other obvious causes. *Late* posttraumatic epilepsy refers to recurrent seizures occurring more than 1 week after head injury. The incidence of early and late epilepsy is estimated at 2.5 to 7.0 percent and 5 to 7 percent, respectively [137, 138].

The risk of early posttraumatic epilepsy is related to the type and severity of head injury. Younger patients (under 5 years) are more susceptible. Up to 25 percent of patients with an early seizure may have a late seizure. However, there is no evidence that prophylactic administration of phenytoin prevents or reduces the incidence of early posttraumatic seizures [139]. If posttraumatic epilepsy does occur, anticonvulsant therapy should be given. Late posttraumatic epilepsy is related to the type and severity of head injury. A mild injury alone, without significant loss of consciousness and no early seizure, is associated with only a 1 to 2 percent risk of late posttraumatic epilepsy. Traumatic intracranial hematomas have a high incidence of posttraumatic seizures, ranging from 20 percent of patients with epidural hematomas to almost 50 percent of patients with subdural or intracerebral hematomas [140]. Once posttraumatic epilepsy is established, there is little change in the attack frequency [141]. There is a significant relationship between seizure frequency and duration. The greater the frequency of seizures, the more likely they are to persist. The efficacy of anticonvulsant therapy in preventing late posttraumatic epilepsy has not been proven [142, 143].

Posttraumatic Hydrocephalus. The suggested incidence of posttraumatic hydrocephalus varies widely [144–146]. It may be of the exvacuo kind (compensatory ventricular dilatation following parenchymal atrophy) or communicating (from impaired CSF absorption due to basal adhesions). The syndrome of normal pressure hydrocephalus (NPH) may be a result of previous head injury.

Postconcussive Syndrome. Postconcussive syndrome may develop following a minor head injury. It includes many "soft" neurologic symptoms: headaches, dizziness, memory difficulties, anxiety, impaired concentration, acoustophobia, and photophobia [147]. It usually resolves gradually but may persist indefinitely, particularly when secondary gain exists. It is rare in children and increases in incidence from early adolescence through middle age. Most patients require little more than reassurance and encouragement. If symptoms are disabling or persist, a neuropsychiatric evaluation, occupational rehabilitative programs, and symptomatic treatment may be helpful.

Carotid-Cavernous Sinus Fistulas

A carotid-cavernous sinus fistula (CCSF) is an abnormal communication (shunt) between the carotid artery or its branches and the cavernous sinus (CS). It may arise spontaneously or secondary to trauma.

Classification

CCSFs are classified according to (1) *etiology,* i.e., traumatic or spontaneous; (2) *hemodynamics,* i.e., high or low flow; and (3) *angiographic anatomy*, i.e., direct (type A) or dural (types B, C, or D) based on arterial supply to the fistula. Type A fistulas are direct communications between the intracavernous internal carotid artery and the CS; they are usually traumatic (severe closed or penetrating head injury) with high-flow characteristics. Type B is a fistula between meningeal branches of the internal carotid artery and the CS; they are rare. Type C is a communication between the meningeal branches of the external carotid and the CS. Type D is a dural shunt from meningeal branches of both the internal and external carotid arteries and the CS. Types B and C are usually spontaneous, low-flow shunts; for unknown reasons they are more common in eldery women [148].

Clinical Presentation

The high-flow fistula is usually associated with a bruit, pulsating exophthalmos, and chemosis from orbital venous hypertension; cranial nerve palsies may result in diplopia, visual loss, and facial dysesthesiae. Types B, C, and D may present insidiously with progressive glaucoma, proptosis, or a "red eye." Angiography is the investigation of choice. The pattern consists of early opacification of the cavernous sinus and the draining veins. The superior ophthalmic vein is often dilated and fills in a retrograde manner.

Treatment

Type A lesions are treated in the first instance by interventional neuroradiologic techniques—a detachable balloon catheter occludes the fistula and preserves flow through the carotid artery [149, 150]. Sometimes this procedure is not feasible, either because the carotid artery has previously been sacrificed or because it cannot be preserved with balloon techniques [151].

The next option is direct surgical repair within the cavernous sinus [152–155]. Types B, C, and D may resolve spontaneously, so that they are initially managed expectantly with periodic evaluation of visual parameters. If symptoms progress, definitive treatment (embolization or surgical repair) may be necessary.

Tic Douloureux (Trigeminal Neuralgia)

Tic douloureux is a painful condition of the trigeminal nerve. Because tic is a clinical diagnosis, particular attention must be paid to the patient's history.

Clinical Features

The pain of tic affects the face within the trigeminal distribution and is usually unilateral. The second or third divisions of the trigeminal nerve are involved more often than the first. Sometimes two divisions are involved. The right side is more frequently involved than the left. The pain is paroxysmal, very brief (seconds to minutes), and excruciating. It has a lancinating or electrical quality. It may recur many times a day or may disappear for months at a time, only to reappear. With successive cycles, the pain tends to recur more often and become more severe. Attacks are evoked by touching the face, shaving, brushing the teeth, eating, speaking, or a gust of cold wind. The pain is more pronounced during the day. Because the pain is often felt in the region of a tooth, many patients seek dental help. Some even have many teeth pulled (to no avail) and are edentulous (or nearly so) by the time the diagnosis is made. Most patients are female and over 50 years. Typically, there is a paucity of clinical signs, unless there is some other underlying disease such as multiple sclerosis (in 3% of cases) or tumor (5–8% of cases). Occasionally, with idiopathic trigeminal neuralgia, there may be a small area of hypesthesia in the trigeminal distribution.

It is currently accepted that the majority of cases of tic douloureux are due to microvascular compression in the root entry zone where the trigeminal nerve enters the pons. Most often a loop of the superior cerebellar artery is responsible [156].

Diagnosis

As already noted, the diagnosis is made clinically. The main purpose of the workup is to exclude other lesions. A contrast-enhanced CT scan or MRI scan is done to exclude schwannomas, meningiomas, or epidermoid tumors in the cerebellopontine angle. If multiple sclerosis is suspected, evoked potentials, CSF analysis, and MRI are helpful in making the diagnosis.

Treatment

Medical Treatment. Currently carbamazepine is the most effective drug in treatment of tic douloureaux [157]. Approximately 70% of patients will obtain significant relief of pain. The drug is started gradually at a dose of 100 mg/day twice a day and increased by 100 mg every 2 days to a dose of 200 mg three times a day. A small number of patients will get relief at a lower dose; the incremental dose should be stopped when pain is relieved. If necessary, the dose may be increased to 1200 to 1800 mg/day. Patients taking carbamazepine require monitoring of hematologic indexes.

The drug can be a gastric irritant and should be taken with liquid or food. Other drugs effective in the treatment of tic douloureux include phenytoin and baclofen; both are less effective than carbamazepine. Approximately 25 percent of patients will get relief with phenytoin. It may be started at a dose of 100 mg three times daily. A serum level should be determined and the dose adjusted to achieve a therapeutic level. Narcotics should not be used in the long-term management of tic douloureux.

Surgical Treatment. Surgery should be reserved for those patients unresponsive or intolerant to medication. Currently three main options are available: (1) microvascular decompression (MVD), (2) percutaneous retrogasserian radiofrequency thermal rhizotomy, and (3) percutaneous retrogasserian glycerol rhizotomy [158]. Peripheral nerve avulsions, alcohol injections, and subtemporal rhizotomy all have been essentially supplanted by gangliolysis and microvascular decompression as primary surgical procedures; however, there are selected patients for whom these procedures may be indicated.

Percutaneous trigeminal RF lesion rhizotomy is a thermally induced gangliolysis and is therefore an ablative procedure. Because of recent reports of intracranial hemorrhages related to the needle-electrode puncture for the RF lesion or glycerol injection, it is advisable to screen for hemorrhagic diathesis in these patients. Preoperative atropine is given to counteract vasovagal reactions, and an anxiolytic and antiemetic agent are recommended.

Morbidity is low and mortality is essentially zero. One trades a sensory deficit for pain relief. There is a risk of corneal anesthesia and anesthesia dolorosa (denervation hyperpathia). Tic within the first division of the trigeminal nerve is a relative contraindication for the procedure because of a risk of corneal anesthesia and subsequent neuroparalytic keratitis.

Success rates are quite high. The procedure can be repeated as necessary if pain recurs. Hospitalization is brief. It is well suited to elderly patients who are poor operative risks for posterior fossa craniectomy (MVD) and who have had an unsuccessful trial of medical treatment [160–162].

Glycerol is a neurotoxic agent fortuitously discovered to be efficacious in the treatment of tic. This method is very similar to the RF procedure. Because it is reputed to carry less risk of corneal anesthesia or anesthesia dolorosa, it is recommended for those patients with trigger areas in the first division of the trigeminal nerve [163, 164].

Posterior fossa retromastoid craniectomy for microvascular decompression of the trigeminal nerve (MVD or Jannetta procedure) is probably the surgical procedure of choice for typical trigeminal neuralgia in an otherwise young, healthy patient [165]. It is a major intracranial procedure; however, it spares the nerve and avoids dysesthetic sequelae and corneal anesthesia. Preoperative evaluation is as for intracranial surgery.

CNS Tumors

Tumors of the CNS account for 5 percent of all neoplastic disease. Tumors in children are most common in the infratentorial (posterior fossa) compartment, whereas in adults the supratentorial compartment is the common location.

Meningiomas

Meningiomas are the most common primary tumor of nonglial origin arising within the CNS. They account for 15 percent of all primary intracranial tumors. Over 90 percent are benign. They are more common in females and have a peak incidence between the fifth through seventh decades. In children, meningiomas are more common in males and have a predilection for the lateral ventricles. Twenty-five percent of patients with meningioma in childhood have neurofibromatosis [166, 167]. Ninety percent of intracranial meningiomas are supratentorial; the remainder are infratentorial. The intracranial location determines the clinical presentation and the operative approach. Approximately 30 percent arise along the superior sagittal sinus or the falx (parasagittal); 30 percent arise over the convexity; and 30 percent arise from basal regions such as the sphenoid and petrous ridges, the tuberculum sella, and the olfactory groove. Other locations include the cerebellopontine angle and the lateral ventricle. Although there are several histologic subtypes of meningioma (syncytial, fibroblastic, transitional, angioblastic, and sarcomatous), the prognostic significance of tumor histology is controversial. Traditionally, angioblastic meningiomas have been considered the most aggressive variety.

Diagnosis COMPUTED TOMOGRAPHY. On nonenhanced CT, there may be areas of increased density or calcification within an isodense tumor usually adjacent to the duras. The tumor is frequently associated with mass effect or shift. Peritumoral edema is common. With contrast-enhanced CT, there is usually a marked homogeneous enhancement of the tumor. CT bone windows may show reactive hyperostosis [168].

MAGNETIC RESONANCE IMAGING. Meningiomas may have a low or isodense signal intensity on both the T1- and T2-weighted images because of the calcified psammomatous component. The surrounding edema appears as an area of increased signal on the T2-weighted images [169]. Postgadolinium contrast infusion T1-weighted MRI results in marked contrast enhancement of meningiomas [344].

PLAIN SKULL X-RAY FILMS. Skull x-ray films are not required for definitive diagnosis. However, findings on skull x-ray film suggesting meningioma include calcification, enlargement or tortuousity of vascular channels related to a mass lesion, and reactive hyperostosis [170].

ANGIOGRAPHY. Meningiomas usually derive their blood supply from the external carotid artery through the middle meningeal artery and its branches; therefore a selective external carotid arteriogram is frequently combined with internal carotid arteriography. Angiography is helpful for surgical planning by defining vascular supply, determining if important vessels are encased by tumor, and establishing the patency of major dural venous sinuses.

In addition, preoperative embolization (interventional radiology) may reduce tumor vascularity and operative blood loss, thereby facilitating complete removal of the tumor [171].

Surgical Treatment. The treatment of choice is surgical resection; with few exceptions it is the sole treatment. Because most meningiomas are benign, total resection is theoretically curative. However, meningiomas do recur. The most important determinant of recurrence is the completeness of the surgical resection [172, 173].

Radiotherapy is of some benefit in partially resected, recurrent, or malignant meningiomas [174, 175].

Preoperative management follows the guidelines for major intracranial surgery.

Lymphomas

Primary malignant CNS lymphomas account for 1.0 to 1.5 percent of intracranial tumors. They are also known as microglioma or reticulum cell sarcomas. There has been an increased incidence of these lesions with the rising tide of AIDS and iatrogenic immunodeficiency states following organ transplantation. They are usually B-cell lymphomas. They are common between ages 55 to 65. They may be found in the cerebral hemisphere (usually frontal), basal ganglia, or posterior fossa and are not commonly multifocal and ill-defined.

Treatment is surgery and radiotherapy. The prognosis is poor. Secondary lymphomas usually result in a diffuse infiltration of the subarachnoid space (meningeal carcinomatosis). Cranial nerve palsies or communicating hydrocephalus may result.

Chordomas

Two percent of CNS tumors are chordomas. Forty percent are located in the vertebral column (sacrococcygeal, lumbosacral, cervical, or thoracic) or in the skull base (clivus and dorsum sella, occipital bone or orbit).

They are slow growing tumors. They cause local bone destruction and compression of cranial or spinal nerves. Their location often precludes successful surgical extirpation.

Gliomas

Approximately 50 percent of all intracranial neoplasms are gliomas, making them the most common intracranial tumors. Gliomas arise from the glial cells of the CNS. Broadly speaking, they are divided into *astrocytomas, oligodendrogliomas,* and *ependymomas* from astrocytes, oligodendrocytes (which myelinate neurons), and ependymal cells (which line the ventricles) respectively.

In order of progressive malignancy, astrocytomas may be classified as:

Kernohan Classification [176]	*WHO Classification [177]*
Astrocytoma grade 1	Astrocytoma
Astrocytoma grade 2	Anaplastic astrocytoma

Astrocytoma grade 3   Glioblastoma multiforme (GBM)
Astrocytoma grade 4   Glioblastoma multiforme (GBM)

Presently both the four- and three-tiered systems are in use, although consensus favors the latter, since there is skepticism regarding the use of subdividing the GBM [178].

Astrocytoma is the more "benign" end of the spectrum. Most lesions in adults arise in the supratentorial cerebral white matter. In children, the brainstem and cerebellum are common sites. Anaplastic astrocytoma has a peak incidence in slightly older (40–50 years of age) patients than does astrocytoma. GBM is the most common glioma. It has a predilection for men aged 50 to 60 years. The tumor grows rapidly and, left untreated, is almost uniformly fatal. Most patients die within 24 months of diagnosis. Gliomas tend to spread along white matter fiber tracts, are sometimes multiple, and may present in both hemispheres by spreading across the corpus callosum ("butterfuly glioma"). About 1 to 5 percent are multifocal [179], and microscopic remote foci may be found quite often with careful postmortem search.

The tumor margins are notoriously ill-defined, making "total surgical resection" all but impossible. Distant tumor metastasis is rare [180].

Oligodendrogliomas account for about 5 percent of intracerebral gliomas. They occur most frequently in the frontal lobes and often calcify. They are found principally in adults. Approximately 50 percent of oligodendrogliomas are actually mixed tumors, containing elements of astrocytoma and oligodendroglioma. Seziures are the common presentation.

Ependymomas are found throughout the CNS. They arise from cells lining the ventricles and central canal of the spinal cord. They are common in childhood (peak 10–15 years). They are the most common hemispheric glioma of childhood. The fourth ventricle is a common site; here they are often exophytic masses that may obstruct CSF pathways. The spinal lesions, especially those of the filum terminale, are usually seen in adults.

Choroid plexus papillomas are uncommon tumors. They are most often found in the fourth ventricle (adult) or lateral (children) ventricles. For unknown reasons, lateral ventricle papillomas tend to occur on the left side. They may present with hydrocephalus, probably due to overproduction of CSF. They tend to seed the CSF pathways and often recur.

Colloid cysts of the third ventricle are found on the roof of the third ventricle. They frequently obstruct the foramen of Monro and cause hydrocephalus. Their origin may be related to the embryonic paraphysis (a glandular structure derived from a telencephalic pouch). The cysts are unilocular and contain a viscid mucoid substance.

Intermittent positional headaches are a common presenting symptom.

Treatment options include excision, stereotactic aspiration, or ventricular shunting.

Diagnosis CLINICAL FEATURES. Clinical features of gliomas are of two varieties: (1) focal findings dependent on the intracranial site (e.g., hemiparesis or dysphasia, visual defects, and seizures) and (2) nonspecific signs and symptoms from raised ICP and diffuse cerebral dysfunction (e.g., headaches, altered mental status, papilledema, vomiting, and, later, coma). A new onset seizure in a patient over 40 years of age is the signature of a brain tumor until proved otherwise.
COMPUTED TOMOGRAPHY AND MAGNETIC RESONANCE IMAGING. Nonenhanced CT usually demonstrates a poorly defined low-density area with associated mass effect. There may be scattered areas of calcification or hemorrhage. The presence of calcification suggests a slowly growing mass. With contrast-enhanced CT, there is an irregular pattern of enhancement with a hypodense center (necrosis or cyst) and a varying amount of surrounding edema. In general, CT changes roughly correlate with histologic grading. Masses that are sharply marginated, homogenous in intensity, and show little enhancement are more likely to be "benign." On the other hand, poor margination, inhomogeneous dense enhancement, and irregular outline are associated with malignancy. Double-dose contrast-enhanced CT and delayed scanning can be useful when subtle lesions are suspected.

MRI is very sensitive and may demonstrate a low-grade glioma even when the CT is normal or shows only minimal abnormality. T1-weighted sequences show decreased signal intensity or an isointense signal in the region of the tumor; mass effect may be evident. The tumor and surrounding edema show up as areas of increased signal intensity on T2-weighted sequences. Contrast enhancement may be beneficial in segregating tumor from edema. Calcified portions are poorly visualized as areas of low signal intensity.
ANGIOGRAPHY. Angiography is rarely necessary in the diagnosis of gliomas. Malignant gliomas produce a tumor stain and neovascularity. There may be an early draining vein.
Surgical Treatment. Surgery has a central diagnostic and palliative role in the management of gliomas. Preoperative preparation should include steroids continued through the perioperative period to reduce edema. In patients with significant neurologic deficit, there may be profound improvement with preoperative steroids. Anticonvulsants may be given prophylactically if not therapeutically.

Surgical management may be biopsy or resection. Biopsy by *open* or *closed (stereotactic)* methods provides tissue for histodiagnosis.

Since gliomas are generally infiltrating tumors and sometimes multicentric, surgical "resection" is almost never complete. Resection of tumor accomplishes the following goals: (1) adequate sampling of tissue for histodiagnosis, (2) cytoreduction of tumor bulk to increase the success of adjunctive therapy, and (3) immediate relief of raised ICP.

The selection of surgical treatment depends on many factors, including tumor location and surgical risk, the patient's medical condition, neurologic status, and prognosis for useful recovery.

Surgical treatment for most gliomas is only palliative. Radiotherapy is an important part of the treatment for malignant gliomas. Without surgery or radiation, the mean survival for glioblastomas from the time of diagnosis is about 4 months; with surgery alone, it is approximately 6 months; with both surgery and radiation, mean survival is about 12 months.

Patients who are too ill for formal craniotomy and those with lesions in deep locations such as the basal ganglia or brainstem may benefit from stereotactic CT–guided biopsy with or without laser resection and radiotherapy [181, 182].

Late deterioration in patients with gliomas may be due to tumor expansion, radiation-induced encephalopathy and necrosis, intratumoral hemorrhage, or medical complications. Even the most histologically malignant gliomas rarely ever metastasize outside the CNS.

Metastatic Tumors

Parenchymal Metastases

Some 15 to 20 percent of cancer patients develop brain metastases [183], most of which originate, in descending order, from lung, breast, melanoma, colon, kidney, and lymphoma. The route of spread is usually hematogenous; tumor deposits have a predilection for the parenchyma at the grey-white matter junction. In some series, a predominance of the middle cerebral artery, explained on the basis of laminar flow. Carcinoma of the lung accounts for 35 to 40 percent of brain metastases, and squamous cell is the commonest variety. Choriocarcinomas have a peculiar preference for vascular invasion and may produce degeneration of the vessel wall, dilatation, aneurysm formation, and parenchymal or subarachnoid hemorrhage [345]. Melanomas are also associated with a significant risk of hemorrhage.

Clinical features are similar to those of an intracranial mass. The tumor grows rapidly, and neurologic deterioration is frequently as much a result of edema as it is of the lesion per se. Steroids are usually of striking benefit in the treatment of edema.

The typical picture of CT is a round, subcortical mass that even when small is surrounded by a large amount of edema. Most of these tumors are hypodense on nonenhanced CT and the majority show enhancement [184].

Resective surgery is best suited to patients with a single brain metastasis who do not have widespread or rapidly progressive cancer. Biopsy may be preferable for the very ill patient unable to undergo formal craniotomy. For patients with carcinomatous meningitis, it may be useful to place an Ommaya reservoir to deliver intrathecal chemotherapy. This is done through a burr hole [185], usually with the catheter placed in a frontal horn. Radiotherapy is usually required as adjunctive treatment.

Systemic tumors may metastasize to the skull, dura, or leptomeninges (meningeal carcinomatosis). *Meningeal carcinomatosis* occurs frequently with acute leukemias and adenocarcinomas of the gastrointestinal tract. The onset is often insidious, presenting with symptoms of meningeal irritation, cranial nerve lesions, mental changes, diffuse headaches, nausea, and vomiting. The CSF shows increased protein, low glucose, and neoplastic cells.

Skull Metastases

Skull metastases are particularly common in carcinoma of the breast and neuroblastoma. Skull metastases are usually asymptomatic and sometimes require treatment. Occasionally they grow to a large size, invade the epidural space, and compress the brain.

Spinal Metastases

Spinal cord compression by metastases may be a cause of significant morbidity in the patient with cancer. The most frequent primary sites are the breast, lung, prostate, and hematopoietic system, or a direct extension from an adjacent primary. These sources jointly account for about two-thirds of the cases [346]. Epidural metastases are the commonest location. Symptoms include neck, back, or radicular pain and neurologic deficit. Once neurologic symptoms develop, progression is often quite rapid—a patient can go from normal function to complete paraplegia in a matter of hours or days. Success of treatment depends to a great extent on neurologic status at the time of treatment.
Diagnosis. *Plain x-ray* films of the spine may show vertebral collapse, erosion of pedicles, or a paravertebral mass without bony changes. *Myelography* usually demonstrates a partial or complete block to the flow of dye.
Treatment. High-dose steroids, dexamethasone, or an equivalent should be given intravenously. In patients with widespread metastases, radiotherapy and corticosteroids may provide palliative treatment. Surgical decompression may be undertaken in patients with localized disease, uncertain diagnosis, or tumors known to be radioresistant. Surgical treatment includes decompressive laminectomy for lesions located dorsal or lateral to the spinal cord. Ventral lesions may be approached by vertebral body resection with methyl methacrylate-pin stabilization. One advantage of this apporach is that patients resume ambulation early and usually do not require prolonged use of rigid external orthoses [347].

Cerebellopontine Angle Tumors

The commonest tumor (80–90%) arising in the cerebellopontine angle (CPA) is the acoustic neuroma (neurilemoma, neurinoma, schwannoma). Others include meningiomas, cholesteatomas, arachnoid cysts, gliomas, and trigeminal neuromas. Acoustic neuroma is one of the more common intracranial tumors; it constitutes 5 to 10 percent of most large series.

Most patients are between 30 and 60 years of age. In young patients with acoustic neuromas, other evidence of neurofibromatosis (von Recklinghausen's disease) should be sought. Five percent of patients with peripheral neurofibromatosis and 95 percent of patients with central neurofibromatosis will harbor acoustic neuromas.

Bilateral acoustic neuromas are virtually pathognomonic of central neurofibromatosis and frequently coexist with other CNS lesions (e.g., meningiomas, optic gliomas, and neurofibromas). In such patients, deafness is a distinct possibility, so if surgery is contemplated they should be taught to lip-read beforehand. Acoustic neuromas arise from the neurilemmal sheath of the vestibular division of the eighth cranial nerve, usually within the porus acousticus, just distal to the Schwann-glial junction. The tumor expands the porus, initially remains intracanalicular, and later intrudes into the CPA. Early enlargement compresses the cochlear nerve. Unilateral hearing loss and tinnitus are common early symptoms. Difficulty in speech recognition often precedes pure tone deficit, and patients first become aware of their hearing loss while using the telephone. Later, fifth and seventh nerve symptoms such as facial numbness or corneal hypesthesia and facial weakness may be present. Meningiomas, however, are associated with early involvement of the seventh and fifth cranial nerves. Cerebellar signs are a late presentation with acoustic neuromas.

Diagnosis

The diagnosis of acoustic neuromas is currently being made at an early stage, partly because of the sensitivity of radiographic and neurophysiological tests.

Otologic Evaluation. A complete otologic evaluation is necessary. This may include pure-tone audiometry for air and bone conduction, speech reception threshold, speech discrimination, impedance audiometry, and brainstem auditory evoked potentials.

Vestibular Testing. Vestibular testing in the form of caloric stimulation, electronystagmography (ENG), and Bárány chair rotation completes the evaluation.

Computed Tomography. CT has been the mainstay of radiologic diagnosis. Large lesions cause effacement of the cerebellopontine angle cistern and displace the fourth ventricle. The tumor is almost isodense with the parenchyma. Calcification is rare with acoustic neuroma but more common with meningioma. After contrast, most acoustic neuromas enhance and have well-defined margins. Thin sections are necessary to find small tumors. Using bone window technique, widening of the porus acousticus and erosion of the internal auditory canal can be demonstrated. This bony change aids in the differentiation of acoustic neuromas from meningiomas and neurinomas of other nerves in the cerebellopontine angle.

Gas Computed Tomography Cisternography. This is useful for detecting small intracanalicular acoustic tumors that are beyond the resolution of intravenous contrast CT. In a healthy person, gas enters the internal auditory canal and clearly defines the neurovascular bundle. In the patient with a small acoustic neuroma, a filling defect is present [187].

Epidermoid tumors (cholesteatomas) appear as low-density irregularly contoured lesions with little mass effect. The tumor usually does not enhance with contrast. There may be some bony erosion. These tumors are relatively large before they are discovered because of their minimal mass effect [188].

Magnetic Resonance Imaging. Acoustic neuromas are readily visualized on MRI. They are best demonstrated on T1-weighted images in the axial and coronal planes. Effacement of the brainstem by the extracanalicular part of the tumor is seen on the coronal view. The tumors are often of higher intensity than the surrounding brain. The natural contrast of the low-signal intensity of the petrous bone and the high-signal intensity of the CSF on T2-weighted images outlines the internal auditory canal, showing up an intracanalicular tumor.

Angiography. Angiography is rarely necessary for the patient with classic clinical, audiometric, and CT or MRI findings. Typically, acoustic neuromas are hypovascular; they may displace the anterior-inferior cerebellar artery and obliterate the petrosal vein by mass effect [189].

Surgical Treatment

The usual neurosurgical approach to acoustic tumors is suboccipital retromastoid (posterior fossa) craniectomy. Other options include combined posterior and middle fossa and translabyrinthine approaches (suitable for small tumors with minimal intracranial extension). The preoperative evaluation follows the scheme for major intracranial surgery. Preoperative anticonvulsants are not necessary. Steroids may be used if cerebral edema is prominent or cerebellar retraction has been long and difficult. However, in posterior fossa craniectomy, steroids have been associated with poor wound healing and postoperative CSF leaks. For those who prefer the sitting position, the usual intraoperative precautions should be applied.

Hemangioblastoma

Hemangioblastoma of the cerebellum is the commonest primary adult intraaxial posterior fossa tumor. Although the cerebellar hemisphere is the commonest location, lesions may occur in the brainstem and spinal cord. They account for 1.0 to 1.5 percent of all intracranial tumors. Hemangioblastomas are vascular tumors and are usually cystic with a mural nodule; the tumor often grows into and infiltrates the leptomeninges. Multiple lesions are found in 10 percent of patients, especially in association with von Hippel-Lindau disease [191].

Diagnosis

Computed Tomography. The *nonenhanced CT* shows an eccentric mass of isodense solid tumor or a mural nodule with a cyst. There is often surrounding hypodensity representing edema. On *contrast-enhanced CT* there is marked enhancement, often with a central hypodensity representing a cyst [192].

Angiography. Angiography shows a very vascular tumor with large, early-draining veins.

Treatment

Complete removal of the tumor nodule is usually curative. About 25 percent of hemangioblastomas are solid and are particularly difficult to remove if they invade the brainstem or cord. Tumor recurrence may be from residual or undetected lesions and usually carries a higher mortality and morbidity. Patients with evidence of residual tumor postoperatively should receive radiation treatment to the tumor bed. Tumor growth may be monitored by follow-up CT scans [193, 194].

Pineal Region Tumors

Pineal region tumors are a heterogeneous group of lesions originating in and around the pineal gland. Some 10 to 15 percent are benign, while the remainder are malignant. The main types are: (1) germ cell tumors (in descending order of malignancy: germinomas, teratomas, embryonal carcinomas, endodermal sinus tumor, and choriocarcinomas), (2) dermoid and epidermoid cysts, (3) pineal cell tumors (pineocytomas and pineoblastomas), and (4) tumors of the supporting elements (astrocytomas and meningiomas).

Germ Cell Tumors

Germ cell tumors are mostly germinomas (over 60%). Ninety-five percent of intracranial germinomas arise in the midline from the suprasellar cistern to the pineal gland, and a small number involve both sites. The majority of germinomas arise in the suprasellar cistern (57%), while most nongerminomatous germ cell tumors preferentially occur in the pineal gland (68%) [348].

Although the majority of germinomas arise in the suprasellar cistern, germinomas are the most common tumors (over 50%) of the pineal region. The majority of germinomas occur in the second and third decades of life, and mostly in males. They are histologically malignant and infiltrative [195].

Diagnosis

Symptoms arise from compression of (1) CSF pathways (obstructive hydrocephalus), with headaches, altered level of consciousness, and (2) neural structures (superior colliculi and pretectal area) with impairment of upward gaze and convergence, retractory nystagmus, and pupillary abnormalities (Parinaud's syndrome). Hydrocephalus and raised ICP may also present with sixth nerve paresis. Impingement on the rostral midline cerebellum may cause dysmetria, ataxia, and intention tremor.

Parasellar germinomas commonly present with diabetes insipidus, visual field deficits, and hypothalamic-pituitary failure. Cytologic examination of the CSF may show malignant cells and so establish the nature of the lesion. Seeding of the CSF is characteristic of germinomas.

Immunoassay for alpha-fetoprotein (AFP) and the beta subunit of human chorionic gonadotrophin (beta hCG) assists in the diagnosis of germ cell tumors. Forty to fifty percent of germinomas and embryonal cell carcinomas elaborate beta hCG. AFP is secreted by malignant teratomas.

Endocrinologic evaluation may unearth subclinical diabetes insipidus, suggesting anterior extension of tumor.

Neuroophthalmologic evaluation establishes visual defects and serves as a baseline for subsequent evaluations.

On nonenhanced CT, germinomas are well-defined, hypodense masses; on contrast CT the pattern of enhancement is moderate and homogenous.

MRI may effectively rule out aneurysms of the great cerebral vein of Galen.

Treatment

When the patient is symptomatic from hydrocephalus and raised ICP, a ventricular shunt may be placed to relieve symptoms. Biopsy or resection may be performed later. There are several operative approaches to the pineal region. The most common options include the *posterior fossa (supracerebellar-infratentorial)* and the *occipital transtentorial* approaches [196]. Approximately 25 to 30 percent of all tumors are encapsulated; these can be safely removed by microneurosurgical techniques. The more malignant tumors are treated on the basis of histologic type [197].

Germinomas are very radiosensitive [198]; surgical biopsy is therefore followed by 4000 rad to the whole brain and a 1000-rad boost to the tumor bed; some neurosurgeons advocate surgical debulking before radiotherapy [199].

Chemotherapy works well for highly malignant germ cell tumors such as choriocarcinomas, yolk sac tumors, and also embryonal carcinomas.

Hydrocephalus and Cerebrospinal Fluid Diversion Procedures

Hydrocephalus is an abnormal, usually progressive accumulation of CSF within the ventricular system that distends the ventricles and often raises ICP. In children hydrocephalus is often due to congenital lesions or posterior fossa tumors. There is progressive enlargement of the head, papilledema, and a bulging, tense, enlarged fontanele.

Etiology

Congenital hydrocephalus may be due to malformations (forking or atresia) of the aqueduct of Sylvius or atresia of the foramina of Magendie and Luschka. Hydrocephalus is associated with myelomeningocele, and the Arnold-Chiari malformation. CT scan or cranial ultrasound (in infants with patent anterior fontanelles) is the initial investigation and shows enlargement of all or some ventricular spaces. From this, one may be able to establish the most likely site of obstruction.

Treatment

The classic treatment is CSF diversion (shunt) from the ventricle into the peritoneal cavity (VP shunt) or right atrium (VA shunt). Shunts are made from Silastic tubes and their connections, collectively referred to as shunt hardware. Infection and malfunction are the most frequent complications. As the child grows, the tubes may become disconnected or pull out of their intended cavity, requiring a revision procedure.

A variety of shunt systems are available (Fig. 5-1). Generally, each set is composed of three basic parts: (1) proximal or ventricular catheter, (2) valve, and (3) distal catheter. Ancillary devices may be inserted in line with this basic system to augment shunt function. They include reservoirs, on-off devices, filters, and antisiphon devices [200].

Ventricular Catheter. This is the proximal end of the system. It is introduced into the ventricule through a burr hole. Almost all are made of Silastic and are made radiopaque by barium impregnation. They may have tantalum markings along their length and at the tip. A number of tip designs are available.

Valve. Flow is unidirectional (away from the ventricle) with these differential pressure valves; i.e., the valve opens and closes whenever its hydrostatic opening or closing pressure is reached. Variations in design allow for different pressure and flow characteristics. Some examples include the Pudenz-Schulte, Holter, Hakim, and Denver valves (Fig. 5-1). Valves are described in terms of their closing pressures, except for the Denver shunt, which varies according to its flow rate. Closing pressure figures vary with each valve manufacturer. Typical values are 90 to 140 mm of water (high), to 50 to 90 mm of water (medium), and 20 to 50 mm of water (low).

Distal (Drainage) Catheter. This enters the cavity to which CSF is being shunted, usually the peritoneal cavity or the right atrium. The distal catheter is also made of Silastic. The ends may be open or have a slit valve. One design has a spring-embedded tubing to reduce the likelihood of kinking.

Reservoir (Antechamber). This is usually attached to the ventricular catheter, as with the Rickham reservoir, or it may be inserted more distally in the system. Reservoirs can be accessed by needle puncture to withdraw CSF or to instill antibiotics or chemotherapeutic agents (see the section on shunt tap).

On-Off Device (Percutaneously Reversible Occlusion Valve). As the name suggests, the on-off device allows the shunt system to be activated or deactivated to provide intermittent shunting. The switch is a button that is depressed percutaneously.

Antisiphon Device. The antisiphon device is designed to stop the flow of CSF when there is negative pressure in the ventricle compared with the shunting cavity. It is usually positioned just distal to the valve. It is meant to prevent problems of overshunting (e.g., low pressure headaches, subdural hematomas, shunt craniosynostosis, and slit-ventricles) [201–203]. Overdrainage is liable to occur in the upright position since the pressure in the ventricle can become subatmospheric in the upright position [204].

Filter. Filters are incorporated in line with the shunt system to prevent tumor cells from spreading through CSF from the ventricular system to distant sites. They may be useful when shunting is performed to relieve hydrocephalus secondary to tumor but have the distressing tendency to become obstructed and cause shunt malfunction.

Prophylactic Antibiotics. Since intraoperative inoculation of the shunt is the commonest mode of shunt infection, many pediatric neurosurgeons use perioperative prophylaxis.

Shunt Infections

Shunt infections are not uncommon in infants. The incidence varies among reported series [205–207]. Most shunt infections become apparent within 6 months of the operative procedure. The most common causative organism is *Staphylococcus epidermidis. Streptococcus viridans, Staphylococcus aureus,* and diphtheroids are responsible for most of the remainder. In newborns, genera of the enterobacteriaceae family and the enterococci are common etiologic agents. *S. epidermidis* infection is insidious; *S. aureus* tends to be more fulminant. Since most infections occur soon after surgery and are caused by organisms that reside on the skin, contamination of the prosthesis at surgery is the likely source [208].

A number of technical factors seem to influence the rate of infection:

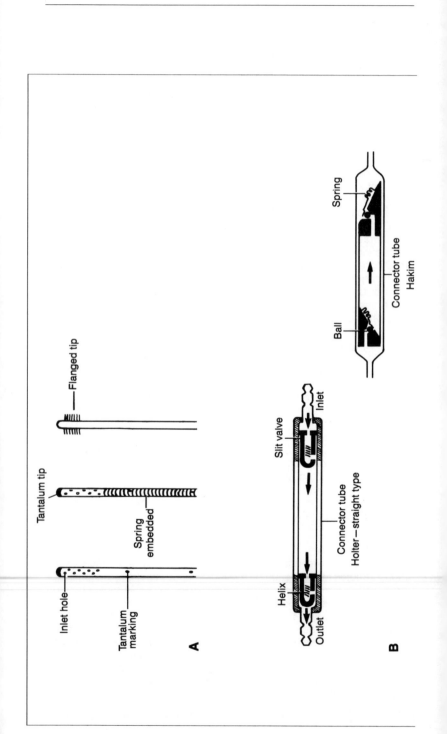

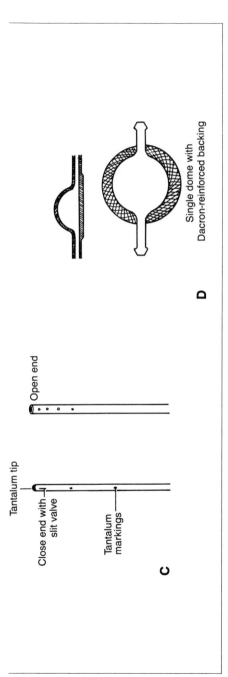

Fig. 5-1. Shunt hardware. A. Proximal catheter B. Valves. C. Distal catheter. D. Reservoir.

skin preparation, experience of the surgeon, and duration of the procedure. The presence of shunt components appears to impair host defenses and to enhance microbial survival.

Diagnosis. Clinical features include fever, irritability, altered level of consciousness, nausea, vomiting or a failure to thrive. Nuchal rigidity is not common in these patients. In children, these symptoms may be difficult to differentiate from gastrointestinal disturbance, urinary tract infection, or otitis media. If an identifiable source of infection is not apparent, CSF should be obtained for culture. Shunt infection may lead to shunt malfunction. Ventriculoatrial shunt infection may be complicated by an immune-complex nephritis with fever, hematuria, and proteinuria. Pulmonary hypertension and cor pulmonale have also been described with VA shunt infections.

Because of the more serious sequelae of shunt infection in VA over VP shunts and the greater ease of placement of VP shunts, the peritoneal cavity is the more favored shunt cavity.

Treatment. The usual approach to management of shunt infection is removal of the infected hardware. A number of algorithms employ varying degrees of antibiotic therapy and removal of shunt hardware [209, 210]. Some advocate aggressive medical management of shunt infections without removal of shunt components [211]. A major problem in treating shunt infection is the need for continuing ventricular drainage in most patients during and after eradication of the infection.

One approach for the treatment of shunt infection is as follows: immediate removal of the infected shunt, insertion of external ventricular drainage (EVD), administration of intravenous antibiotics, monitoring of CSF cultures, and replacement of the shunt when the CSF is sterile.

External Ventricular Drainage (EVD)

EVD was initially described by Wernicke in 1881 for treatment of hydrocephalus [349].

Indications include the following:

1. Infected shunt-dependent hydrocephalus. EVD removes infected fluid, allowing CSF turnover, and provides ICP control while awaiting sterilization of CSF. Intrathecal antibiotics can also be delivered [212–214].
2. Posthemorrhagic hydrocephalus in premature infants [215].
3. When definitive shunt operation must be delayed for medical or other reasons in a patient with symptomatic hydrocephalus [216].
4. Myelodysplasia. For temporary control of hydrocephalus in the presence of an open myelomeningocele [217].

The procedure is the same as for ventriculostomy (see Chap. 2). When inserted for CSF shunt infection, EVD is maintained until the infection has cleared, usually after three consecutive sterile CSF cultures have been obtained.

Evaluation of Shunt Function

Several methods have been proposed to evaluate the functional status of shunts, including digital compression, radionuclide or contrast media as tracers, thermosensitive techniques, and ultrasonic Doppler probes. One disadvantage of most of these techniques is the need for equipment that may not be available in the emergency or ambulatory setting where these problems are initially evaluated. Shunt chamber palpation is a simple method of evaluating shunt function. The pumping chamber is compressed; normally, it should readily return to its original shape. If it compresses and does not refill, proximal catheter occlusion is likely. When there is undue resistance to compression, there may be obstruction at the valve or distal catheter. The test is by no means infallible and false-positive results are just as likely as false-negative ones [218]. Demonstrating flow through the tube with an ultrasonic flow probe is 90 percent accurate, with 5 percent false-positive and 5 percent false-negative results [219]. A manometric method using valve or reservoir puncture is less accurate (75%).

The definitive method of evaluating the shunt system is intraoperative examination.

Shunt Taps

Proximal and distal flow can be evaluated by tapping the shunt reservoir (Fig. 5-2). The procedure is as follows:

1. If the type of hardware is unknown, it is best to obtain "shunt series" x-ray films. This includes anteroposterior and lateral views of the skull and anteroposterior and lateral views of the neck, chest, and abdomen. Type of hardware, disconnections, and tube migrations can be seen.
2. The patient should be recumbent.
3. Shave a circular area around the reservoir.
4. Prepare the skin with 70% alcohol or providone-iodine solution. Sterile technique is essential to prevent shunt infection. The region of interest is covered with a Steridrape.
5. Select a point on the dome of the reservoir and introduce a 23-gauge or 25-gauge butterfly needle percutaneously.
6. Open the hub of the tubing and watch for egress of CSF. Failure to obtain CSF may indicate ventricular catheter obstruction or low CSF pressure.
7. If fluid is obtained, manometric studies to determine ventricular pressure, valve competence, and distal runoff can be performed. Attach a manometer filled with sterile 0.9% NaCl or water to the hub of the tubing. The patency of the distal component can be evaluated by watching the fluid column descend in the manometer. A rapid descent to the closing pressure of the valve suggests patency of the valve and distal catheter. If there is no drop of fluid, depress the pumping chamber of the valve a few times.

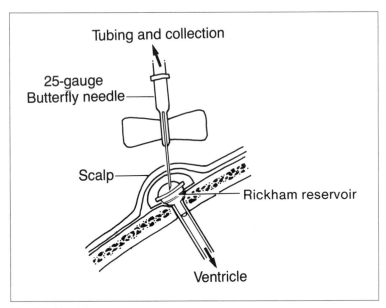

Fig. 5-2. Shunt tap.

If the column falls only with pumping, presume failure of absorption or pseudocyst. If the column fails to drop even with pumping, then the valve is probably obstructed.

8. If finger pressure does not cause flow to resume, inject small amounts of sterile 0.9% NaCl (1–2 ml) in a tuberculin syringe into the reservoir while applying digital finger pressure to the tubing just distal to it. This tends to force fluid through the ventricular catheter and may dislodge small amounts of debris or choroid plexus. If this does cause flow to resume, it is dangerous to inject larger volumes or employ higher injection pressure to attempt dislodgment [350] (Fig. 5-2).

Subdural Collections of Infancy

Subdural collections may be arbitrarily classified as acute, subacute, or chronic depending on the stage of evolution and CT appearance.

Clinical Assessment

Once considered idiopathic and probably related to nutrition or the dehydration attendant upon gastroenteritis, subdural collections must be considered a sign of child abuse until proved otherwise. Other conditions such as recently shunted-hydrocephalus, blood dyscrasias, and

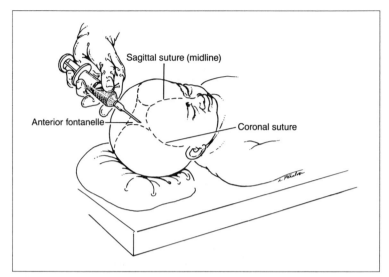

Fig. 5-3. Sudural tap in an infant.

hemophilus meningitis may be the cause. With chronic effusions, the child may fail to thrive and have progressive increase in head size or tense fontanelle, irritability, or seizures. In acute subdural hemorrhages, retinal hemorrhages and symptoms of raised ICP are likely. A search for other injuries is mandatory and the child should be referred to the child-abuse team. Head circumference should be followed. Serial hemoglobin and hematocrit determinations are necessary because subdural bleeding may be enough to render the child anemic.

Subdural Tap

Indication. The usual indication for subdural tap is treatment of subdural collections. Fig. 5-3 shows a subdural tap. A hypnotic such as chloral hydrate or a procedural cocktail should be given to ensure cooperation.

Positioning and Landmarks. The infant is positioned supine, brow-up with the arms restrained. Palpate the anterior fontanelle and its lateral corner (entry point), which is at the level of the coronal suture.

Procedure. The step-by-step procedure is as follows:

1. Shave the scalp to expose fully the anterior fontanelle.
2. Prepare the scalp with 70% alcohol or povidone-iodine solution; drape with sterile towels.
3. Introduce a 23-gauge or 25-gauge butterfly needle through the anterior fontanelle at its lateral corner where it meets the coronal suture.
4, Enter in a zigzag trajectory to prevent a tract that may later leak fluid.

First puncture the skin and then move the skin with the needle in place. Next, penetrate the pericranium perpendicularly in a sagittal plane. Advance deliberately until the dura is traversed. A characteristic "give" is felt as this occurs.

5. Watch for egress of fluid while steadying the needle in position to prevent dislodgment. The ICP may be measured by manometer.
6. Collect fluid for analysis (sugar, protein, cells, gram's stain, and culture). Allow the collection to drain spontaneously; do not aspirate.
7. To facilitate drainage, it may be necessary to rotate the head to promote displacement of fluid toward the puncture site. Continue until dry.
8. If there is a contralateral collection, the tap may be repeated in the contralateral corner at the same sitting.
9. Lightly touch puncture sites with a collodion-impregnated cotton tip. Apply a Band-Aid.

Interpretations/Results. Because the subdural space is only a potential space, in the absence of a pathologic condition only a few drops of serous fluid are obtainable. More than 3 or 4 ml should make one suspect a collection or penetration beyond the subdural space. The collection usually reaccumulates, and it may be necessary to repeat the tap a few times. In time the volume and the protein content gradually decrease, and taps usually can be discontinued in several days. A negative tap should be verified by CT scan to confirm resolution of the collection. If the collection persists after this regimen, a subdural-peritoneal shunt may be needed.

Complications. Complications of a subdural tap include bleeding from improper needle insertion, cortical injury, and infection. These risks are minimal in experienced hands.

Brain Tumors in Children

Posterior Fossa

Certain tumors of childhood have a penchant for the posterior fossa. They include medulloblastoma, astrocytoma, ependymoma, and brainstem glioma. With exception of the brainstem glioma, their clinical presentations are similar. Head tilt and neck stiffness are common, but often ignored, early warning signs.

Elevated ICP may be from peritumoral edema or obstructive hydrocephalus. Peritumoral edema responds well to steroid therapy, which should be continued postoperatively, and then gradually tapered as clinical conditions allow. There is controversy as to whether or not a CSF shunting procedure for hydrocephalus should be performed before definitive removal of the tumor [220]. Generally, if the child is sick from hydrocephalus, it is wiser to shunt first.

Medulloblastomas. Medulloblastomas are *midline (cerebellar vermis)* posterior fossa masses. They are more common in males than females and have a high incidence in the first decade of life. They are the most common pediatric midline tumor.

The cell of origin continues to be a matter of controversy [351]. Medulloblastomas are malignant tumors and readily seed the CSF pathways.

CLINICAL FEATURES. Clinical features include headache, vomiting, papilledema, ataxia, frequent falls, and clumsiness.

DIAGNOSIS. On nonenhanced CT, the lesion is hyperdense or isodense, usually partially intraventricular, and surrounded by edema. Obstructive hydrocephalus is usually evident, and the fourth ventricle is enlarged or obliterated by tumor. Contrast-enhanced CT shows an irregular pattern of enhancement [221].

MRI shows low signal intensity on T1-weighted images and high signal intensity on T2-weighted images. Myelography is being supplanted by MRI of the spine for demonstrating spinal metastases [352]. Cytologic examination reveals abnormal cells in about 50 percent of patients, and elevated polyamines in the CSF may predict recurrence [353].

TREATMENT. The goal of surgery is gross total removal of tumor. The usual approach is a posterior fossa craniectomy. There is improved 5-year survival in patients undergoing radical resection (40–60%) versus those having subtotal resections (30%) [222, 223]. If the child is symptomatic from hydrocephalus, there is usually a good response to the insertion of a ventricular shunt. CSF shunting decompresses the posterior fossa and facilitates subsequent craniectomy and tumor resection.

Ventricular shunting has been implicated in tumor spread along and beyond the neuraxis; therefore some surgeons advocate the use of millipore-type filters in line with the shunt hardware. This may lead to shunt malfunction as the filter becomes obstructed by tumor cells [226].

Medulloblastomas are radiosensitive; therefore, postoperative radiotherapy is generally given. Because of the concern for intellectual and growth impairment in young children, the radiation dose is limited in this group of patients to 2500 rad following gross total tumor removal. Some protocols forego radiation until about age $3\frac{1}{2}$, using chemotherapy instead.

Children aged less than 2 years do particularly poorly, partly because their disease tends to be more widespread at the time of diagnosis, and partly because radiation adequate to control the tumor carries a high risk of damage to the developing brain [354].

In adults and older children, approximately 3500 rad is given to the spinal cord, 4000 rad to the brain, and 1500 rad boost to the posterior fossa (tumor bed) [224, 225].

Medulloblastomas tend to recur in the posterior fossa and often metastasize via the CSF pathways to the spinal cord and roots. With optimal treatment, the 5-year survival rate is approximately 40 to 50 percent, and the 10-year survival is about 30 percent. The role of adjuvant chemotherapy remains controversial. Follow-up CT or MRI studies at regular intervals are helpful for monitoring recurrence of tumor.

Cerebellar Astrocytoma. Cerebellar astrocytomas constitute 10 to 20 percent of childhood brain tumors. They have a peak incidence about the middle of the first decade and are infrequent in adults. Astrocytomas are usually low-grade neoplasms.

CLINICAL FEATURES. Most children present with symptoms of raised ICP, with morning headaches and vomiting. There may be a history of "clumsiness," representing cerebellar dysfunction. Examination may reveal diplopia, papilledema, head tilt, dysmetria, and abnormal gait.

DIAGNOSIS. These tumors may be solid or cystic and associated with a mural nodule. On CT the solid tumor is usually of mixed density and may show areas of calcification. Midline lesions are predominantly solid, and lateral lesions are predominantly cystic. There may be tumor extension into the cerebellar peduncles. On contrast-enhanced CT, solid lesions show diffuse, focal, or ringlike enhancement. Cystic tumors show enhancement of the cyst wall or of a mural nodule [228].

TREATMENT. Posterior fossa craniectomy and resection, as near total as feasible, is the optimal surgical treatment. With solid tumors and brainstem extension it may be difficult, if not impossible, to achieve total resection. In patients with cystic astrocytomas, removal of the mural nodule alone may be sufficient for cure, and removal of the cyst wall is usually not necessary. The prognosis of children with cerebellar astrocytoma is generally good. There is a 5-year survival rate of about 85 percent with adequate surgical treatment [229]. Some subtypes carry an even more favorable prognosis—a 10-year survival rate of up to 94 percent [230]. Follow-up CT or MRI studies may detect asymptomatic recurrence. Postoperative radiation therapy is reserved for patients with histologically malignant lesions or for lesions in inaccessible sites (e.g., brainstem).

Ependymomas Ependymomas constitute about 5 percent of gliomas. Ependymomas may arise from any ependymal surface, but the commonest location is within the fourth ventricle, especially in patients under 10 years of age. Fourth-ventricle ependymomas account for approximately 10 percent of pediatric posterior fossa tumors. They are less common than either medulloblastomas or astrocytomas. Posterior fossa ependymomas grow from the floor of the fourth ventricle and extend into the cerebellum. Paraventricular tumors may spread by CSF pathways. Another common site of origin is the central canal of the spinal cord.

CLINICAL PRESENTATION. Clinical presentation is similar to that of the other posterior fossa tumors; it may include symptoms and signs of increased ICP from hydrocephalus (e.g., nausea, vomiting, papilledema, and lethargy). There may also be features from local compression (e.g., gait ataxia, nystagmus, and cranial nerve palsies). Children are usually younger than 5 years of age.

DIAGNOSIS. On nonenhanced CT, ependymomas are of variable density. Generally, hydrocephalus is present to some degree, and calcification is not unusual. Small internal lucencies, cysts, or necrosis are common. On contrast-enhanced CT there is solid or ring enhancement.

MRI demonstrates an intraventricular mass on T1-weighted images, and the tumor has a high signal intensity on the T2-weighted image.

TREATMENT. Although they usually arise in the fourth ventricle, ependymomas may extend into the brainstem, cerebellar hemispheres, cerebellopontine angle, or protude into the upper cervical canal, requiring an upper cervical laminectomy in addition to a posterior fossa craniectomy. These lesions all too often are intimately adherent to the floor of the fourth ventricle, and complete removal may not be possible. Ependymomas are quite radiosensitive.

Postoperative adjunctive radiotherapy is useful when surgical excision is incomplete or tumor recurs. Radiation dosage is usually 4500 rads of whole brain radiation delivered over 5 to 6 weeks, followed by a boost to 5000 rads in the area of tumor involvement. In children under 3 years of age, this dose is reduced proportionately. Subarachnoid metastases occur in 5 to 10 percent of patients; this is associated with a poorer prognosis and may be detected by examining the CSF for malignant cells. The 5-year survival rate with posterior fossa ependymomas is about 20 to 30 percent with surgery and postoperative radiotherapy [232, 375]. Follow-up CT or MRI studies at regular intervals following resection are useful for detecting asymptomatic recurrences [233].

Spinal cord ependymomas comprise 40 to 70 percent of intramedullary, intraspinal tumors; they are uncommon in children under 5 years of age, but frequent in adults between 35 and 45 years of age. The myxopapillary cauda equina ependymoma is a common variety of spinal ependymoma.

Presenting features include weakness and dysesthesias, bladder and bowel dysfunction, and pain (low back or radicular). MRI is the imaging modality of choice. Treatment is surgical excision; radiotherapy may be required when resection is incomplete or tumor recurs.

Brainstem Gliomas Brainstem gliomas represent 10 to 20 percent of all primary brain tumors in children, with a peak incidence between 5 to 8 years of age. These tumors usually involve the pons or midbrain. The majority are astrocytomas with varying degrees of anaplasia. They may have an exophytic component that intrudes into the cerebellum or the cerebellopontine angle.

CLINICAL FEATURES. Multiple (often bilateral) cranial nerve involvement and long tract signs are common features. Obstructive hydrocephalus may occur but is usually late. Astrocytomas of the mesencephalon, especially the tectal plate, may cause early hydrocephalus from aqueductal compression.

DIAGNOSIS. MRI has become the imaging modality of choice for brainstem gliomas; it shows a smoothly contoured swelling of the pons (less commonly of the midbrain and medulla with areas of hypointense signal on T1-weighted images). There may be cystic components; T2-weighted images usually demonstrate areas of increased signal intensity. These lesions are more difficult to diagnose on CT because of surrounding bone artifact. On CT scan, there may be an isodense enlargement of the pons with irregular enhancement.

Glucocorticoid therapy often provides temporary symptomatic relief and may transiently reverse neurological dysfunction.

SURGICAL TREATMENT. Options include stereotactic biopsy for diagnosis or aspiration of an associated cyst. Subtotal excision of some exophytic lesions extending into the fourth ventricle may be undertaken. CSF shunting is usually necessary when patients present with hydrocephalus.

RADIATION THERAPY. In conventional or hyperfractionated regimens, radiation therapy has resulted in a slight increase in survival. However, the outlook is grim even with optimal treatment; 5-year survival rates in most series is about 30 percent [355, 356].

Suprasellar Tumors

The suprasellar area is another common location for pediatric brain tumors. The region includes the optic apparatus, pituitary-hypothalamic axis, and the anterior portion of the third ventricle.

As a group, these lesions produce visual symptoms (visual acuity or field deficits), hydrocephalus from obstruction of the foramina of Monro, endocrinopathies, and cranial nerve palsies. Common tumors encountered here are *craniopharyngiomas, optic pathway gliomas, and suprasellar germinomas.*

Craniopharyngiomas. Craniopharyngiomas are common in the first and second decades of life and account for 5 to 9 percent of childhood brain tumors. The craniopharyngioma is the most common supratentorial tumor of primary nonglial origin in childhood. A second peak incidence is seen in the fourth and fifth decades of life. Although the origin of these tumors is somewhat controversial, many accept that they originate from the remnants of Rathke's pouch, an ectodermal outgrowth from the roof of the primitive oral cavity that joins with a caudal outpouching from the floor of the third ventricle to form the hypophysis.

Craniopharyngiomas are predominantly suprasellar and occasionally intrasellar. In children, about 70 percent of craniopharyngiomas are calcified, whereas only 30 percent of the adult tumors demonstrate this feature. The tumor is cystic in approximately 55 percent of cases and is mixed or predominantly solid in 45 percent of cases. The cyst usually contains "motor oil or crankcase dirty yellow-green fluid" with cholesterol crystals.

CLINICAL PRESENTATION. In children, clinical presentation is usually from symptoms of increased intracranial pressure and, secondly, compression of the visual pathways. Endocrine and hypothalamic disturbances such as retarded growth, hypopituitarism, and temperature lability are also encountered. In adults visual symptoms are the commonest presenting feature.

DIAGNOSIS. Preoperative evaluation should include an endocrine panel. CT features suggestive of craniopharyngioma include calcification, cystic hypodense areas, and variable degree of contrast enhancement in the solid areas of the tumor. On MRI, signal intensity may be variable on T1-weighted images; on T2-weighted images, marked increased signal intensity is common. Sagittal and coronal images are helpful in surgical planning by delineating the extent of the lesion and its relationship to surrounding structures.

TREATMENT. Craniopharyngiomas grow aggressively, often invading brain tissue. They are adjacent to arterial, visual, and hypothalamic structures in the suprasellar area and often adhere to them, making surgical extirpation difficult.

Cyst drainage alone is palliative, but invariably the cyst recurs. If the patient is very ill from acute hydrocephalus, a CSF shunting procedure is the initial priority.

The lesion may be removed by craniotomy through the subfrontal, pterional, or transcallosal approaches. During surgery, spillage of cyst contents should be prevented since the fluid is very irritating and may cause a chemical meningitis. Dense adhesions and tumor extension may limit tumor resection. Diabetes insipidus is often encountered in the postoperative period. Radiotherapy is a useful adjunct to surgery, especially since tumor recurrence following apparent gross total removal is not uncommon.

Optic Nerve Glioma. The majority (75%) of optic nerve gliomas occur within the first decade of life. The sex incidence is approximately equal. An association of optic nerve glioma with neurofibromatosis has long been recognized, and at least 25 percent of patients will have neurofibromatosis. The tumor may spread contiguously along the optic nerve posteriorly to the chiasm or arise multicentrically ("skip lesions").

CLINICAL PRESENTATION. Gliomas arising in the orbital portion of an optic nerve present with proptosis, visual loss, gliosis of the optic nerve head, and enlargement of the optic canal. Tumors that originate in the chiasm produce visual field deficit (usually central scotomata) without proptosis; larger tumors in this region may cause hypothalamic or pituitary dysfunction and hydrocephalus.

DIAGNOSIS. CT and MRI show enlargement, irregularity, and nodularity of the optic nerve that enhances with contrast. The MRI signal may be isointense on T1-weighted images and isointense or hyperintense on T2-weighted images. These tumors are low-grade astrocytomas.

There is controversy regarding the biologic behavior and proper management of these lesions. In fact, they were long considered to be hamartomas, but they have an unpredictable course.

TREATMENT. Surgical treatment depends on the clinical presentation. Lesions with proptosis and visual impairment may be approached by combined transcranial and orbital exploration and resection. Chiasmal gliomas may be treated by a combination of surgical debulking and radiotherapy or chemotherapy. However, tumors that obstruct the foramen of Monro and cause hydrocephalus usually require CSF shunting before radiotherapy.

Germinomas. See the section on pineal region tumors.

Craniosynostosis

Craniosynostosis is the premature closure of one or more cranial sutures. Primary craniosynostosis is an intrinsic abnormality of the developing skull; secondary craniosynostosis may be due to inadequate growth of the underlying brain (microcephaly) or overshunting. Here we are concerned with the primary variety.

Enlargement of the infantile cranium is due to the growth of the enclosed brain. Premature closure of a suture restricts growth perpendicular to the fused suture but allows growth in other directions, resulting in characteristic skull configurations. Craniosynostosis encompasses a broad range of syndromes, from a single suture to the complex craniofacial dysostoses.

Clinical problems associated with craniosynostosis include cerebral compression and raised ICP with multiple suture involvement, other congenital malformations (e.g., syndactylism, cleft lip and palate, facial hypoplasia, hydrocephalus, and spina bifida), and esthetic displeasure. In general, when there is single suture involvement, the problem is mainly cosmetic; with the involvement of two or more sutures, the problems of brain growth and raised ICP become more pressing [234, 358].

Types

Sagittal Synostosis. Sagittal synostosis is the commonest type of primary craniosynostosis; 80 percent of cases are males. The deformity is distinctive; there is skull lengthening in an occipitofrontal direction, resulting in a long, narrow head (*dolicocephaly*). *Scaphocephaly* is a form of dolicocephaly with bulging of the bregma. The sagittal suture can be palpated as a hyperostotic ridge, much like the keel of a boat. It is rarely associated with other anomalies.

Coronal Synostosis. Coronal synostosis occurs preferentially in females (60 percent). Associated congenital malformations (facial dysostosis, myelomeningocele, congenital heart disease) are present in one-third of those with unilateral and two-thirds of those with bilateral suture involvement. The skull tends to expand superiorly and laterally (*brachycephaly*). The orbits are apt to be shallow and hyperteloric with variable proptosis. If the defect is unilateral, the cranial deformity is asymmetric; the ipsilateral anterior fossa is foreshortened and the orbit is retracted upwards and laterally, with flattening of the anterolateral surface of the skull (*anterior or frontal plagiocephaly*).

Metopic Synostosis. Metopic synostosis may result in a prominent triangulation of the forehead (*trigonocephaly*) and hypotelorism. There is a strong male predominance. There are two forms of trigonocephaly. The first is the more common and has few abnormalities except for the abnormal shape of the forehead and orbits. The second type is associated with holoprosencephaly.

Multiple Suture Synostosis. Multiple suture synostosis may occur in various combinations. The skull tends to expand toward the vertex, resulting in a pointed, turret-shaped head (*oxycephaly*). There is usually raised ICP, hypotelorism, shallow orbits, exophthalmos, and choanal atresia.

Lambdoidal Synostosis. Lambdoidal synostosis is less common. It produces flattening of the back of the head (*plagiocephaly*) with the ear on the ipsilateral side being displaced superiorly and anteriorly. Lambdoidal synostosis must be differentiated from positional moulding that results in occipital flattening.

Diagnosis

The clinical diagnosis of craniosynostosis is confirmed by plain skull x-ray films. Sutures are not visible and there is parasutural sclerosis.

Radioisotope bone scanning with technetium (^{99M}Tc) may be required if plain skull x-ray findings are equivocal. An area of hyperactivity indicates a closing suture; when the suture is completely closed no isotope is picked up.

CT scan or MRI should be obtained to rule out associated intracranial malformations in clinically suspected cases. Further evidence of suture closure may also be gleaned from the CT scan [359].

Treatment

Indications for surgery include correction of deformity and relief or prevention of intracranial hypertension.

Patients with stenosis of two or more sutures should be operated on as soon as possible after birth. Operations for single suture stenosis are done electively but generally after 6 weeks. It is inadvisable to delay surgery since the rapid growth of the brain in the first 6 to 12 months of life is the major determinant of skull remodeling following corrective surgery.

Operative treatments vary—they may be suture removal (strip craniectomy) or a more involved bone resection and craniofacial reconstruction. The bony margins may be lined with a Silastic film to retard fusion; the same delay can be achieved by a wider craniectomy. In coronal synostosis, craniotomy and removal of the suture(s) may be combined with unilateral or bilateral canthal advancement. Blood loss is of major concern during these procedures, and availability of banked blood should be ensured preoperatively. Cosmetic improvement is soon apparent. Although there is usually significant postoperative soft tissue swelling, it recedes quickly [360, 361, 362].

The Dysraphic States

Types

Spina Bifida. Spina bifida is an incomplete fusion of one or more laminae of the vertebral column. The spinal cord or its membranes may protrude through the defect (spina bifida aperta).
Spina Bifida Occulta. Spina bifida occulta differs from the above in that no intraspinal contents extrude. The anomaly per se is usually asymptomatic but may be accompanied by a cutaneous lesion (dimple, angiomas, sinus, hypertrichosis or subcutaneous lipomas) or may be the signature of a sublime dysraphism.
Dermal Sinus. Dermal sinus is epithelial-lined tract that extends from the skin with variable penetration into the deeper structures and spinal canal. Externally, there is a pinpoint ostium that is usually tethered to the underlying tissue. Infection of the sinus may lead to meningitis or deep abscess [235]. In uncomplicated cases, the treatment is removal of the sinus tract.
Lumbosacral Lipoma. Lumbosacral lipoma may be a pure subcutaneous lipoma or one that infiltrates into the cord with tethering adhesions (lipomeningocele or lipomyelomeningocele) [363].
Meningocele. Meningocele is the condition of herniation of dura mater and arachnoid through a spinal defect without neural elements. It is usually found in the lumbar area; it may be associated with hydrocephalus.
Myelomeningocele. Myelomeningocele is condition in which anomalous neural and glial elements of the nerves and spinal cord and their overlying meninges herniate through a spina bifida. These lesions may occur anywhere along the spinal axis but are more common in the lumbosacral region. Depending on location of the defect and the extent of neural involvement, there may be varying degrees of paralysis, sensory loss, and sphincter disturbances. Other CNS lesions (hydrocephalus, Chiari II malformation) and genitourinary and skeletal malformations are frequently associated with these lesions. There is a higher incidence among females, and there are marked geographic and demographic variations. Parents who have a child with a meningomyelocele are at increased risk of having other children born with similar malformations. The risk of recurrence (spina bifida and anencephaly) after one affected offspring is approximately 5 percent [364, 365, 366].
Diastematomyelia (split cord). The spinal cord is divided longitudinally into two portions by a bony, cartilaginous, or fibrous septum arising from the anterior aspect of the spinal canal. The anomaly is common in the lower thoracic and upper lumbar regions. The septum divides the neural canal partially or completely for a distance of one or more segments and transfixes the cord, which is unable to ascend with growth of the vertebral column; traction on the cord may result in pro-

gressive neurologic deficit. There may be hypertrichosis in the midline or a dermal sinus.

Diagnosis may be established by plain x-ray films of the spine, myelography, or MRI.

Tethered Cord. There are two varieties of tethered cord: primary and secondary. *Primary tethering* is associated with an anatomic anomaly (e.g., the tight filum terminale that results from a failure of ascent of the conus with abnormal shortening and thickening of the filum). *Secondary tethering* commonly follows the repair of myelomeningocele; the dorsal aspect of the cord adheres to the overlying dura [367].

Diagnosis

The intrauterine diagnosis of neural tube defects by biochemical (fetal-specific alpha-1-globulin) and radiologic methods is a means of screening potential high-risk pregnancies.

Treatment

A multidisciplinary concept is required for successful management. Neurosurgical treatment aims at coverage of the protruding mass to prevent infection and facilitate nursing care. Neurologic improvement may occur, but is not particularly a function of early closure. The closure of broad-based myelomeningoceles may raise problems of skin coverage, requiring plastic surgery methods. The unoperated sac must be protected from trauma, rupture, and infection by keeping the infant prone, applying topical moist dressing, and preventing soilage with urine or feces.

Orthopedic care is designed to correct deformities and obtain the best possible ambulatory function and posture [236].

Bladder Dysfunction

Some degree of bladder dysfunction is present in most children with myelomeningocele. Urinalysis and radiography of the upper urinary tract may detect infection and changes in urinary tract morphology and function. Control of urinary incontinence is of major concern. There has been more success in managing rectal incontinence, with regular periods of defecation, taking advantage of the gastrocolic reflex. High-fiber diets and enemas are helpful [237].

Chiari Malformations

The Chiari malformations are a series of four types of disordered morphogenesis involving the hindbrain.

Type I. The adult type, it is the mildest form. The cerebellar tonsils are displaced through the foramen magnum into the upper cervical canal.

Associated conditions include hydromyelia (50%), arachnoid adhesions and dural bands, Klippel-Feil syndrome (37%), cervicomedullary kinking, and hydrocephalus (3%).

Type II. Also known as the Arnold-Chiari malformation, it is seen mostly in childhood. In this subtype, there is elongation and caudal displacement of the brainstem and fourth ventricle, herniation of the cerebellar tonsils through the foramen magnum, and enlargement of the foramen magnum. Associated anomalies include beaking of the tectum, kinking of the cervicomedullary junction, upward angulation of the upper cervical roots, myelomeningocele, agenesis of the corpus callosum, dysplasia of the falx with interdigitation of the cerebral hemispheres, and hydromyelia. The cerebellum (superior vermis) towers through an abnormally widened incisura and produces a heart-shaped density on CT scan.

TYPE III. Consists of a high cervical or occipital encephalocele with displacement of the cerebellum, medulla, and fourth ventricle.

Type IV. This form involves extreme cerebellar hypoplasia and caudal displacement of the posterior fossa contents.

Clinical Features

The clinical features are varied and dependent on type and age at presentation. Chiari II malformations in infancy may present with nystagmus, apneic attacks, fixed retrocollis, weak or absent cry, and inspiratory stridor from tenth nerve paresis. Long tract signs (i.e., spasticity, exaggerated reflexes, and hypertonia) may also be noted. When there is coexistent myelodysplasia, the spectrum of associated malformations should also be looked for.

Chiari I malformations may present in adolescence and adulthood with spastic paresis or unsteady gait, nystagmus, a suspended dissociated sensory loss from syringomyelia, and paroxysmal intracranial hypertension (headache related to coughing or neck movements).

Diagnosis

Plain x-ray films of the skull and cervical spine may reveal associated anomalies, (e.g., segmentation errors [Klippel-Feil syndrome], basilar impression, and spina bifida). CT scan demonstrates the spectrum of anomalies, but MRI is superior to other imaging modalities for anomalies of the cervicomedullary junction and posterior fossa. Myelography has less of a role with the expanding use of MRI.

Treatment

Surgical treatment may include (1) shunting for hydrocephalus, (2) suboccipital craniectomy and upper cervical laminectomy for decompression, and (3) shunting of a syrinx.

Dandy-Walker Syndrome

The Dandy-Walker syndrome is a developmental anomaly of the rostral embryonic roof of the rhombencephalon. It consists of a posterior fossa cyst and a varying amount of hypoplasia of the cerebellar vermis and the medial aspects of the cerebellar hemispheres. The posterior fossa is enlarged and the tentorium cerebelli is elevated. There may be hydrocephalus and agenesis of the corpus callosum. In the Dandy-Walker variant, the cyst communicates with the fourth ventricle through the vallecula.

Diagnosis is by CT or MRI. Treatment may be monocompartmental or multicompartmental, shunting for both the cyst and ventricles if they do not communicate.

Carotid Endarterectomy

The goal of carotid endarterectomy (CEA) is the reduction of stroke risk in patients with extracranial carotid atherosclerotic vascular disease. For the procedure to be effective and justifiable, the operative risk should not outweigh the natural history of the disease. The case for CEA is currently the subject of medical investigation [238].

Patients most likely to benefit from CEA are those with carotid transient ischemic attacks (TIAs) in whom severe carotid stenosis or ulceration is demonstrated on angiography [239–241]. Studies of the natural history of untreated TIAs suggest that such patients have an annual risk of stroke of about 10 percent [242, 243]. Similar data on the natural history in patients with asymptomatic carotid disease are less well defined [244–246]. The procedure is also performed in patients who have had a stable nondevastating stroke [247, 248]. CEA for asymptomatic bruit remains controversial.

Noninvasive Studies

Noninvasive tests provide virtually risk-free methods for detecting hemodynamically significant carotid stenosis. Some are direct (examine the carotid bifurcation); others are indirect (measure the distal circulation). No one test is self-sufficient, and a combination of tests is used in evaluating patients.

Direct Noninvasive Studies. CAROTID PHONOANGIOGRAPHY. This can be done if a bruit is present. It estimates residual lumen diameter by frequency analysis of the bruit (*quantitative spectral phonoangiography*). Spectral phonoangiography is particularly useful in the follow-up of asymptomatic carotid bruits [249, 250].

ULTRASOUND IMAGING. There are two types of ultrasound imaging techniques: one uses the Doppler principle, and the other uses B-mode ultrasonography. Both modalities have been combined into a single instrument called a Duplex scanner. Doppler ultrasound arteriography estimates flow velocity by detecting signals reflected from moving red blood cells. Analysis of the flow velocities by audiofrequency or color coding allows identification of regions of high or low velocity, suggesting varying degrees of stenosis [251–253]. Real-time B-mode ultrasonography is used to study the morphology of the arterial wall and estimate the degree of stenosis [254, 255]. By combining B-mode scanning with range-gated Doppler ultrasound, the Doppler sampling volume can be placed at any location within the blood vessel imaged by the B-mode scanner. Duplex scanning has been found to be very sensitive and specific in evaluating carotid occlusive disease [256, 257].

Indirect Noninvasive Studies. Indirect tests are the most commonly used and least expensive tests for noninvasive evaluation of patients with carotid disease. Generally, a hemodynamically significant lesion must exist proximal to the area being evaluated. However, if there is good collateral flow, some of these tests may remain negative in the face of severe occlusive disease. Therefore, they should generally be combined with a direct study.

OPHTHALMODYNAMOMETRY. Ophthalmodynamometry is a measurement of pressure in the retinal artery that reflects ophthalmic artery pressure. Both eyes are compared, and established criteria are used for interpretation [258].

OCULOPLETHYSMOGRAPHY. This technique measures flow and pressure in the ophthalmic artery. In the presence of carotid occlusive disease, there are alterations in distal ophthalmic flow and pressure [259]. Of the currently available indirect tests, oculoplethysmography measuring pressure appears to be the most sensitive and accurate and provides quantitative values.

PERIORBITAL DIRECTIONAL DOPPLER ULTRASONOGRAPHY. This uses the Doppler principle to determine the direction of flow in the periorbital blood vessels. In the presence of hemodynamically significant internal carotid occlusion, the direction of flow is reversed, moving from branches of the external carotid into the supraorbital and frontal arteries (branches of the ophthalmic artery) [260].

Invasive Studies

Carotid angiography remains the benchmark for the evaluation of carotid artery disease. The patient should be well hydrated before the procedure; coagulation indexes as well as BUN and creatinine are needed. Common lesions include atherosclerotic narrowing and subintimal plaque hemorrhage, associated with hemodynamic TIA, and plaque ulceration, associated with embolic TIA. Symptomatic carotid disease is usually located at the origin of the internal carotid artery.

Biophysically, a single carotid stenosis must narrow the artery by 90 percent or more to cause significant reduction of flow. Ulcerated plaques may produce embolic TIAs without carotid narrowing.

Spinal Cord Injuries

Cervical spinal cord injury occurs frequently in young male patients, usually as a result of motor vehicle accidents or water sports. Head injuries are the most common associated injury, followed by chest injury.

Diagnosis

The extent of spinal cord injury is determined by neurologic examination. It is crucial to document findings when the patient is first received and at regular intervals thereafter to monitor the evolution of neurologic status. The injury may be a complete (i.e., no sensory or motor function distal to the lesion) or incomplete (preservation of some function) lesion. Evidence of sacral sparing such as perianal skin sensation, toe flexion, or sphincter control indicates an incomplete lesion with a possibility for recovery. Spinal shock refers to the state of bradycardia, arterial hypotension, and increased venous capacitance due to an interruption of sympathetic outflow and responses [261]. Many patients are also poikilothermic. There is flaccidity and an absence of reflexes below the level of injury. The period of "spinal shock" is variable.

Mechanical injuries are varied. Some of the more common ones are discussed below.
Atlantooccipital Dislocation. This is frequently due to severe hyperextension. There are at least three varieties (anterior, posterior, and longitudinal). The commonest variety is anterior atlantooccipital dislocation in which the occiput is subluxed anteriorly on the lateral masses of C1. Atlantooccipital dislocation is a rare and often fatal injury [368].
Jefferson Fracture. This is a "burst" fracture of the atlas (C1) caused by vertical compression force (axial loading) transmitted through the occipital condyles to the lateral masses of C1. The ring of C1 (i.e., anterior and posterior arches) is fractured bilaterally, anteriorly, and posteriorly. The fragments are thrust outward from the spinal canal. Significant neurologic injury is rare. The anteroposterior cervical x-ray film shows lateral displacement of both lateral masses with respect to the dens. Axial cervical spine CT demonstrates this fracture.

These fractures are managed according to the degree of displacement of the lateral masses. Those with less than 7.0 mm dislocation on the anteroposterior cervical x-ray film are effectively treated with a Philadelphia collar for 8 to 12 weeks. Halo vest immobilization is used for those patients with C1 fractures with over 7.0 mm dislocation [262].
Odontoid Fractures. These may be divided into three types. *Type I* are avulsions of the tip of the odontoid. They represent about 5 percent of all odontoid fractures and are usually the result of avulsion of the alar ligaments. It is generally a stable injury. Complete healing is almost invariable. *Type II* fractures account for 50 to 60 percent of all odontoid fractures. The fracture is at the neck of the odontoid (i.e., at the junction of the odontoid process and the body of C2). This is relatively avascular cortical bone, and consequently the fractures are slow to heal and prone to nonunion. Anterior or posterior subluxation is common; these frac-

tures are generally unstable and require treatment by posterior C1–C2 cervical fusion. *Type III* fracture is a fracture of the superior portion of the axis body that extends into the base (subdental fracture) [369]. They represent 30 percent of all odontoid fractures. While they may be unstable, the majority heal well with halo vest immobilization.

Hangman's Fracture. This is a fracture of the posterior elements of C2 (lamina, pedicle) with subluxation of C2 forward on C3 (anterolisthesis). It is an extension injury of the upper cervical spine classically resulting from judicial hanging but frequently produced in motor vehicle accidents by rapid deceleration of the head and neck on the dashboard. The spectrum of hangman's fracture extends from only a pedicle fracture of C2 to anterolisthesis of C2 on C3 with spinal cord compromise. Hangman's fracture with significant subluxation and instability may be treated by reduction (in skeletal traction) and immobilization in a halo vest; if there is no subluxation or instability, a Philadelphia collar may suffice. Most fractures will heal adequately over 8 to 12 weeks. A few patients with hangman's fractures and severe C2–C3 instability will require fusion [263, 370, 371].

Clayshoveler's Fracture. This fracture is the result of sudden contracture of the trapezius and rhomboid muscles on the spinous processes during heavy lifting or when shoveling clay. There is an avulsion fracture of the spinous process(es) near the laminal line, usually at C6, C7, T1, or T2.

Unilateral Facet Dislocation. This is a result of flexion rotation, with tearing of the interspinous ligaments and the facet capsule unilaterally. There is dislocation of the facet joint opposite the direction of rotation; the dislocated articular mass is displaced anterior to the subjacent facet and becomes wedged in the inferior portion of the intervertebral foramen. On cervical spine lateral views, there is less than 50 percent anterior displacement between the involved vertebral bodies, and anteroposterior views show the spinous processes rotated toward the side of the fracture. Oblique views demonstrate the jumped facets and narrowing of the intervertebral foramina. Unilateral facet dislocation is associated with segmental nerve root compression and, less frequently, myelopathy.

Bilateral Locked Facets (Bilateral Interfacetal Dislocation). This is the result of a major hyperflexion distractive force. The inferior articular facets of the dislocated vertebra pass superiorly and anteriorly over the adjacent superior articulating facet of the vertebra below and come to lie in the inferior portion of the corresponding intervertebral foramina. The lateral cervical spine x-ray film shows anterior displacement of at least 50 percent of the anteroposterior diameter of the body of the upper cervical vertebra upon the lower vertebra. On cervical spine CT, the central canal is markedly narrowed. This injury is associated with a high incidence of spinal cord injury. It is generally unstable.

Wedge Compression Injury. This is a flexion-compression injury. The spine may be unstable if there is associated posterior ligamentous disruption. *Teardrop fractures* and *comminuted fractures* are part of this spectrum. The latter fractures may result in displacement of bone fragments into the central canal.

Thoracolumbar Injuries. Thoracolumbar spine injuries are commonly one of two types. *Burst fractures* (comminuted) result from axial loading and compression of the vertebral body. Bony fragments may be retropulsed into the spinal canal. CT of the spine with multiplanar reconstructions is the best imaging modality for these fractures.

Flexion-compression (wedge) fractures may have the added feature of distraction injury to the posterior elements, in which case they are potentially unstable.

Wedge fractures may be anterior or lateral and may result in kyphosis (anterior wedge compression) or scoliosis (lateral wedge compression). Associated pelvic and extremity injuries are common.

To diagnose thoracolumbar injuries, obtain anteroposterior and lateral x-ray films of the thoracolumbar spine. Vertebral body compression is a common abnormality; however, the degree of cord compression cannot be estimated on plain x-ray films. Disruption of the posterior elements may be inferred by an increase in the distance between the spinous processes. CT with intrathecal contrast is useful for assessing spinal canal compromise.

Most patients do not require surgery. The priorities of *nonoperative treatment* are to maintain spinal alignment, avoid weight bearing, and begin early rehabilitation. A period of bed rest and gradual ambulation in a lumbar corset will usually achieve these goals. While on bed rest, prevention of deep vein thrombosis is important.

Operative treatment consists of decompression and stabilization, which may be required in patients with significant spinal canal compromise (and associated neurological deficit) or instability.

Chance Fracture. This is a distraction fracture of the lumbar spine. It usually results from motor vehicle accidents in which seat belts without shoulder harnesses are worn; rapid deceleration with hyperflexion results in a fracture through the pedicles, lamina, and spinous processes. The fracture line may extend anteriorly to include the vertebral body.

Generally, these fractures can be reduced and heal well with immobilization.

Clinical Syndromes

Spinal cord injury can be divided into two broad categories: complete and incomplete. Incomplete lesions include the following:

Central Cord Syndrome. This is characterized by motor impairment of the upper rather than the lower extremities. It is common in elderly patients with spondylotic cervical spines who suffer sudden hyperextension injuries as a result of a fall. A vascular etiology may be involved in this injury since the distribution of deficit corresponds to the territory of the midline anterior spinal artery and its perforating branches.

Anterior Cord Syndrome. In anterior cord injuries, there is motor paresis and loss of pain and temperature sensation below the level of injury; deep touch, position, and vibratory sense remain intact. It may be seen with hyperflexion injuries, posterior displacement of fragments of a comminuted vertebral body, or extrusion of intervertebral disk material.

Brown-Séquard Syndrome. This syndrome consists of ipsilateral paresis and loss of proprioception, touch, and vibratory sense and contralateral loss of pain and temperature sensation. It is associated with penetrating injuries of the spinal canal, severing one-half of the cord.

Pediatric Spinal Injuries

Spinal cord injury is uncommon in the pediatric population (1–10% of all spine injuries). The pediatric spine presents differences in anatomic and biomechanical properties, resulting in patterns of spinal injury different from those of adults.

Some of these differences relate to the ossification of the atlas and axis and ligamentous laxity with resultant hypermobility. Ossification of the atlas is incomplete at birth; neither the anterior nor the posterior arches are fused. The posterior arch becomes completely fused by 4 years of age, while fusion of the anterior arch is delayed until the seventh to tenth year. The body of the axis is ossified at birth but the posterior arches only partly, so they fuse posteriorly by the second or third year and unite with the body by the seventh year. The os terminale unites with the body of the dens by age 11 or 12. The neurocentral synchrondosis that separates the dens from the lateral masses fuses between the third and sixth years. The subdental synchrondosis between the dens and the axis centrum (body of C2) also fuses between age 3 and 6 years; it is readily visible as a transverse lucent line between the axis centrum and the dens on a lateral x-ray film simulating a fracture.

The width of retropharyngeal prevertebral space in children shows a physiologic variation between inspiration and expiration because of the laxity of the tissues. In expiration the space is wider and may be mistaken for a prevertebral hematoma from a fracture. Therefore the lateral x-ray film should be taken during maximal inspiration. A similar effect is obtained during flexion and extension; the space is wider in flexion.

Ligamentous laxity also allows for a greater range of motion at the atlantoaxial level during flexion compared with extension. The variation in the atlantodental interval (the space between the anterior arch of C1 and the dens) is from 2 to 5 mm with the greater width in flexion.

Finally, there is a physiologic anterolisthesis of C2 on C3 or C3 on C4 in children under 8 years of age—another result of ligamentous laxity [372]. A helpful indicator as to whether an observed anterior displacement is physiologic or due to traumatic anterolisthesis of C2 is the posterior cervical line. This is an imaginary line drawn through the posterior lamina line of C1 to the posterior lamina line of C3. On a lateral cervical x-ray film in the neutral postion, the posterior lamina line of C2 lies on or within 1 to 3 mm anterior or posterior to the imaginary posterior cervical line. When C2 is intact, C2 translates as a whole, anteriorly in flexion or posteriorly in extension but always with its posterior laminal line within 1 to 3 mm anterior or posterior to the imaginary posterior cervical line. If the positional relationship between the body of C2 and C3 in neutral, flexion, and extension is the same as that of the posterior laminal line to the imaginary posterior cervical line, one may reasonably exclude a traumatic anterolisthesis of C2 [373, 374].

Some pediatric spinal cord injuries include the following:

1. SCIWORA syndrome (spinal cord injury without radiographic abnormality) occurs in 20 to 30 percent of pediatric spinal cord injuries.
2. Vertebral column injuries. Cervical spine injuries are more common in children aged 0 to 9 years than in children aged 10 to 16 years. The pattern of vertebral column injury in the younger group favors the occiput to C2 level, whereas older children have a more even spread in the location of spinal injuries. When they do sustain injury, younger children have a higher incidence of neurologic compromise and a worse prognosis than do their older counterparts [264–266].

Diagnostic Studies

Plain Cervical Spine X-Ray Films. Studies should include lateral, anteroposterior, open-mouth odontoid views, and right and left obliques. The C7–T1 junction *must* be visualized. If necessary, a downward pull on both shoulders or a swimmer's view should be performed to enhance visualization.

An organized approach to the evaluation of spine radiographs makes it less likely that abnormalities will be missed.

Helpful hints in the cervical spine x-ray film include the following:

1. *The skull base and craniocervical junction* presents a number of abnormalities that may be determined by radiographic measurements.

   On the lateral cervical spine x-ray film, *Welcker's basal angle* is formed by a line from the nasion to the tuberculum sella, joining another from the tuberculum sella to the anterior margin of the foramen magnum. The angle ranges from 125 to 143 degrees.

   The basal angle is a measurement of platybasia or flattening of the skull base.

   On the lateral cervical spine x-ray film, *Chamberlain's line* joins the hard palate to the posterior lip of the foramen magnum. The tip of the odontoid process of C2 usually lies at or below this line. Protrusion of the odontoid above this line indicates basilar invagination.
2. The *predental space* extends from the posterior margin of the anterior arch of C1 to the anterior surface of the odontoid process of C2. The

width of this space should not exceed 3 mm in adults or 5 mm in children.

3. The *anterior soft tissue line* that bounds the *prevertebral* space, consisting of the retropharyngeal region above and the retrotracheal space at C6 measures 10 to 20 mm (in adults) and up to 14 mm in children.

4. The *oblique view of the cervical spine x-ray film* displays the neural foramina, superior and inferior articular facets, pedicles, and the intervertebral articulations. The articular facets are oriented obliquely like shingles.

Changes that may indicate cervical spine injury include (1) loss of the normal lordotic curve (may be due to spasm or positioning), (2) angular deformity of the cervical spine (kyphosis of the cervical spine is associated with disruption of the posterior ligaments), (3) anterior or posterior displacements of the vertebral bodies, (4) increased separation between the spinous processes, and (5) increased width of the preverterbral space.

Flexion and Extension Lateral Cervical X-Ray Films. These studies should only be done under a physician's direction and in a conscious patient. These views are useful in the diagnosis of ligamentous injury and spinal instability.

Spondylolysis refers to a defect in the pars interarticularis. It may be bilateral and predispose to anterior displacement of the vertebral body (spondylolisthesis). The etiology of the pars defect may be congenital, traumatic, or degenerative.

Spondylolisthesis is graded according to the degree of displacement of the vertebral body (e.g., spondylolisthesis of L5 is referenced to the sacrum). On the lateral x-ray film, the rostral surface of the sacrum is divided into four equal segments. Grade I is less than 25 percent displacement, grade II is up to 50 percent forward on the sacrum, grade III is up to 75 percent, and grade IV is greater than 75 percent displacement.

Computed Tomography. Thin-section CT of the region of a presumed fracture or subluxation should be obtained to clarify suspicious findings on cervical spine x-ray film. CT scanning may show narrowing of the spinal canal or impingement by bone fragments. Metrizamide myelography in conjunction with the CT scan is of value in patients with persistent neurologic deficit unexplained by the radiographic studies already obtained.

Three-dimensional CT allows rotation of the images about any axis and transection of the image along axial, coronal, or sagittal planes. Complex anatomic relationships and injuries may be better comprehended when visualized three dimensionally.

Magnetic Resonance Imaging. MRI can directly visualize the acutely traumatized cord. In a recent study of MRI in patients with acute spinal trauma, a variety of pathologic findings were detected: anatomic cord transections, spinal cord deformity secondary to extrinsic compression, focal cord enlargement and swelling, hyperintense intramedullary lesions, and disk herniations. Practical limitations in obtaining an MRI in this group of patients include maintaining spinal stability and scan times in unmonitored patients [267].

Treatment

Goals of management include (1) correction of bony malalignment (reduction), (2) decompression—i.e., removal of bone fragments in the spinal canal or root foramen or diskectomy, since any of these may result in neurologic deficit that could improve with surgical decompression, and (3) stabilization in an orthotic device or with surgery (bony fusion or instrumentation).

Immediate Management. Immediate management requires that the patient be supine on a firm flat surface. Lateral motion is restricted by a Philadelphia collar and sandbags on both sides of the head. If the patient cannot lie supine for any reason (e.g., vomiting), the lateral position is acceptable. The neutral position must be maintained throughout the physical examination, resuscitative procedures, and x-ray evaluation. Lift or roll the head and trunk as one unit (logroll). Secure the airway by clearing the mouth and upper airway of obvious foreign material and inserting a nasal airway if necessary. Assess the quality of respiratory effort, obtain ABGs, and provide supplemental oxygen by prongs or mask. Pulmonary dysfunction and acute respiratory failure is a major cause of mortality in patients with spinal cord injury. Intercostal muscles are often ineffective, and respiratory effort is provided almost solely by the diaphragm. These patients tire easily and may become hypoxic and hypercapnic. Repeat ABGs are necessary to monitor changes in respiratory status and to direct the need for intubation and ventilation [268]. Patients with weak intercostal and diaphragmatic muscles cannot mount a strong cough to clear secretions and will require frequent suctioning. Some improvement in vital capacity tends to occur with time [269].

Generally, in the patient with spinal cord injury, nasotracheal intubation is safer than orotracheal intubation. Nasotracheal intubation is technically more difficult; if it fails, orotracheal intubation with flexible fiberoptic bronchoscopy is a reasonable alternative. Spinal alignment should be maintained throughout by traction.

Although many patients require mechanical ventilation at first, most can be successfully weaned. In patients who are likely to require prolonged ventilatory support, a tracheostomy should be considered. This facilitates patient comfort, eating, and pulmonary toilet. Subsequently, it may allow patients to talk.

Poor sympathetic tone associated with "spinal shock" may lead to bradycardia and hypotension, requiring volume expansion. Insert large-bore intravenous catheters and begin fluid infusion; take care not to

overload the circulation, since these patients are also at risk for congestive heart failure. Moving or tilting the patient suddenly may worsen
hypotension because compensatory postural reflexes are lost.

Gastrointestinal complications occur in acute cervical spine injury.
Gastric atony and adynamic ileus accompany spinal shock. A nasogastric tube should be placed for decompression. Enteral feeding
should begin when bowel sounds return. Stool softeners, laxatives, or
disimpaction may be necessary. Gastrointestinal hemorrhage may
occur in 1 to 5 percent of patients; prophylaxis with antacids and his-
tamine-receptor blockers reduces this risk [270].

Urinary retention and bladder distension should be managed by catheterization. Once the patient is stable, remove the catheter and begin
a program of intermittent bladder catheterization. The incidence of urolithiasis is increased in the spinal cord–injured patient. These patients
are commonly hypercalciuric, which contributes to urolithiasis; this, together with urinary tract infections, places the patient at risk for renal
failure, which is a major cause of mortality in the chronic spinal cord–
injured patient.

As with all immobilized patients, one should consider prophylaxis for
deep venous thrombosis and pulmonary embolism with pneumatic
compression boots and low-dose heparin [271, 272]. Patients with
quadriplegia may develop symptoms of acute sensory deprivation,
even to the point of psychosis. The sudden loss of peripheral sensory
input including splanchnic stimuli in combination with a totally alien
environment (white walls and ceiling, rhythmic-sounding machines, severely restricted field of view) may overwhelm the psyche. Sensible
precautions include early ambulation, radio and TV, and generous vis-
itation.

Cervical Skeletal Traction. Cervical skeletal traction is applied to re-
store or maintain the normal alignment of the cervical spine (reduction
and immobilization). It is not indicated for thoracic or lumbar fracture
or dislocation. Several types of skull tongs (calipers) are available, representing evolution in design from the initial presentation by Crutchfield
in 1933 [273]. These modifications have largely eliminated the use of
Crutchfield tongs. The indications for their use are similar; however,
techniques of application vary.

Gardner-Wells tongs (Fig. 5-4) consist of a metal frame that follows the
coronal contour of the skull. At each end is a screw with cone-shaped
points. The points are tilted in the direction of pull so that with traction
they tend to press in rather than pull out. One point is spring loaded
to indicate when sufficient force has been applied to penetrate just the
outer table of the skull [274]. A small metal plate with application in-
structions is permanently attached to the traction link, which floats on
the tong arms. The pins are long enough to be adaptable to a variety
of head sizes. The patient should be supine when the tongs are applied
(Fig. 5-5):

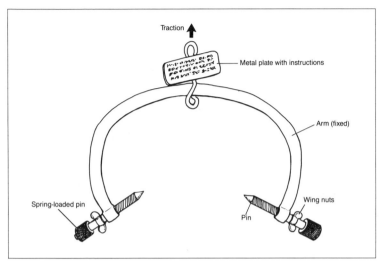

Fig. 5-4. Gardner-Wells skull traction tongs.

1. Clean the hair and scalp in the temporal regions with antiseptic solution. Hair removal is optional but may allow for easier application. Inject about 1 ml of 1% lidocaine into the area.
2. Have the patient's head supported by an assistant.
3. Because of the fixed arms, first determine that the tongs will fit adequately and clear the head.
4. Place tongs in the temporal region, about 2.5 to 3.0 cm above the ear, or just below the temporal ridges in the longitudinal axis of the spine.
5. Turn down the screws on either side of the device simultaneously. Watch the indicator over the spring-loaded pin; the spring yields on encountering bone. Tighten until it protudes 1 mm beyond its flat surface. At this point approximately 30 lb of pressure exists between the two pins. Tilt the tongs back and forth to ensure proper seating, and retighten if the indicator has recessed. The pins may advance slightly after the initial setting; they stabilize in 24 hours, after which no further adjustments of the points are needed.
6. Tighten the nuts external to the arms to lock the pins in position. The "wing nuts" can be tightened by hand [275].
7. Attach traction line through the eye of the traction link and over a pulley and be sure it hangs free. Check the patient for position (i.e., neither being pulled out of or sliding down the bed; if so, adjust the elevation of the head of the bed as necessary to provide the correct amount of counter-traction) and comfort.
8. The direction of traction (i.e., slight flexion or extension or neutral) is dictated by x-ray findings. The patient's weight acts as counter-traction.

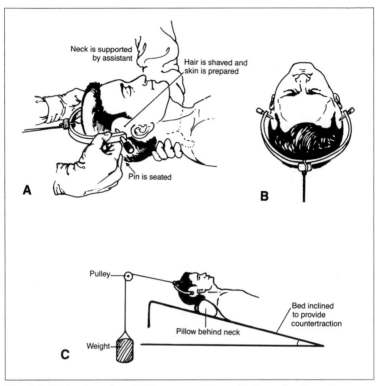

Fig. 5-5. Skeletal traction. A. Placement of tongs. B. Tongs in place. C. Position of patient in traction.

9. The general rule for applying weights is 5 lb for each level below the occiput, so that at C2 one would require 10 lb, progressing to a maximum of 35 lb at C7. Always start traction with a small amount, such as 10 lb, and obtain an initial x-ray film to make sure there is no overdistraction before progressing to the desired weight.
10. Obtain x-ray films to determine reductions, alignment, and position of the tongs.
11. Inspect pin sites frequently. They may be cleaned with a peroxide-soaked cotton-tipped applicator if traction is to be maintained for a long time. Regular turning will prevent the development of occipital decubiti, especially in comatose patients.

University of Virginia tongs (Fig. 5-6) provided improvement in tong design from the Gardner-Wells tongs by allowing for variation in breadth to suit smaller skull sizes (as in children and adolescents). Also, the reduced lateral mass of the arms allows for easier patient turning and nursing care [276].

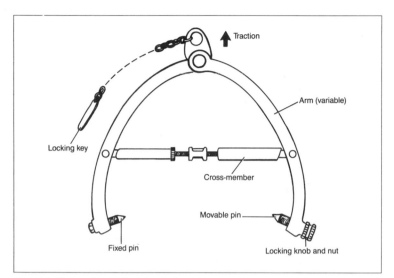

Fig. 5-6. University of Virginia skull traction tongs.

The tongs are applied as follows:

1. Follow steps 1 and 2 on page 201.
2. Approximate the interpin distance to the skull size by turning the central locking knob on the cross-member. Turn the central locking nut away from the cross-member shoulder to allow sufficient room for free adjustment.
3. Adjust the movable pin until it protrudes slightly less than the fixed pin.
4. Place the tongs on the skull (just below the temporal ridge). Adjust the fit by turning the central knob of the cross-member to close the tongs; turn until the pressure on the pins first begins to move the fixed nut slightly away from the arm shoulder.
5. Tighten the movable pin until the ring indicator beneath the nut of the fixed pin protrudes approximately 2 mm. The pins are now exerting about 30 lb of pressure between the points.
6. Lock the unit by turning the central locking nut until it is against the shoulder of the cross-member. Tighten the central locking knob against the nut and shoulder securely using the key. This maneuver ensures the unit will not spontaneously unravel.
7. Follow steps 7 through 11 on pages 201–202.

Management of cervical spine injuries has been improved by use of the *halo traction immobilization apparatus* (Fig. 5-7) [277–281].

The halo brace consists of three main parts: (1) a steel ring with openings for the placement of skull pins, (2) an adjustable metal superstruc-

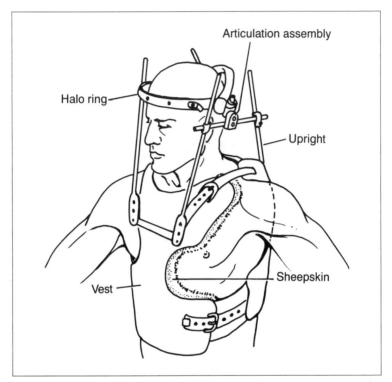

Fig. 5-7. Halo apparatus.

ture that connects the halo ring to the vest, and (3) a plastic vest to support the superstructure (Fig. 5-7). Compared with skull tongs, the direction of the traction force can be better controlled with the halo because there is no movement between the skull and the fixation pins. The principal advantage of the halo apparatus is that it allows the patient to get out of bed while traction is maintained (mobile traction). The halo may be applied in the first instance or later in place of skull tong traction when the patient is ready for ambulation.

Trippi-Wells dual-purpose cranial tongs [282] have been developed for cervical spine traction and can be easily incorporated into a halo apparatus without disturbing skeletal traction. The dual-purpose tongs use four-point fixation with spring-loaded pins. Once reduction has been accomplished, and if long-term management in a halo apparatus is desired, the vest portion can be attached directly to the tongs. This can be done only after the tongs have been in place for 24 hours. After the vest is attached, the weights used in reduction are removed.

The halo may also be used as an adjunct to cervical fusion before, during, and after surgery. Placing the patient in a halo jacket preoperatively provides safety when turning and positioning under general anesthesia. The halo has also been used in the treatment of malignancies, infectious processes, congenital abnormalities of the cervical spine, and degenerative cervical spine disease.

Halo application is described below [283–285].

1. The halo ring is available in several sizes. Select the appropriate one so that there is a 1.5-cm clearance on all sides of the head. The ring is positioned just inferior to the equator of the skull (the greatest circumference of the head) to prevent cephalad displacement. The ring has threaded holes for placement of skull fixation pins. The ring is arched upward posteriorly to clear the occipital area for surgical access.
2. Traction should be maintained during halo application; this may be done manually by an assistant or by an existing halter or tongs.
3. The head should extend slightly beyond the edge of the bed. An assistant supports the head while allowing room for the ring to be positioned around the patient's head. Alternately, one may use the Hershey halo jig [286].
4. Skin areas beneath the holes selected are shaved, if necessary, and cleaned with povidone-iodine and then infiltrated with 1% lidocaine.
5. Four fixation pins are used—two anterior and two posterior. The anterior pins are placed about 1 cm above the lateral third of the supraorbital ridge, preferably behind the hairline. The posterior pins are best positioned posterior and superior to the external ear. Positioning pins are placed in holes adjacent to those selected for the skull pins.
6. The pins are turned with finger pressure until they just touch the scalp. After the skull pins are secured finger tight, the positioning pins are removed. Do the final tightening of the skull pins with torque screwdrivers; generally 6 in.-lb of pressure is required for adults, but for children with thin skulls 3 to 4 in.-lb of torque may be sufficient for fixation. To keep the ring centered, tighten diagonally opposite pins simultaneously. Finally, tighten the set screws to lock the halo pins in place and prevent loosening. Retorque the skull pins only once, 24 to 36 hours after application.
7. The patient is now ready to be placed in traction or in a plastic jacket. a. If traction is required, select the appropriate position (flexion or extension) by directing the traction line more anteriorly for extension or more posteriorly for extension. Fit the halo bail and cord and attach the traction weight. Be sure the weight hangs free. A head rest or skate attachment may be applied to the ring to decrease direct ring pressure, allowing more head movement. This also prevents the pins from catching in the bedsheet. b. Alternately, the halo ring may be attached to a sheepskin-lined, plastic body jacket (halo brace) with shoulder straps. The size of the vest required is determined by measuring the circumference of the chest

at the level of the xiphoid. The back section of the vest is slid under the patient and is positioned to fit snugly on the shoulders. The anterior portion is positioned and loosely secured to its fellow by straps. The metal framework is attached to the vest and halo ring. Adjusting the height of the upright bars regulates the amount of traction applied. Positioning can be altered to provide extension or flexion as needed. Attached to one of the vertical support bars is a linkage assembly that gives a third point of fixation on the halo ring, eliminating any hinge action between the halo and the support bars. With the patient sitting, tighten the unit with the head and neck in the desired position.

9. Once the halo brace has been applied, the patient may sit or ambulate as neurologic condition and general health allow. Since the halo brace weighs about 10 lb, balance may be a problem initially; the patient must also become accustomed to a decreased peripheral field of vision. A wrench should be kept by the patient at all times, since if the patient suffers cardiac arrest, rapid access to the chest wall is necessary. The anterior vest can be removed by unlocking the two bolts that attach the anterior uprights to the anterior vest and unbuckling all four straps.

10. Pin cleaning is as with skull tongs. It may be done by a family member after the patient is discharged. Routine hygiene should not be neglected; the sheepskin may be changed as often as necessary [287, 288].

11. The patient should return at intervals for inspection of the apparatus and pin sites and for follow-up x-ray films. Removal of the halo pins is performed on an outpatient basis, and pin sites generally heal uneventfully.

There are several *complications of skeletal traction.* Scars over the eyebrows may be aesthetically displeasing and occasionally need surgical revision. Inflammation around the pin sites may result in seropurulent drainage; the material should be cultured and the patient treated with appropriate antibiotics. If drainage persists, it may be necessary to remove the pins and insert them at another site. Occasionally it will be necessary to curet that area of the skull for local debridement.

If pins become loose, the pin sites may have to be changed. Rarely pins may penetrate through both bony tables and produce a CSF leak [289]. The pins should be removed; such leaks generally seal spontaneously.

Tangential views of the skull may demonstrate perforation of the inner table.

Decubitus ulcers may develop beneath a halo brace, particularly if the patient has sensory impairment over the thoracic region.

A serious complication of skull tong traction is overdistraction, which itself may cause cord dysfunction [290]. In older patients with cervical spondylosis, overdistraction is particularly likely. Simple traction on the

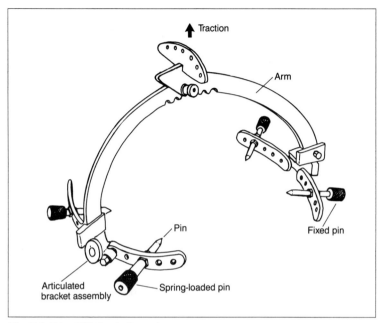

Fig. 5-8. Trippi-Wells skull traction tongs.

patient's shoulders for a portable cervical x-ray film while he or she is in traction has resulted in distraction [291]. These patients may require less than the usual weight. Figure 5-8 shows an example of skull traction tongs.

Immediate follow-up x-ray films are necessary after tongs are applied or weights are added and at regular intervals while the patient is in traction. The amount of weight required for reduction may be reduced if muscle spasm is treated with diazepam.

Rarer complications include osteomyelitis of the skull, epidural hematoma, epidural abscess, and cerebral abscess [292].
Cervical Halter Traction. Halter traction (Fig. 5-9) was first employed for the treatment of fracture dislocation of the cervical spine [293]. This form of cervical traction is currently most commonly used for the conservative management of cervical radiculopathy from disk disease or spondylosis but may also be effective in some cases of cervical trauma. Usually, in the case of cervical spine injury, it serves as a temporary measure and may be the only available device in an emergency.

It consists of two strips of padded canvas connected by two loops of cord. The anterior pad sits under the mandible, while the posterior one supports the occiput. The traction loops are hung over a metal spreader

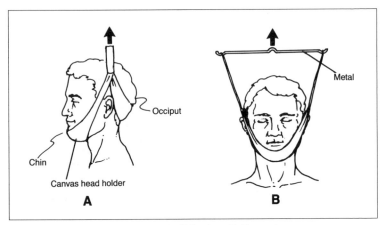

Fig. 5-9. Cervical halter traction. A. Side view. B. Front view.

and connected to a water-bag weight (7–10 lb). Halter traction kits may be purchased for use at home. The traction system is placed over the head of the bed with the head slightly elevated so that the direction of traction is in line with the cervical spine. Some models use a door frame as the suspending mechanism; the patient sits on a chair during treatment.

Generally, the patient uses traction for 30 to 45 minutes 3 to 4 times a day. Excess weight may cause discomfort in the jaw or pressure sores on the skin. Sometimes traction will aggravate neck pain or brachialgia, particularly if there is muscle spasm; if so, it should be discontinued, although use of a muscle relaxant before traction may avoid the problem.

Surgery in Cervical Spine Trauma. The major role of surgery is in the stabilization of unstable cervical injuries. There are many operative approaches, and there is controversy over which method to apply, in which situations, and when. The options include bone graft; posterior fusion with wires, plates, and screws; and various internal orthoses [294, 295, 296]. A further role for surgery is the decompression of intraspinal contents to improve both root and cord function.

Cervical Disk Disease

Cervical disk herniation is often referred to as "soft" cervical disk, as opposed to the "hard" cervical disk of cervical spondylosis (see below).

Diagnosis

Patients may complain of neck pain and brachialgia (usually unilateral and in a radicular distribution). The pain tends to wax and wane. There may be voluntary restriction of neck movement. Neck extension or lateral flexion to the side of the lesion often exacerbates the pain. The C5–C6 level is most frequently involved, followed by the C6–C7 level.

Symptoms and signs correspond to the segmental level involved and include paresthesia, pain, motor deficit, and loss of reflexes:

C5–C6 disk herniation results in a C6 radiculopathy with pain radiating down the lateral side of the arm and forearm, often into the thumb and index finger. There may be weakness of the biceps muscle and depression of the biceps reflex. C6–C7 disk herniation results in a C7 radiculopathy with pain radiating down the middle of the forearm, usually to the middle finger, although the index and ring fingers may be involved. There is weakness of the triceps muscle and depression of the triceps reflex.

Long tract syndromes from "soft" cervical disk herniation are uncommon but not unknown. They are common in cervical spondylosis.

Radiological diagnosis usually is by *myelography,* with follow-up thin slice *CT* cuts through the regions of interest. There may be anterior defects from posterior vertebral body osteophyte formation and intervertebral disk herniation or lateral nerve root amputation. MRI now offers increased sensitivity.

Treatment

Nonsurgical Treatment. The hallmark of conservative treatment is cervical halter traction, which is described on page 207. Other treatments of benefit include mild analgesics, muscle relaxants, nonsteroidal antiinflammatory drugs, and various local applications. Many patients with cervical disk disease recover spontaneously and never require surgery; others improve only to have recurrent attacks. Where pain is the only symptom and there is no neurologic deficit, it becomes a matter of individual tolerance whether to undergo surgery. For those patients who exhibit clear-cut neurologic deficit, have a corresponding structural lesion demonstrated on radiologic studies, and have failed a satisfactory trial of conservative treatment, surgical treatment should be considered. Myelopathy is virtually an absolute indication for surgical intervention, since the likelihood of recovery otherwise is slim; delay only serves to reduce the chances of reversibility.

Surgical Treatment. These lesions may be approached by one of two methods: (1) posterolateral ("keyhole") laminotomy, foraminotomy, and diskectomy; and (2) anterior cervical diskectomy (with or without fusion). The relative merits and limitations of both approaches are considered on pages 210–211.

Cervical Spondylosis

Chronic disk degeneration with posterior osteophyte formation (cervical spondylosis) is a common cause of spinal cord or root dysfunction in patients over 55 years of age.

Diagnosis

A *radicular* syndrome, caused by root irritation from osteophytic spurs, is the most common presentation. The pain may be bilateral. Neck pain, often episodic, periscapular, or between the shoulders and stiffness persist between bouts of radicular pain and dysesthesias. Pain may yield to the wearing of a soft collar or cervical traction. The *myelopathic* syndrome often develops insidiously and without pain. The hallmark here is spasticity; later weakness of the lower extremities develops, seldom with sphincter involvement. There may be radicular symptoms in the arms. Very occasionally, a specific cord syndrome may be seen. Myelopathy, especially the central cord syndrome, may be precipitated by minor trauma.

Cervical Spine X-Ray Films. A significant percentage of healthy adults over 50 years of age will show features considered characteristic of cervical spondylosis on cervical x-ray study, and, therefore, x-ray changes of cervical spondylosis are only relevant when they can be correlated with clinical signs and symptoms. Typical findings include foraminal encroachment on the oblique view and posterior spondylotic "spurs" and narrowing of the disk space on the lateral view.

The average anteroposterior diameter of the cervical canal from C3–C7 is about 17 mm; it is generally agreed that cervical spinal cord compression is very likely when the diameter is less than 11 mm. In patients with cervical spondylosis, there is usually some reduction in the anteroposterior diameter of the spinal canal; when it is associated with a congenitally narrow canal, myelopathy is likely to develop.

Myelography. As with plain x-ray films, myelograms must be interpreted in light of clinical evidence. There may be anterior defects from osteophyte compression; infolding of a hypertrophied, sometimes calcified ligamentum flavum; or lateral nerve root defects. Not infrequently there is a myelographic block of sluggish flow of dye. The contrast carries only a certain distance along the nerve root sleeve; therefore, laterally placed lesions may not be visualized on the myelogram. Cervical spine MRI is becoming an excellent diagnostic tool and is much less troublesome to the patient.

Electromyography and Nerve Conduction Studies. These may aid the differential diagnosis when clinical findings are equivocal.

Two main operative approaches are in use: anterior cervical diskectomy and posterior cervical lamnectomy. Selection of one or the other is based in part on scientific fact and in part on the surgeon's training and experience [296, 296a].

Myelopathy carries the least favorable prognosis. Surgery is primarily designed to halt disease progression; although existing symptoms are sometimes eliminated, this cannot be ensured. Radiculopathy is frequently improved when satisfactory decompression has been accomplished.

Anterior Cervical Diskectomy (With or Without Fusion). This approach allows removal of the disk and anterior osteophytes without retraction of the spinal cord or nerves. Placement of a bone graft distracts the neural foramina and vertebral bodies and stabilizes the spine. However, in time, instability and disk degeneration may develop above or below the fused segment because of the differential stress on these joints. A minor limitation is the fact that the nerve root is not visualized directly for a part of its length, and so intraoperative assessment of the adequacy of decompression is done indirectly [297–299].

The availability of cadaver grafts has reduced the need for autogenous iliac crest bone, which caused much postoperative discomfort for many patients. Some neurosurgeons do not perform interbody fusion [300, 301].

Posterior Cervical Laminectomy. This approach gives the surgeon a good view of cord and roots and allows for a wide decompression when performed for spondylotic myelopathy. The posterior laminotomy and foraminotomy for soft cervical disk herniation is a more limited exposure and is directed to the affected nerve root. It does not require fusion [302, 303].

Lumbar Disk Herniation

Lumbar disk herniation is an exceedingly common lesion. The L5–S1 is the commonest involved level, followed by L4–L5. L5–S1 disk herniation causes pain and paresthesias in the S1 distribution, with loss of the ankle jerk. weakness of plantar flexion, and positive straight leg raising.

Disk herniation of L4–L5 produces radicular pain in the L5 distribution, with weakness of dorsiflexion. Sensory disturbance is present in the L5 dermatome. Straight leg raising is positive.

L3–L4 disk herniation causes pain and paresthesias in an L4 distribution. There may be depression of the knee jerk and weakness of the quadriceps muscle. Reverse straight leg raising may be positive.

Diagnostic Studies

The nonenhanced CT scan may demonstrate disk protrusion and nerve root compression. Myelography may be done if CT findings are equivocal, although some surgeons perform the study routinely. Herniated intervertebral disks appear as a focal deformity of the contrast column at the intervertebral disk level or amputation of the nerve root sleeve. MRI is becoming more widely used and is very sensitive. It is better than CT in demonstrating soft tissue pathology within the spinal canal since the bone signal is dampened.

Treatment

Most patients should be treated initially by a conservative regimen of at least 2 weeks of complete bed rest, analgesics, and muscle relaxants. The exception to this is a patient with a rapidly advancing deficit or with cauda equina syndrome. For those patients who do not improve with bed rest, lumbar diskectomy may be considered electively. Considerations for surgery should include the patient's life-style, degree of incapacitation, and a psychological assessment.

Lumbar Spinal Stenosis

Patients with lumbar spinal stenosis present with a long history of intermittent low back pain. They are usually elderly. Standing and walking (neurogenic claudication) usually accentuate the pain. The pain may follow a radicular pattern; more often it is described as aching in the calf with dysesthetic qualities. Discomfort begins in the buttocks and spreads into the posterior thigh and calf. There is usually a paucity of neurologic signs; often reflexes are symmetrically depressed.

Diagnostic Tests

Lumbar X-Ray Films. Lumbar x-ray films show degenerative changes including osteophytes, disk space narrowing, and spondylolisthesis. These of themselves are not bothersome in the elderly patient except in the context of clinical signs and symptoms.
Computed Tomography. CT shows narrowing of the sagittal diameter or the lateral recesses. Stenosis may involve multiple levels. There is facet hypertrophy and neural foraminal encroachment.
Myelography. Myelography is very useful, showing a reduction of the sagittal diameter of the spinal canal and multiple filling defects ("hourglass" deformities); there may be a partial or complete block to the flow of dye. The myelogram delineates the rostrocaudal extent of the disease and pinpoints which nerve roots may require decompression.
TREATMENT The treatment of choice is a wide decompressive laminectomy with foraminotomies as necessary. Multiple levels are usually involved. Blood should be available since intraoperative blood loss can be significant. Pain may limit early ambulation, especially in elderly patients. Adequate pain control is necessary to prevent prolonged recumbency and the problems of immobility.

References

1. Seeger J. F., Weinstein P. R., Carmody R. F., et al. Digital video subtraction angiography of the cervical and cerebral vasculature. *J. Neurosurg.* 56:173, 1982.
2. Kelly W. M., Brant-Zawadzki M. N., Pitts L. H. Arterial injection-digital subtraction angiography. *J. Neurosurg.* 58:851, 1983.
3. Brant-Zawadzki M., Gould R., Norman D., et al. Digital subtraction cerebral angiography by intraarterial injection. *A.J.R.* 140:347, 1983.
4. Levin D. C., Schapiro R. M., Boxt L. M., et al. Digital subtraction angiography. *A.J.R.* 143:447, 1984.

5. Brant-Zawadzki M., Miller E. R., Federle M. P. CT in the evaluation of spine trauma. *A.J.R.* 136:369, 1981.
6. Carrera G. F., Williams A. L., Haughton V. M. Computed tomography in sciatica. *Radiology* 137:433, 1980.
7. Bydder G. M. Magnetic resonance imaging of the brain. *Radiol. Clin. North Am.* 22:770, 1984.
8. Brant-Zawadzki M. N., Davis P. L., Crooks L. E., et al. NMR demonstration of cerebral abnormalities: Comparison with CT. *A.J.N.R.* 4:117, 1983.
9. Burrows E. H. Myelography with iohexol (Omnipaque): Review of 300 cases. *A.J.N.R.* 6:349, 1985.
10. Dublin A. B., McGahan J. P., Reid M. H. Value of computed tomographic metrizamide myelography in the neurological evaluation of the spine. *Radiology* 146:79, 1983.
11. Phelps M. E., Mazziotta J. C., Schelbert H. R. (eds.). *Positron Emission Tomography and Autoradiography: Principles and Application to the Brain and Heart*. New York: Raven Press, 1986.
12. Frackowiak R. S. J., Lenzi G., Jones T., et al. Quantitative measurement of regional cerebral blood flow and oxygen metabolism in man using ^{15}O and positron emission tomography: Theory, procedure, and normal values. *J. Comput. Assist. Tomogr.* 4:727, 1980.
13. Sarner M., Rose F. C. Clinical presentation of ruptured intracranial aneurysm. *J. Neurol. Neurosurg. Psychiatry* 30:67, 1967.
14. Okawara S. H. Warning signs prior to rupture of intracranial aneurysm. *J. Neurosurg.* 38:575, 1973.
15. Pakarinen S. Incidence, etiology, and prognosis of primary subarachnoid hemorrhage: A study based on 589 cases diagnosed in a defined urban population during a defined period. *Acta Neurol. Scand.* 29(Suppl.):1, 1967.
16. Hunt W. E., Hess R. M. Surgical risk as related to time of intervention in the repair of intracranial aneurysms. *J. Neurosurg.* 28:14, 1968.
17. Davis K. R., New P. F., Ojemann R. G., et al. Computed tomographic evaluation of hemorrhage secondary to intracranial aneurysm. *A.J.R.* 127:143, 1976.
18. Ghoshhajra K., Scotti L., Marasco J., et al. CT detection of intracranial hemorrhage in subarachnoid hemorrhage. *A.J.R.* 132:613, 1979.
19. Liliequist B., Lindqvist M., Valdimarssan E. Computed tomography and subarachnoid hemorrhage. *Neuroradiology* 14:21, 1977.
20. Adams H. P. Jr., Kassell N. F., Torner J. C., et al. CT and clinical correlations in recent aneurysmal subarachnoid hemorrhage: A preliminary report of the cooperative aneurysm study. *Neurology* 33:981, 1983.
21. Fisher C. M., Kistler J. P., Davis J. M. Relation of cerebral vasospasm to subarachnoid hemorrhage visualized by computed tomographic scanning. *Neurosurgery* 6:1, 1980.
22. van Gijn J., Hijdra A., Wijdicks E. F. M., et al. Acute hydrocephalus after aneurysmal subarachnoid hemorrhage. *J. Neurosurg.* 63:355, 1985.
23. Kistler J. P., Crowell R. M., Davis K. R., et al. The relation of cerebral vasospasm to the extent and location of subarachnoid blood visualized by CT scan: A prospective study. *Neurology* 33:424, 1983.
24. Perret G., Nishioka H. Report on the cooperative study of intracranial aneurysms and subarachnoid hemorrhage. VI. Arteriovenous malformations. *J. Neurosurg.* 25:467, 1966.
25. Andrews R. J., Spiegel P. K. Intracranial aneurysms. Age, sex, blood pressure, and multiplicity in an unselected series of patients. *J. Neurosurg.* 51:27, 1979.

26. Nehls D. G., Flom R. A., Carter L. P., et al. Multiple intracranial aneurysms: Determining the site of rupture. *J. Neurosurg.* 63:342, 1985.
27. Béguelin C., Seiler R. Subarachnoid hemorrhage with normal panangiography. *Neurosurgery* 13:409, 1983.
28. Eskesen V., Sorensen E. B., Rosenorn J., et al. The prognosis in subarachnoid hemorrhage of unknown etiology. *J. Neurosurg.* 61:1029, 1984.
29. Perret G., Nishioka H. Report on the cooperative study of intracranial aneurysms and subarachnoid hemorrhage. IV. Cerebral angiography, an analysis of the diagnostic value and complications of carotid and vertebral angiography in 5,484 patients. *J. Neurosurg.* 25:98, 1966.
30. DeLaPaz R. L., New P. F. J., Bounanno F. S., et al. NMR imaging of intracranial hemorrhage. *J. Comput. Assist. Tomogr.* 8:599, 1984.
31. Gomori J. M., Grossman R. I., Bilaniuk L. T., et al. High-field MR imaging of superficial siderosis of the central nervous system. *J. Comput. Assist. Tomogr.* 9:972, 1985.
32. Jane J.A., Winn H. R., Richardson A. E. The natural history of intracranial aneurysms: Rebleeding rates during the acute and long-term period and implication for surgical management. *Clin. Neurosurg.* 24:176, 1977.
33. Farhat S. M., Schneider R. C. Observations on the effect of systemic blood pressure on intracranial circulation in patients with cerebrovascular insufficiency. *J. Neurosurg.* 27:441, 1967.
34. Solomon R. A., Post K. D., McMurtry J. G. III. Depression of circulating blood volume in patients after subarachnoid hemorrhage: Implications for the management of symptomatic vasospasm. *Neurosurgery* 14:354, 1984.
35. Tovi D., Nilsson I. M., Thulin C. A. Fibrinolytic activity of the cerebrospinal fluid after subarachnoid hemorrhage. *Acta Neurol. Scand.* 49:1, 1973.
36. Wilkins R. H. Attempts at prevention or treatment of intracranial arterial spasm: An update. *Neurosurgery* 18:808, 1986.
37. Wijdicks E. F. M., Vermeulen M., Ten Haaf J. A., et al. Volume depletion and natriuresis in patients with a ruptured intracranial aneurysm. *Ann. Neurol.* 18:211, 1985.
38. Kassel N. F., Peerless S. J., Durward Q. J., et al. Treatment of ischemic deficits from vasospasm with intravascular volume expansion and induced arterial hypertension. *Neurosurgery* 11:337, 1982.
39. Allen G. S., Ahn H. S., Preziosi T. J., et al. Cerebral arterial spasm—a controlled trial of nimodipine in patients with subarachnoid hemorrhage. *N. Engl. J. Med.* 308:619, 1983.
40. Philippon J., Grob R., Dagreou F., et al. Prevention of vasospasm in subarachnoid hemorrhage. A controlled study with nimodipine. *Acta Neurochir.* 82:110, 1986.
41. Auer L. M. Acute operation and preventive nimodipine improve outcome in patients with ruptured cerebral aneurysms. *Neurosurgery* 15:57, 1984.
42. Ljunggren B., Brandt L., Saveland H., et al. Outcome in 60 consecutive patients treated with early aneurysm operation and intravenous nimodipine. *J. Neurosurg.* 61:864, 1984.
43. Petruk K. C., West M., Mohn G., et al. Nimodipine treatment in poor-grade aneurysm patients: Results of a multicenter double-blind placebo-controlled trial. *J. Neurosurg.* 68:505, 1988.
44. Zubkov Y. N., Nikiforov B. M., Shustin V. A. Balloon catheter technique for dilatation of constricted cerebral arteries after aneurysmal SAH. *Acta Neurochir.* 70:65, 1984.
45. Nornes H., Magnaes B. Intracranial pressure in patients with ruptured saccular aneurysm. *J. Neurosurg.* 36:537, 1982.
46. Torner J. C., Kassell N. F., Wallace R. B., et al. Preoperative prognostic

factors for rebleeding and survival in aneurysm patients receiving antifibrinolytic therapy: Report of the cooperative aneurysm study. *Neurosurgery* 9:506, 1979.

47. Andreoli A., di Pasquale G., Pinelli G. Subarachnoid hemorrhage: Frequency and severity of cardiac arrhythmias. A survey of 70 cases studied in the acute phase. *Stroke* 18:558, 1987.

48. Marion D. W., Segal R., Thompson M. E. Subarachnoid hemorrhage and the heart. *Neurosurgery* 18:101, 1986.

49. Melin J., Fogelholm R. Electrocardiographic findings in subarachnoid hemorrhage. *Acta Med. Scand.* 213:5, 1983.

50. Ciongolu A. K., Poser C. M. Pulmonary edema secondary to subarachnoid hemorrhage. *Neurology* 22:867, 1972.

51. Weir B. Medical aspects of the preoperative management of aneurysms: A review. *Can. J. Neurol. Sci.* 6:441, 1979.

52. Takaku A., Shindo K., Tanaka S., et al. Fluid and electrolyte disturbances in patients with intracranial aneurysms. *Surg. Neurol.* 11:349, 1979.

53. Robinson A. G., DDAVP in the treatment of central diabetes insipidus. *N. Engl. J. Med.* 294:507, 1976.

54. Kassel N. F., Torner J. C., Adams H. P. Antifibrinolytic therapy in the acute period following aneurysmal subarachnoid hemorrhage. Preliminary observations from the cooperative aneurysm study. *J. Neurosurg.* 61:225, 1984.

55. Mizukami M., Kawase T., Usami T., et al. Prevention of vasospasm by early operation with removal of subarachnoid blood. *Neurosurgery* 10:301, 1982.

56. Chyatte D., Fode N. C., Sundt T. M. Early versus late intracranial aneurysm surgery in subarachnoid hemorrhage. *J. Neurosurg.* 69:326, 1988.

57. Kassel N. F., Boarini D. J., Adams H. P., et al. Overall management of ruptured aneurysm. Comparison of early and late operation. *Neurosurgery* 9:120, 1981.

58. Robins M., Baum H. M. Incidence. *Stroke* 12(Suppl. 1):145, 1981.

59. Fisher C. M. Clinical syndromes in cerebral thrombosis, hypertensive hemorrhage, and ruptured saccular aneurysm. *Clin. Neurosurg.* 22:117, 1974.

60. Kaneo M., Tokomi K., Yokoyama T. Early surgical treatment for hypertensive intracerebral hemorrhage. *J. Neurosurg.* 46:579, 1977.

61. Kanno T., Sano H., Shinomiya T. Role of surgery in hypertensive intracerebral hematoma. *J. Neurosurg.* 61:1091, 1984.

62. Pallias J. E., Alliez B. Surgical treatment of spontaneous intracerebral hemorrhage: Immediate and long-term results in 250 cases. *J. Neurosurg.* 39:145, 1973.

63. Kandel E. I., Peresedov V. V. Stereotaxic evacuation of intracerebral hematomas. *J. Neurosurg.* 62:206, 1985.

64. Heros R. C. Cerebellar hemorrhage and infarction. *Stroke* 13:106, 1982.

65. Wilkins R. H. Natural history of intracranial vascular malformations: A review. *Neurosurgery* 16:421, 1985.

66. Pressman R. D., Kirkwood J. R., Davis D. O. Computerized transverse tomography of vascular lesions of the brain. I. Arteriovenous malformations. *A.J.R.* 124:208, 1975.

67. Lee B. C. P., Herzberg L., Zimmerman R. D., et al. MR imaging of cerebral vascular malformations. *A.J.N.R.* 6:863, 1985.

68. Drake C. G. Arteriovenous malformations of the brain. The options for management. *N. Engl. J. Med.* 309:308, 1983.

69. Kunc Z. Surgery for arteriovenous malformations in the speech and motor-sensory regions. *J. Neurosurg.* 40:293, 1974.

70. Wolpert S. M., Stein B. M. Catheter embolization of intracranial arteriove-

nous malformations as an aid to surgical excision. *Neuroradiology* 10:73, 1975.
71. Kjellberg R. N., Hanamura T., Davis K. R., et al. Bragg-peak proton-beam therapy for arteriovenous malformations of the brain. *N. Engl. J. Med.* 309:269, 1983.
72. Annegers J. F., Hauser W. A., Elveback L. R., et al. Remission and relapse of seizures in epilepsy. In Wada J. A., Penry J. K. (eds.) *Advances in Epileptology. The Tenth Epilepsy International Symposium.* New York: Raven Press, 1980. Pp. 143–47.
73. Commission on Classification and Terminology of the International League Against Epilepsy. Proposal for revised clinical and electroencephalographic classification of epileptic seizures. *Epilepsia* 22:489, 1981.
74. Augustine F. A., Novelly R. A., Mattson R. H., et al. Occupational adjustment following neurosurgical treatment of epilepsy. *Ann. Neurol.* 15:68, 1984.
75. Lieb J. P., Engel J. Jr., Brown W. J., et al. Neuropathological findings following temporal lobectomy related to surface and depth EEG patterns. *Epilepsia* 22:539, 1982.
76. Lüders H., Hahn J., Lesser R., et al. Localization of epileptogenic spike foci: Comparative study of closely spaced scalp electrodes, nasopharyngeal, sphenoidal, subdural and depth electrodes. In Akimoto H., et al. (eds.). *Advances in Epileptology. The Twelfth Epilepsy International Symposium.* New York: Raven Press, 1982. pp. 185–189.
77. Penfield W., Jasper H. H. *Epilepsy and the Functional Anatomy of the Human Brain.* Boston: Little, Brown, 1954.
78. Meyer F. B., Marsh W. R., Laws E. R., Jr., et al. Temporal lobectomy in children with epilepsy. *J. Neurosurg.* 64:371, 1986.
79. Ojemann G. A. Surgical therapy for medically intractable epilepsy. *J. Neurosurg.* 66:489, 1987.
80. Dodrill C. B., Wilkus R. J., Ojemann G. A., et al. Multidisciplinary prediction of seizure relief from cortical resection surgery. *Ann. Neurol.* 20:2, 1986.
81. Engel J. Jr., Sutherling W., Cahan L., et al. The role of positron emission tomography in the surgical therapy of epilepsy. In Porter R. J., Mattson R. H., Ward A. A. Jr., et al (eds.). *Advances in Epileptology. The Fifteenth Epilepsy International Symposium.* New York: Raven Press, 1984. Pp. 427–432.
82. Gloor P., Olivier A., Ives J. Prolonged seizure monitoring with stereotaxically implanted depth electrodes in patients with bilateral interictal temporal epileptogenic foci: How bilateral is bitemporal epilepsy? In Wada J. A., Penry J. K. (eds.). *Advances in Epileptology. The Tenth Epilepsy International Symposium.* New York: Raven Press, 1980. Pp. 83–88.
83. King D., So E., Marcus R., et al. Techniques and applications of sphenoidal recording. *J. Clin. Neurophysiol.* 3:51, 1986.
84. Wiesser H. G. Selective amygdalohippocampectomy: Indications, investigative technique and results. In Symon L (ed.). *Advances and Technical Standards in Neurosurgery,* vol. 13. Berlin: Springer-Verlag, 1986, Pp. 39–133.
85. Spencer S. S. Depth Electroencephalography in selection of refractory epilepsy for surgery. *Ann. Neurol.* 9:207, 1981.
86. Engel J. Jr., Suthreling W., Cahan L., et al. The role of positron emission tomography in the surgical therapy of epilepsy. In Porter R. J., Mattson R. H., Ward A. A. Jr., et al. (eds.). *Advances in Epileptology. The Fifteenth Epilepsy International Symposium.* New York: Raven Press, 1984. Pp. 427–432.
87. Oakley J., Ojemann G. A., Ojemann L. M., et al. Identifying epileptic foci

on contrast-enhanced computerized tomographic scans. *Arch. Neurol.* 36:669, 1979.
88. Kuhl D. E., Engel J. Jr., Phelps M. E., et al. Epileptic patterns of local cerebral metabolism and perfusion in humans determined by emission computed tomography of [18]FDG and [13]NH$_3$. *Ann. Neurol.* 8:348, 1980.
89. Landolt A. M. Ultrastructure of human sellar tumors. Correlations of clinical findings and morphology. *Acta Neurochir.* 22(Suppl.):1, 1975.
90. Kovacs K., Horvath E. Pathology of pituitary adenomas. *Bull. Los Angeles Neurol. Soc.* 42:92, 1979.
91. Kovacs K., Horvath E., Ryan N., et al. Null cell adenoma of the human pituitary. *Virchows Arch. Pathol. Anat.* 387:165, 1980.
92. Sapziante R., deDivitiis E., Stella L., et al. The empty sella. *Surg. Neurol.* 16:418, 1981.
93. Sage M. R., Blumberg P. C., Mulligan B. P., et al. The clinical and radiological features of the empty sella syndrome. *Clin. Radiol.* 31:513, 1980.
94. Doppman J. L., Oldfield E. H., Cruddy A. G., et al. Petrosal sampling for Cushing's syndrome: Anatomical and technical considerations. *Radiology* 150:99, 1984.
95. Mohr G., Hardy J. Hemorrhage, necrosis, and apoplexy in pituitary adenomas. *Surg. Neurol.* 18:181, 1982.
96. Roppolo H. M. N., Latchaw R. E. Normal pituitary gland. I. Microscopic anatomy–CT correlation. *Am. J. Radiol.* 4:927, 1983.
97. Roppolo H. M. N., Latchaw R. E., Meyer J. D. Normal pituitary gland. II. Microscopic anatomy–CT correlation. *Am. J. Radiol.* 4:937, 1983.
98. Davis P. C., Hoffman J. C. Jr., Tindall G. T., et al. Prolactin-secreting microadenomas: Inaccuracy of high-resolution CT imaging. *A.J.R.* 144:151, 1985.
99. Bilaniuk L. T., Zimmerman R. A., Wehrle F. W., et al. Magnetic resonance imaging of pituitary lesions using 1.0 to 1.5 T field strength. *Radiology* 153:415, 1984.
100. Kaufman B. Magnetic resonance imaging of the pituitary gland. *Radiol. Clin. North Am.* 22:795, 1984.
101. DiChiro G., Nelson K. B. The volume of the sella turcica. *A.J.R.* 87:989, 1962.
102. Lloyd H. M., Meares J. D., Jacobi J. Effects of oestrogen and bromocriptine on in vivo secretion and mitosis in prolactin cells. *Nature* 255:497, 1975.
103. Wass J. A. H., Moult P. J. A., Thorner M. O., et al. Reduction of pituitary tumor size in patients with prolactinoma and acromegaly treated with bromocriptine with or without radiotherapy. *Lancet* 2:66, 1979.
104. Thorner M. O., Perryman R. L., Rogul A. D., et al. Rapid changes of prolactinoma volume after withdrawal and reinstitution of bromocriptine. *J. Clin. Endocrinol. Metab.* 53:480, 1981.
105. Molitch M. E., Elton R. L., Blackwell R. E. Bromocriptine as primary therapy for prolactin-secreting macroadenomas: Results of a prospective multicenter study. *J. Clin. Endocrinol. Metab.* 60:698, 1985.
106. Wass J. A. H., Thorner M. O., Morris D. V., et al. Long-term treatment of acromegaly with bromocriptine. *Br. Med. J.* 1:875, 1977.
107. Besser G. M., Wass J. A. H., Thorner M. O. Acromegaly—results of long term treatment with bromocriptine. *Acta Endocrinol.* 216(Suppl.):187, 1978.
108. Parkes D. Drug therapy: Bromocriptine. *N. Engl. J. Med.* 301:873, 1979.
109. Bergh T., Nillius S. J., Wide L., et al. Clinical course and outcome of pregnancies in amenorrheic women with hyperprolactinemia and pituitary tumors. *Br. Med. J.* 1:875, 1978.
110. Wilson C. B. Neurosurgical management of large and invasive pituitary

tumors. In Tindall G. T., Collins W. F. (eds.). *Clinical management of Pituitary Disorders.* New York: Raven Press, 1979. Pp. 335–342.

111. Wilson C. B. A decade of pituitary microsurgery: The Herbert Olivecrona lecture. *J. Neurosurg.* 61:814, 1984.

112. Faria M. A. Jr., Tindall G. T. Transphenoidal microsurgery for prolactin-secreting pituitary adenomas. Results in 100 women with the amenorrhea-galactorrhea syndrome. *J. Neurosurg.* 56:33, 1982.

113. Randall R. V., Laws E. R., Abboud C. F., et al. Transphenoidal microsurgical treatment of prolactin-producing pituitary adenomas. Results in 100 patients. *Mayo Clin. Proc.* 58:108, 1983.

114. Domingue J. N., Richmond I. L., Wilson C. B. Results of surgery in 114 patients with prolactin-secreting adenomas. *Am. J. Obstet. Gynecol.* 137:102, 1980.

115. Burch W. A survey of results with transsphenoidal surgery in Cushing's disease. *N. Eng J. Med* 308:103, 1983.

116. Masters S. J., McClean P. M., Arcarese J. S., et al. Skull x-ray examinations after head trauma. Recommendations by multidisciplinary panel and validation study. *N. Engl. J. Med.* 36:84, 1987.

117. Kingsley D., Till K., Hoare R. Growing fractures of the skull. *J. Neurol. Neurosurg. Psychiatry* 41:312, 1978.

118. Zimmerman R. A., Bilaniuk L. T., Gennarelli T. Computed tomography of shearing injuries of the cerebral white matter. *Radiology* 127:393, 1978.

119. Zimmerman R. A., Bilaniuk L. T., Bruce D., et al. Computed tomography of pediatric head trauma: Acute general cerebral swelling. *Radiology* 126:403, 1978.

120. Barnett G. H., Ropper A. H., Johnson K. A. Physiological support and monitoring of critically ill patients during magnetic resonance imaging. *J. Neurosurg.* 68:246, 1988.

121. Molofsky W. J. Steroids and head trauma. *Neurosurgery* 15:424, 1984.

122. Clifton G. L., Robertson C. S., Grossman R. G., et al. The metabolic response to severe head injury. *J. Neurosurg.* 60:687, 1984.

123. Gaddisseux P., Ward J. D., Young H. F., et al. Nutrition and the neurosurgical patient. *J. Neurosurg.* 60:219, 1984.

124. Turner W. W. Nutritional considerations in the patient with disabling brain disease. *Neurosurgery* 16:707, 1985.

125. Norton J. A., Oh L. G., McClain C., et al. Intolerance to enteral feeding in the brain injured patient. *J. Neurosurg.* 68:62, 1988.

126. Rapp R. P., Young B., Twyman D., et al. The favorable effect of early parenteral feeding on survival in head-injured patients. *J. Neurosurg.* 58:906, 1983.

127. Klastersky J., Sadeghi M., Brihaye J. Antimicrobial prophylaxis in patients with rhinorrhea or otorrhea: A double blind study. *Surg. Neurol.* 6:111, 1976.

128. Oberson R. Radioisotopic diagnosis of rhinorrhea. *Radiol. Clin. Biol.* 41:28, 1972.

129. Spetzler R. F., Wilson C. B. Dural fistulae and their repair. In Youmans J. R. (ed.). *Neurological Surgery,* ed. 2. Philadelphia: Saunders, 1982. PP. 2209–2227.

130. Rimel R. W., Giordani B., Barth J. T., et al. Disability caused by minor head injury. *Neurosurgery* 9:221, 1981.

131. Jennet B. The problem of mild head injury. *Practitioner* 221:77, 1978.

132. Feuerman T., Wackym P. A., Gade G. F., et al. Value of skull radiography, head computed tomographic scanning, and admission for observation in cases of minor head injury. *Neurosurgery* 22:449, 1988.

133. El Gindi S., Salama M., Tawfik E. N., et al. A review of 2,000 patients with

craniocerebral injuries with regard to intracranial hematomas and other vascular complications. *Acta Neurochir.* 48:237, 1979.

134. Yamada S., Kindt G. W., Youmans J. R. Carotid artery occlusion due to nonpenetrating injury. *J. Trauma* 7:333, 1967.

135. Batzdorf U., Bentson J., Machleder H. I. Blunt trauma to the high cervical carotid artery. *Neurosurgery* 5:195, 1979.

136. Caldicott W. J. H., North J. B., Simpson D. A. Traumatic cerebrospinal fluid in children. *J. Neurosurg.* 38:1, 1973.

137. Annegers J. F., Grabow J. D., Groover R. V., et al. Seizures after head trauma: A population study. *Neurology* 30:683, 1980.

138. Jennett B. *Epilepsy after Non-Missile Head Injuries*, ed. 2. Chicago: Year Book, 1975.

139. Young B., Rapp R. P., Norton J. A., et al. Failure of prophylactically administered phenytoin to prevent early posttraumatic seizures. *J. Neurosurg.* 58:236, 1983.

140. Jennett B. Epilepsy and acute traumatic intracranial hematoma. *J. Neurol. Neurosurg. Psychiatry* 38:378, 1974.

141. Caveness W. F., Meirowsky A. M., Rish B. L., et al. The nature of posttraumatic epilepsy. *J. Neurosurg.* 50:545, 1979.

142. Penry J. K., White B. G., Brackett C. E. A controlled prospective study of the pharmacologic prophylaxis of posttraumatic epilepsy. *Neurology* 29:600, 1979 (abstr.).

143. Young B., Rapp R. P., Norton J. A., et al. Failure of prophylactically administered phenytoin to prevent late posttraumatic seizures. *J. Neurosurg.* 58:236, 1983.

144. Beyerl B., Black P. Posttraumatic hydrocephalus. *Neurosurgery* 15:257, 1984.

145. Kishore P. R. S., Lipper M. H., Miller J. D., et al. Post-traumatic hydrocephalus in patients with severe head injury. *Neuroradiology* 16:261. 1978.

146. Levin H. S., Meyers C. A., Grossman R. G. Ventricular enlargement after closed head injury. *Arch. Neurol.* 38:623, 1981.

147. Levin H. S., Grossman R. G., Rose J. E., et al. Long term neuropsychological outcome of closed head injury. *J. Neurosurg.* 50:412, 1979.

148. Barrow D. L., Spector R. H., Braun I. F., et al. Classification and treatment of spontaneous carotid-cavernous sinus fistulas. *J. Neurosurg.* 62:248, 1985.

149. Serbinenko F. A. Balloon catheterization and occlusion of major cerebral vessels. *J. Neurosurg.* 41:125, 1974.

150. Debrun G. M., Vinuela F., Fox A. J., et al. Indications for treatment and classification of 132 carotid-cavernous fistulas. *Neurosurgery* 22:285, 1988.

151. Barrow D. L., Fleischer A. S., Hoffman J. C. Complications of detachable ballon catheter technique in the treatment of traumatic intracranial arteriovenous fistulas. *J. Neurosurg.* 56:396, 1982.

152. Parkinson D. A surgical approach to the cavernous portion of the carotid artery. Anatomical studies and case report. *J. Neurosurg.* 23:474, 1965.

153. Parkinson D. Carotid cavernous fistula: Direct repair with preservation of the carotid artery. Technical note. *J. Neurosurg.* 38:99, 1973.

154. Dolnec V. Direct microsurgical repair of intracavernous vascular lesions. *J. Neurosurg.* 58:824, 1983.

155. Isamat F., Ferrer E., Twose J. Direct intracavernous obliteration of high-flow carotid-cavernous fistulas. *J. Neurosurg.* 65:770, 1986.

156. Jannetta P. J. Arterial compression of the trigeminal nerve at the pons in patients with trigeminal neuralgia. *J. Neurosurg.* 26:159, 1967.

157. Rasmussen P., Riishede J. Facial pain treated with carbamazepine (Tegretol). *Acta Neurol. Scand.* 46:385, 1970.
158. Lundsford L. D., Apfelbaum R. I. Choice of surgical therapeutic modalities for treatment of trigeminal neuralgia: Microvascular decompression, percutaneous retrogasserian thermal or glycerol rhizotomy. *Clin. Neurosurg.* 32:319, 1985.
159. Burchiel K., Steege T. D., Howe J. F., et al. Comparison of percutaneous radiofrequency gangiolysis and microvascular decompression for the surgical management of tic douloureux. *Neurosurgery* 9:111, 1981.
160. Sweet W. H., Wepsic S. G. Controlled thermocoagulation of trigeminal ganglion and results for differential destruction of pain fibers. *J. Neurosurg.* 39:143, 1969.
161. Tew J. M., Keller J. T. The treatment of trigeminal neuralgia by percutaneous radiofrequency technique. *Clin. Neurosurg.* 24:557, 1976.
162. Nugent G. R. Technique and results of 800 percutaneous radiofrequency themocoagulations for trigeminal neuralgia. *Appl. Neurophysiol.* 45:504, 1982.
163. Häkanson S. Trigeminal neuralgia treated by the injection of glycerol into the trigeminal cistern. *Neurosurgery* 9:638, 1981.
164. Lunsford L. D. Treatment of tic douloureux by percutaneous retrogasserian glycerol injection. *J.A.M.A.* 45:504, 1982.
165. Jannetta P. J. Microsurgical approach to the trigeminal nerve for tic douloureux. *Prog. Neurol. Surg.* 7:180, 1976.
166. Deen H. G., Scheithauer B. W., Ebersold M. J. Clinical and pathological study of meningiomas of the first two decades of life. *Neurosurgery* 56:317, 1982.
167. Sano K., Wakai S., Ochiai C., et al. Characteristics of intracranial meningiomas in childhood. *Childs Brain* 8:98, 1981.
168. New P. F., Aronow S., Hesslink J. R. National Cancer Institute Study: Evaluation of computed tomography in the diagnosis of intracranial neoplasms. IV. Meningiomas. *Radiology* 136:665, 1980.
169. Zimmerman R. D., Fleming C. A., Saint-Louis L. A., et al. Magnetic resonance imaging of meningiomas. *A.J.N.R.* 6:149, 1985.
170. Gold L. H. A., Kieffer S. A., Peterson H. O. Intracranial meningiomas: A retrospective analysis of the diagnostic value of plain skull films. *Neurology* 19:873, 1969.
171. Rutka J., Muller P. J., Chui M. Preoperative Gelfoam embolization of supratentorial meningiomas. *Can. J. Surg.* 28:441, 1985.
172. Cromptom M. R., Gautier-Smith P. C. The prediction of recurrence in meningiomas. *J. Neurol. Neurosurg. Psychiatry* 33:80, 1970.
173. Simpson D. The recurrence of intracranial meningiomas after surgical treatment. *J. Neurol. Neurosurg. Psychiatry* 20:22, 1957.
174. Solan M. J., Kramer S. The role of radiation therapy in the management of intracranial meningiomas. *Int. J. Radiat. Oncol. Biol. Phys.* 11:675, 1985.
175. Carella R. J., Ransohoff J., Newall J. Role of radiation therapy in the management of meningioma. *Neurosurgery* 10:332, 1982.
176. Kernohan J. W., Mabon R. F., Svien H. J., et al. A simplified classification of the gliomas. *Mayo Clin. Proc.* 24:71, 1949.
177. Zülch K. J. *Histological Typing of Tumors of the Central Nervous System.* Geneva: World Health Organization, 1979.
178. Burger P. C. Malignant astrocytic neoplasms: Classification, pathologic anatomy, and response to treatment. *Semin. Oncol.* 13:16, 1986.
179. Jellinger K. Glioblastoma multiforme: Morphology and biology. *Acta Neurochir.* 42:5, 1978.

180. Roth J. G., Elvidge A. R. Glioblastomas multiforme: A clinical survey. *J. Neurosurg.* 17:736, 1960.
181. Kelly P. J., Alker G. J. Jr. A stereotactic approach to deep-seated CNS neoplasms using the carbon dioxide laser. *Surg. Neurol.* 15:331, 1981.
182. Kelly P. J., Alker G. J. Jr., Goerss S. Computer assisted stereotactic laser microsurgery for the treatment of intracranial neoplasms. *Neurosurgery* 10:324, 1982.
183. Posner J. B., Chernik N. L. Intracranial metastases from systemic cancer. *Adv. Neurol.* 19:579, 1978.
184. Deck M. D. F., Messina A. V., Sackett J. F. Computed tomography in metastatic disease of the brain. *Radiology* 119:115, 1976.
185. Ransohoff J. Surgical management of metastatic tumors. *Semin. Oncol.* 2:21, 1975.
186. Bradac G. B., Schramm J., Grumme T., et al. CT of the base of the skull. *Neuroradiology* 17:1, 1978.
187. Solti-Bohman L. G., Magram D. L., Lo W. M., et al. Gas–CT cisternography for detection of small acoustic tumor. *Radiology* 150:403, 1984.
188. Latack J. T., Kartush J. M., Kemink J. L., et al. Epidermoidomas of the cerebellopontine angle and temporal bone: CT and MR aspects. *Radiology* 157:361, 1985.
189. Davis D. O., Roberson G. H. Angiographic diagnosis of posterior fossa mass lesions. *Semin. Roentgenol.* 6:89, 1971.
190. Kingsley D. P. E., Brooks G. B., Leung A. W-L., et al. Acoustic neuromas: Evaluation by magnetic resonance imaging. *A.J.N.R.* 6:1, 1986.
191. Jeffreys R. Pathologic and haematological aspects of posterior fossa: Hemangioblastoma. *J. Neurol. Neurosurg. Psychiatry* 38:112, 1975.
192. Ganti S. R., Silver A. J., Hilal S. K., et al. Computed tomography of cerebellar hemangioblastomas. *J. Comput. Assist. Tomogr.* 6:912, 1982.
193. Jeffreys R. Clinical and surgical aspects of posterior fossa: Hemangioblastoma. *J. Neurol. Neurosurg. Psychiatry* 38:112, 1975.
194. Sung P. I., Chang C. H., Harisiadis L. Cerebellar hemangioblastoma. *Cancer* 49:553, 1982.
195. Neuwelt E. A., Glasberg M., Frenkel E., et al. Malignant pineal tumors: A clinicopathological study. *J. Neurosurg.* 51:597, 1979.
196. Stein B. M. The infratentorial supracerebellar approach to pineal lesions. *J. Neurosurg.* 35:197, 1971.
197. Jooma R., Kendall B. E. Diagnosis and management of pineal tumors. *J. Neurosurg.* 58:654, 1983.
198. Sung D. I., Harisiadis L., Chang C. H. Midline pineal tumors and suprasellar germinomas: Highly curable by radiation. *Radiology* 128:745, 1978.
199. Sano K., Matsutani M. Pinealoma (germinoma) treated by direct surgery and postoperative irradiation: A long term follow-up. *Childs Brain* 8:81, 1981.
200. Post E. M. Currently available shunt systems: A review. *Neurosurgery* 16:257, 1985.
201. Portnoy H. D., Schulte R. R., Fox J. L., et al. Anti-siphon and reversible occlusion valves for shunting in hydrocephalus and preventing post-shunt subdural hematomas. *J. Neurosurg.* 38:729, 1973.
202. Gruber R., Jenny P., Herzog B. Experiences with the antisiphon device (ASD) in shunt therapy of pediatric hydrocephalus. *J. Neurosurg.* 61:156, 1984.
203. Kloss J. L. Craniosynostosis secondary to ventriculoarterial shunt. *Am. J. Dis. Child* 116:315, 1968.
204. Fox J. L., McCullogh D. C., Green R. C. Effect of cerebrospinal fluid shunts

on intracranial pressure and on cerebrospinal fluid dynamics: A new technique of pressure measurement. Results and concepts. *J. Neurol. Neurosurg. Psychiatry* 36:302, 1973.

205. McLaurin R. L. Infected cerebrospinal fluid shunts. *Surg. Neurol.* 1:191, 1973.

206. Schoenbaum S. C., Gardner P., Shillito J. Infections of cerebrospinal fluid shunts. Epidemiology, clinical manifestations and therapy. *J. Infect. Dis.* 131:543, 1975.

207. George R., Leibrock L., Epstein M. Long term analysis of cerebrospinal fluid shunt infections: A 25 year experience. *J. Neurosurg.* 51:804, 1979.

208. Venes J. L. Control of shunt infections report of 150 consecutive cases. *J. Neurosurg.* 45:311, 1976.

209. James H. E., Walsh J. W., Wilson H. D., et al. Prospective randomized study of therapy in cerebrospinal fluid shunt infection. *Neurosurgery* 7:459, 1980.

210. Guertin S. R., Cerebrospinal fluid shunts. Evaluation, complications, and crisis management. *Pediatr. Clin. North Am.* 34:203, 1987.

211. Frame P. T., McLaurin R. L. Treatment of CSF shunt infections with intrashunt plus oral antibiotic therapy. *J. Neurosurg.* 60:354, 1984.

212. Mori K., Raimondi A. J. An analysis of external ventricular drainage as a treatment for infected shunt. *Childs Brain* 1:243, 1975.

213. Rekate H., Yonas H., Colombi, et al. Ventricular drainage and intraventricular antibiotics in the treatment of CNS infections associated with hydrocephalus. Paper presented at the International Society of Pediatric Neurosurgery, Toronto 1975.

214. Scarff T. B., Nelson P. B., Reigel D. H. External drainage for ventricular infection following cerebrospinal fluid shunts. *Childs Brain* 4:129, 1978.

215. Harbaugh R. E., Saunders R. L., Edwards W. H. External ventricular drainage for control of posthemorrhagic hydrocephalus in premature infants. *J. Neurosurg.* 55:766, 1981.

216. White R. J., Dakters G. J., Yashon D. et al. Temporary control of cerebrospinal fluid volume and pressure by means of an externalized valve-drainage system. *J. Neurosurg.* 30:264, 1969.

217. Habal M. B., Vries J. K. Tension free closure of large meningomyelocoele defects. *Surg. Neurol.* 8:172, 1977.

218. Osaka K., Yamasaki S., Hirayama A., et al. Correlation of the response of the flushing device to compression with the clinical picture in the evaluation of the shunting system. *Childs Brain* 3:25, 1977.

219. Brereton R. The value of an ultrasonic flowmeter in assessing the function of CSF shunts. *J. Pediatr. Surg.* 15:73, 1980.

220. Epstein F., Mural R. Pediatric posterior fossa tumors: Hazards of the preoperative shunt. *Neurosurgery* 3:348, 1978.

221. Zimmerman R. A., Bilaniuk L. T., Pahlajani H. Spectrum of medulloblastomas demonstrated by computed tomography. *Radiology* 126:137, 1978.

222. Park T. S., Hoffman H. J., Hendrick E. B., et al. Medulloblastoma: Clinical presentation and management. Experience at the Hospital for Sick Children, Toronto, 1950–1980. *J. Neurosurg.* 30:226, 1983.

223. Hoffman H. H., Hendrick E. B., Humphreys R. P. Management of medulloblastoma in childhood. *Clin. Neurosurg.* 30:226, 1983.

224. Berry M. P., Jenkin D. T. Radiation treatment for medulloblastoma: A 21-year review. *J. Neurosurg.* 55:43, 1981.

225. Tomita T., McClone D. G. Medulloblastoma in childhood: Results of radical resection and low-dose neuraxis radiation therapy. *J. Neurosurg.* 64:238, 1986.

226. Hoffman H. H., Hendrick E. B., Humphreys R. P. Metastasis via ventricu-

loperitoneal shunt in patients with medulloblastoma. *J. Neurosurg.* 44:562, 1976.

227. Gol A. Cerebellar astrocytomas in children. *Am. J. Dis. Child* 106:21, 1963.
228. Zimmerman R. A., Bilianiuk L. T. Computed tomography of cerebellar astrocytoma. *A.J.R.* 130:929, 1978.
229. Carmel P. W. Cerebellar tumors in childhood. *Dev. Med. Child Neurol.* 14:809, 1972.
230. Winston K., Gilles F. H. Leviton A., et al. Cerebellar gliomas in children. *J. Natl. Cancer Inst.* 58:833, 1977.
231. Barone B. M., Elvidge A. R. Ependymomas: A clinical study. *J. Neurosurg.* 33:428, 1970.
232. Dohrmann G. J., Farwell J. R., Flannery J. T. Ependymomas and ependymoblastomas in children. *J. Neurosurg.* 45:273, 1976.
233. Enzmann D. R., Norman D., Levin V., et al. Computed tomography in the follow-up of medulloblastomas and ependymomas. *Radiology* 128:57, 1978.
234. Foltz E. L., Loeser J. D. Craniosynostosis. *J. Neurosurg.* 43:48, 1975.
235. Matson D. D., Jerva M. J. Recurrent meningitis associated with congenital lumbosacral dermal sinus tract. *J. Neurosurg.* 25:288, 1966.
236. Sharrad W. J. W. The orthopedic surgery of spina bifida. *Clin. Orthop. Rel. Res.* 92:195, 1973.
237. Forsythe W. I., Kinely J. G. Bowel control of children with spina bifida. *Dev. Med. Child Neurol.* 12:27, 1970.
238. Winslow C. M., Solomon D. H., Chassin M. R., et al. The appropriateness of carotid endarterectomy. *N. Engl. J. Med.* 318:721, 1988.
239. Shaw D. A., Venables G. S., Cartilage N. E. F., et al. Carotid endarterectomy in patients with transient cerebral ischemia. *J. Neurol. Sci.* 64:45, 1984.
240. Byer J. A., Easton J. D. Transient cerebral ischemia: Review of surgical results. *Prog. Cardiovasc. Dis.* 22:389, 1980.
241. Whisnant J. P., Sandok B. A., Sundt T. M. Carotid endarterectomy for unilateral carotid system transient cerebral ischemia. *Mayo Clin. Proc.* 58:171, 1983.
242. Committee on health care issues, American Neurological Association. Does carotid endarterectomy decrease stroke and death in patients with transient ischemic attacks? *Ann. Neurol.* 22:72, 1987.
243. The Canadian Cooperative Study Group. A randomized trial of aspirin and sulfinpyrazone in threatened stroke. *N. Engl. J. Med.* 299:53, 1978.
244. Chambers B. R., Norris J. W. Outcome in patients with asymptomatic neck bruits. *N. Engl. J. Med.* 315:860, 1986.
245. Wolf P. A., Kannel W. B., Sorlie P., et al. Asymptomatic carotid bruit and risk of stroke: The Framingham study. *J.A.M.A.* 245:1442, 1981.
246. Quiñones-Baldrich W. J., Moore W. S. Asymptomatic carotid stenosis: Rationale for management. *Arch. Neurol.* 42:378, 1985.
247. Takolander R. J., Bergentz S-E, Ericsson B. F. Carotid artery surgery in patients with minor stroke. *Br. J. Surg.* 70:13, 1983.
248. Whittemore A. D., Ruby S. T., Couch N. P., et al. Early carotid endarterectomy in patients with small, fixed neurologic deficits. *J. Vasc. Surg.* 1:795, 1984.
249. Duncan G. W., Gruber J. O., Dewey C. F. Jr., et al. Evaluation of carotid stenosis by phonoangiography. *N. Engl. J. Med.* 293:1124, 1975.
250. Kistler J. P., Lees R. S., Miller A., et al. Correlations spectral phonoangiography and carotid angiography with gross pathology in carotid stenosis. *N. Engl. J. Med.* 305:417, 1981.

251. Reid J. M., Spencer M. P. Ultrasonic Doppler technique for imaging blood vessels. *Science* 176:1235, 1972.
252. White D. N. Color-coded Doppler carotid imaging. In Bernstein E. F. (ed.). *Non-invasive Diagnostic Techniques in Vascular Disease*, ed. 2. St Louis: Mosby, 1982. Pp. 258–264.
253. Blackshear W. M. Jr., Phillips D. J., Chikos P. M., et al. Carotid velocity patterns in normal and stenotic vessels. *Stroke* 11:67, 1980.
254. James E. M., Earnest F. IV, Forbes G. S., et al. High-resolution dynamic ultrasound imaging of the carotid bifurcation: A prospective evaluation. *Radiology* 144:853, 1982.
255. Zweibel W. J., Austin C. W., Sackett J. F., et al. Correlation of high-resolution B-mode and continuous wave Doppler sonography with arteriography in the diagnosis of carotid stenosis. *Radiology* 149:523, 1983.
256. Glover J. L., Bendick P. J., Jackson V. P., et al. Duplex ultrasonography, digital subtraction angiography, and conventional angiography in assessing carotid atherosclerosis. *Arch. Surg.* 119:664, 1984.
257. Yao J. S. T., Flinn W. R., Bergan J. J. Non-invasive vascular diagnostic testing: Techniques and clinical applications. *Prog. Cardiovasc. Dis.* 26:459, 1984.
258. Wiebers D. O., Folger W. N., Forbes G. S., et al. Ophthalmodynamometry and ocular pneumoplethysmography for the detection of carotid occlusive disease. *Arch. Neurol.* 39:690, 1982.
259. Gee W. Review of ocular pneumoplethysmography. *Surv. Ophthalmol.* 29:276, 1985.
260. Muller H. R. The diagnosis of internal carotid occlusion by directional Doppler sonography of the ophthalmic artery. *Neurology* 22:816, 1972.
261. Meyer G. A., Berman I. R., Doty D. B., et al. Hemodynamic responses to acute quadriplegia with or without chest trauma. *J. Neurosurg.* 34:168, 1971.
262. Hadley M. N., Dickman C. A., Browmner C. M., et al. Acute traumatic atlas fractures: Management and long-term outcome. *Neurosurgery* 23:31, 1988.
263. Schneider R. C., et al. "Hangman's fracture" of the cervical spine. *J. Neurosurg.* 22:141, 1965.
264. Pang D., Wilberger J. E. Jr. Spinal cord injury without radiographic abnormalities in children. *J. Neurosurg.* 57:114, 1982.
265. Hadley M. N., Zabramski J. M., Browner C. M., et al. Pediatric spinal trauma: Review of 122 cases of spinal cord and vertebral column injuries. *J. Neurosurg.* 68:18, 1988.
266. Ruge J. R., Sinson G. P., McClone D. G., et al. Pediatric spinal injury: the very young. *J. Neurosurg.* 68:25, 1988.
267. Kalfas I., Wilberger J., Goldberg A., et al. Magnetic resonance imaging in acute spinal cord trauma. *Neurosurgery* 23:295, 1988.
268. Ohry A., Molho M., Rozin R. Alterations of pulmonary function in spinal cord injury patients. *Paraplegia* 13:101, 1975.
269. Ledsome J. R., Sharp J. M. Pulmonary function in acute cervical cord injury. *Am. Rev. Respir. Dis.* 124:41, 1981.
270. Berlly M. H., Wilmont C. B. Acute abdominal emergencies during the first four weeks after spinal cord injury. *Arch. Phys. Med. Rehabil.* 65:687, 1984.
271. Myllynen P., Kammonen M., Rokkanen P., et al. Deep venous thrombosis and pulmonary embolism in patients with acute spinal cord injury: A comparison with non-paralyzed patients immobilized due to spinal fractures. *J. Trauma.* 25:541, 1985.
272. Silver J. R., Moulton A. Prophylactic anticoagulant therapy against pulmonary emboli in acute paraplegia. *Br. Med. J.* 2:338, 1973.

273. Crutchfield W. G. Skeletal traction for dislocation of cervical spine. Report of case. *South. Surg.* 2:156, 1933.
274. Gardner W. J. The principle of spring-loaded points for cervical traction. *J. Neurosurg.* 39:543, 1973.
275. Kaufman H. H. Modification for the Gardner-Wells skull traction tongs. *Surg. Neurol.* 6:220, 1976.
276. Rimel R. W., Butler A. B., Winn H. R., et al. Modified skull tongs for cervical traction. Technical note. *J. Neurosurg.* 55:848, 1981.
277. Perry J., Nickel V. L. Total cervical spine fusion for neck paralysis. *J. Bone Joint Surg.* 41A:37, 1959.
278. Nickel V. L., Perry J., Garrett A., et al. The halo. A spinal skeleton traction fixation device. *J. Bone Joint Surg.* 50A:1400, 1968.
279. Prolo D. J., Runnels J. B., Jameson R. M. The injured cervical spine. Immediate and long-term stabilization with the halo. *J.A.M.A.* 224:591, 1973.
280. Cooper P. R., Maravilla K. R., Sklar F. H., et al. Halo immobilization of cervical spine fractures. Indications and results. *J. Neurosurg.* 50:603, 1979.
281. Chan R. C., Schweigel J. F., Thompson G. B. Halo-thoracic brace immobilization in 188 patients with acute cervical spine injuries. *J. Neurosurg.* 58:508, 1983.
282. Trippi A. C. The principle of dual purpose cranial tongs. *Neurosurgery* 11:258, 1982.
283. Nickel V. L., Perry J., Garrett A. L., et al. Application of the halo. *Orthop. Prosthet. App. J.* 14:31, 1960.
284. Murphy D. J., Young R. Step by step procedure for applying the halo vest. *Orthop. Rev.* 4:33, 1975.
285. Thomassen E. H., Young R. Application of the halo ring. *Orthop. Rev.* 3:62, 1974.
286. Schwentker E. P., Skinner S. R., Bowman L. S. The Hershey halo jig. *Orthopedics* 4:8, 909, 1981.
287. Young R., Murphy D. J. Hygiene care in the halo vest. *Orthop. Rev.* 9:73, 1980.
288. Hummelgard A., Martin E. Management of the patient in a halo brace. *J. Neurosurg. Nurs.* 14:113, 1982.
289. Feldman R. A., Khayyat G. F. Perforation of the skull by a Gardner-Wells tong. *J. Neurosurg.* 44:119, 1976.
290. Fried L. C. Cervical spinal cord injury during skeletal traction. *J.A.M.A.* 229:181, 1974.
291. Kaufman H. H., Harris J. H. Jr., Spencer J. A., et al. Danger of traction during radiography for cervical trauma (letter). *J.A.M.A.* 247:2369, 1982.
292. Weisl H. Unusual complications of skull caliper traction. *J. Bone Joint Surg.* 54B: 143, 1971.
293. Taylor A. S. Fracture dislocation of the cervical spine. *Ann. Surg.* 90:321, 1929.
294. Bremer A. M., Nguyen T. Q. Internal metal fixation combined with interbody fusion in cases of cervical spine injury. *Neurosurgery* 12:649, 1983.
295. Cahill D. W., Bellarigue R., Ducker T. B. Bilateral facet to spinous process fusion: A new technique for posterior spinal fusion after trauma. *Neurosurgery* 13:1, 1983.
296. Wagner F. C. Jr., Chehrazi B. Early decompression and neurological outcome in acute cervical spinal cord injuries. *J. Neurosurg.* 56:699, 1982.
296a. Mayfield F. H. Cervical spondylosis: A comparison of the anterior and posterior approaches. *Clin. Neurosurg.* 13:181, 1965.
297. Smith G. W., Robinson R. A. Anterior lateral cervical disc removal and

interbody fusion for cervical disc syndrome. *Bull. Johns Hopkins Hosp.* 96:223, 1955.

298. Cloward R. B. The anterior approach for removal of ruptured cervical discs. *J. Neurosurg.* 15:602, 1958.
299. Robertson J. T. Anterior operations for herniated cervical disc and for myelopathy. *Clin. Neurosurg.* 25:245, 1978.
300. Murphy M. G., Gado M. Anterior cervical discectomy without interbody fusion. *J. Neurosurg.* 37:71, 1972.
301. Wilson D. H., Campbell D. D. Anterior cervical discectomy without bone graft. Report of 71 cases. *J. Neurosurg.* 47:551, 1977.
302. Fager C. A. Rationale and techniques of posterior approaches to cervical disc and spondylosis. *Surg. Clin. North Am.* 56:581, 1976.
303. Scoville W. B., Dohrmann G. J., Corkill G. Late results of cervical disc surgery. *J. Neurosurg.* 45:203, 1976.
304. Mishkin F. Determination of cerebral death by radionuclide angiography. *Radiology* 115:135, 1975.
305. Bowerman R. A., et al. Natural history of neonatal periventricular/intraventricular hemorrhage and its complications: Sonographic observations. *A.J.R.* 143:1041, 1984.
306. Drake C. G. Report of World Federation of Neurological Surgeons Committee on a Universal Subarachnoid Hemorrhage Grading Scale. *J. Neurosurg.* 68:985, 1988.
307. Jennett B, Bond M. Assessment of outcome after severe brain damage. A practical scale. *Lancet* 1:480, 1975.
308. Heros R. C., Tu Y. K. Is surgical therapy needed for unruptured arteriovenous malformations? *Neurology* 37:279, 1987.
309. Oyesiku N. M., Barrow D. L., Eckman J. R., et al. Intracranial aneurysms in sickle cell anemia: A paradigm for acquired aneurysm formation. *Stroke* 21:168, 1990.
310. Kassell N. F., Torner J. C., Adams H. P. Jr. Antifibrinolytic therapy in the acute period following aneurysmal subarachnoid hemorrhage. Preliminary observations from the Cooperative Aneurysm Study. *J. Neurosurg.* 61:225, 1984.
311. Vermeulen M., Lindsay K. W., Murray G. D., et al. Antifibrinolytic treatment in subarachnoid hemorrhage. *N. Engl. J. Med.* 311:432, 1984.
312. Teasdale G., Jennett B. Assessment of coma and impaired conciousness. A practical scale. *Lancet* 1:480, 1975.
313. Deutschman C. S., Haines S. J. Anticonvulsant prophylaxis in neurological surgery. *Neurosurgery* 17:510, 1985.
314. Crawford P. M., West C. R., et al. Arteriovenous malformations of the brain:natural history in unoperated patients. *J. Neurol. Neurosurg. Psychiatry* 49:1, 1986.
315. Brown R. D. Jr., Wiebers D. O., Forbes G., et al. The natural history of unruptured intracranial arteriovenous malformations. *J. Neurosurg.* 68:352, 1988.
316. Spetzler F., Martin N. A. A proposed grading system for arteriovenous malformations. *J. Neurosurg.* 65:476, 1986.
317. Heros R. C., Tu Y. K. Is surgical therapy needed for unruptured arteriovenous malformations? *Neurology* 37:279, 1987.
318. Iansek R., Elstein A. S., Balla J. I. Application of decision analysis to management of cerebral arteriovenous malformation. *Lancet* 1:1132, 1983.
319. Luessenhop A. J., Rosa L. Cerebral arteriovenous malformations. Indications for and results of surgery, and the role of intravascular techniques. *J. Neurosurg.* 60:14, 1984.

320. Betti O. O., Munari C., Rosler R. Stereotactic radiosurgery with the linear accelerator: treatment of arteriovenous malformations. *Neurosurgery* 24:311, 1989.
321. Steiner L., Lindquist C. Radiosurgery in cerebral arteriovenous malformations. In Tasker R. R. (ed.). *Neurosurgery: State of the Art Reviews*. Philadelphia: Hanley & Belfus, Vol 2, No. 1, 1987. Pp. 329–336.
322. Wechsler D., Stone C. P. *Wechsler Memory Scale*. New York: Psychological Corp. Publishers, 1945.
323. Wada J. Rasmussen T. Intracarotid injection of sodium amytal for the lateralization of cerebral speech dominance: experimental and clinical observations. *J. Neurosurg.* 17:266, 1960.
324. Milner B., Branch C., Rasmussen T. Study of short-term memory after intracarotid injection of sodium amytal. *Trans. Am. Neurol. Assoc.* 87:224, 1962.
325. Reichlin S. The prolactinoma problem. *N. Engl. J. Med.* 300:313, 1979.
326. Klibanski A., Neer R. M., Beitins I. Z., et al. Decreased bone density in hyperprolactinemic women. *N. Engl. J. Med.* 303:1511, 1980.
327. McArthur R. G., Cloutier M. D., Hayles A. B., et al. Cushing's disease in children: findings in 13 cases. *Mayo Clin. Proc.* 47:318, 1972.
328. Styne D. M.,Grumbach M. D., Kaplan S. L., et al. Treatment of Cushing disease in childhood and adolescence by transsphenoidal microadenectomy. *N. Engl. J. Med.* 310:889, 1984.
329. Hamilton C. R., Adams L. C., Maloof F. Hyperthyroidism due to a thyrotropin-producing pituitary chromophobe adenoma. *N. Engl. J. Med.* 283:1077, 1970.
330. Nelson D. H., Meakin J. W., Thorn G. W. ACTH-producing pituitary tumors following adrenalectomy for Cushing's syndrome. *Ann. Intern. Med.* 52:560, 1960.
331. Schnall A. M., Kovacs K., Brodkey J. S., et al. Pituitary Cushing's disease without adenoma. *Acta Endocrinol. (Copenh).* 94:297, 1980.
332. Tindall G. T., Kovacs K., Horvath E., et al. Human prolactin producing adenomas and bromocriptine: a histological immunocytochemical, ultrastructural and morphometric study. *J. Clin. Endocrinol. Metab.* 55:1178, 1982.
333. Jackson I. M. D., Barnard L. B., Lamberton P. Role of a long-acting Somatostatin analogue (SMS 201-995) in the treatment of acromegaly. *Am. J. Med.* 81 (Suppl 6B):94, 1986.
334. Barkan A. L., Lloyd R. V., Chandler W. F., et al. Preoperative treatment of acromegaly with long-acting Somatostatin analogue (SMS 201-995): Shrinkage of invasive pituitary macroadenomas and improved surgical remission rate. *J. Clin. Endocrinol. Metab.* 67:1040, 1988.
335. Zimmerman R. D., Leeds N. E., Danziger A. Subdural empyema: CT findings. *Radiology* 150:417, 1984.
336. Renaudin J. W., Frazee J. Subdural empyema: Importance of early diagnosis. *Neurosurgery* 7:477, 1980.
337. Rosenblum M. L., Hoff J. T., Norman D., et al. Decreased mortality from brain abscesses since advent of computed tomography. *J. Neurosurg.* 49:658, 1978.
338. Rosenblum M. L., Mampalam T. J., Pons V. G. Controversies in the management of brain abscesses. *Clin. Neurosurg.* 33:603, 1985.
339. Stephanov S. Surgical treatment of brain abscesses. *Neurosurgery* 22:724, 1988.
340. Leblanc R., Knowles K. F., Melanson D., et al. Neurocysticercosis: Surgical and Medical Management with Praziquantel. *Neurosurgery* 18:419, 1986.

341. Salaki J. S., Louria, Chmel H. Fungal and yeast infections of the central nervous system. *Medicine* 63:108, 1984.
342. Young R. F., Gade G., Grinell V. Surgical treatment for fungal infections of the central nervous system. *J. Neurosurg.* 63:371, 1985.
343. Weiner L. P., Fleming J. O. Viral Infections of the nervous system. *J. Neurosurg.* 61:207, 1984.
344. Bydder G. M. et al. MR imaging of meningiomas including studies with and without gadolinium-DTPA. *J. Comput. Assist. Tomogr.* 9:690, 1985.
345. Weir B., McDonald N., Mukike B. Intracranial vascular complications of choroid carcinoma. *Neurosurgery* 2:139, 1978.
346. Constans J. P., de Divitiis E., Donzelli R., et al. Spinal metastases with neurological manifestations. Review of 600 cases. *J. Neurosurg.* 59:111, 1983.
347. Sundaresan N., Galicich J. H., Lane J. M., et al. Treatment of neoplastic epidural cord compression by vertebral body resection and stabilization. *J. Neurosurg.* 63:676, 1985.
348. Jennings M. T., Gelman R., Hochberg F. Intracranial germ-cell tumors: natural history and pathogenesis. *J. Neurosurg.* 63:155, 1985.
349. Walker A. E. *A History of Neurological Surgery.* New York: Hafner, 1967.
350. Noetzel M. J., Baker R. P. Shunt fluid examination: risks and benefits in the evaluation of shunt malfunction and infection. *J. Neurosurg.* 61:328, 1984.
351. Rorke L. B. The cerebellar medulloblastoma and its relationship to primitive neuroectodermal tumors. *J. Neuropathol. Exp. Neurol.* 42:1, 1983.
352. Deutsch M. The impact of myelography on the treatment results for medulloblastoma. *Int. J. Radiat. Oncol.* 10:999, 1984.
353. Marton L. J., Edwards M. S., Levin V. A. et al. CSF polyamines: A new and important means of monitoring patients with medulloblastoma. *Cancer* 47:757, 1981.
354. Cook B. R., Guthkelch A. N. Modern approaches to the treatment of medulloblastoma. *Dev. Med. Child. Neurol.* 25:245, 1983.
355. Berger M. S., Edwards M. S. B., LaMasters D., et al. Pediatric brain tumors: radiographic, pathological and clinical correlations. *Neurosurgery* 12:298, 1983.
356. Epstein F., McCleary E. L. Intrinsic brain-stem tumors of childhood: surgical indications. *J. Neurosurg.* 64:11, 1986.
357. Eifel P. J., Cassady J. R., Belli J. A. Radiation therapy of tumors of the brainstem and midbrain in children: experience of the Joint Center for Radiation Therapy and Children's Hospital Medical Center (1971–1981). *Int. J. Radiat. Oncol. Biol. Phys.* 13:847, 1987.
358. Whittle J. R., Johnston I. H., Besser M. Intracranial pressure changes in craniostenosis. *Surg. Neurol.* 21:367, 1984.
359. Furuya Y., Edwards M. S. B., Alpers, et al. Computerized tomography of cranial sutures. Part 2: Abnormalities of sutures and skull deformity in craniosynostosis. *J. Neurosurg.* 61:59, 1984.
360. Hoffman H. J., Mohr G. lateral canthal advancement of the supraorbital margin: A new corrective technique in the treatment of coronal synostosis. *J. Neurosurg.* 445:376, 1976.
361. Olds M. V., Storrs B., Walker M. L. Surgical treatment of sagittal synostosis. *Neurosurgery* 18:345, 1986.
362. Salkind G., Sutton L. N., Bruce D. A., et al. Management of trigonocephaly. *Surg. Neurol.* 25:159, 1986.
363. Hoffman H. J., Taecholarn C., Hendrick E. B., et al. Management of lipomyelomeningoceles. Experience at the Hospital for Sick Children, Toronto. *J. Neurosurg.* 62:1, 1985.

364. Shurtleff D. B., Lemire R. J., Warkany J. Embryology, etiology, and epidemiology. In Shurtleff DB (ed.). *Myelodysplasias and Exstrophies: Significance, Prevention and Treatment.* New York: Grune & Stratton, 1986. PP. 39–64.
365. Richards I. D. G., McIntosh H. T., Sweenie S. A genetic study of anencephaly and spina bifida in Glasgow. *Dev. Med. Child. Neurol.* 14:626, 1972.
366. Reigel D. H. Spina Bifida. In Pediatric Neurosurgery: Surgery of the Developing Nervous System. Section of Pediatric Neurosurgery of the American Association of Neurological Surgeons, 2nd ed. Philadelphia: Saunders, 1989. Pp. 35–52.
367. Piatt J. H. Jr., Hoffman H. J., The tethered spinal cord with focus on the tight filum terminale. A review. II. Clinical presentations, diagnostic investigations, radiological features, urological investigations, electrophysiological evaluation, results. *Neuro-Orthopedics* 4:1, 1987.
368. Lee C. et al. Evaluation of traumatic atlantooccipital dislocations. *A.J.N.R.* 8:19, 1987.
369. Anderson L. D., D'Alonzo R. T. Fractures of the odontoid process of the axis. *J. Bone Joint Surg. [Am.]* 56:1663, 1974.
370. Seljeskog E. L., Chou S. N. Spectrum of hangman's fracture. *J. Neurosurg.* 45:3, 1976.
371. Levine A. M., Edwards C. C. Traumatic spondylolisthesis of the axis (Hangman's fracture). *Orthop. Clin. North. Am.* 17:i, 1986.
372. Cattell H. S., Filtzer D. L. Pseudosubluxation and other normal variations of the cervical spine in children. *J. Bone Joint. Surg.* 47-A:1295, 1965.
373. Swischuk L. E. Anterior dislocation of C2 in children: physiologic or pathologic? *Radiology* 122:759, 1977.
374. Caffey's Pediatrics X-Ray Diagnosis: An Integrated Imaging Approach, 8th ed. Edited by Frederic N. Silverman, Chicago: Yearbook, 1985.
375. Rawlings C. E. III, Giangaspero F., Burger P. C., et al. Ependymomas: A clinicopathologic study. *Surg Neurol* 29:271, 1988.

Suggested Readings

Banna M. *Clinical Radiology of the Spine and Spinal Cord,* Rockville, MD: Aspen, 1985.
Brant-Zawadaki M., and David Norman (eds.). *Magnetic Resonance Imaging of the Central Nervous System.* New York: Raven Press, 1987.
Burger P. C., Vogel F. S. *Surgical Pathology of the Nervous System and Its Coverings,* 2nd ed. New York: Wiley, 1982.
Gehweiler J. A. Jr., Osborne R. L., Becker R. F. *The Radiology of Vertebral Trauma.* Philadelphia: Saunders, 1980.
McLaurin R. L., Schut L., Venes J. L., Epstein F. Pediatric Neurosurgery: Surgery of the Developing Nervous System, 2nd ed. Philadelphia: Saunders, 1989.
Orrison W. W., Jr. *Introduction to Neuroimaging.* Boston: Little, Brown, 1989.
Youmans J. R. (ed.). *Neurological Surgery. Vols. 1–6,* 3rd ed. Philadelphia: Saunders, 1990.

6. Intraoperative Care

Intraoperative care is a team effort requiring the cooperation of the neurosurgeon, neuroanesthesiologist, and nursing staff. Foresight and planning are well rewarded; hindsight and afterthought may improve the next performance but do little for the case at hand. Most teams have established routines for various procedures. Intraoperative care is especially important because of the patient's vulnerability during this period. The intraoperative management of the pediatric patient poses problems of hypothermia and anemia (from blood loss), either of which may lead to physiologic derangements.

Neuroanesthesia

In neuroanesthesia, the goals are cerebral protection, analgesia, a "slack" brain, and a patient who can be evaluated at the end of the procedure.

Monitoring

Certain monitoring parameters are common to all major surgery. These include blood pressure (by cuff or intraarterial line), electrocardiogram (ECG), temperature, neuromuscular blockade, pulse oximetry, capnometry, urinary output, and central venous or pulmonary artery pressure (Swan-Ganz catheter) for patients with severe pulmonary or cardiac disease.

For patients in the sitting position, a precordial Doppler and right atrial catheter are placed to manage potential air embolism. Special monitoring may include cerebral blood flow (CBF) in neurovascular procedures, neurophysiologic parameters such as an electroencephalogram (EEG), and evoked potentials (EPs).

Premedication

Premedication is given to allay patient anxiety, blunt vagal response, and facilitate induction. Neurosurgical patients are often obtunded or at risk for intracranial hypertension, and therefore sedatives must be carefully chosen. Usually an antiemetic, a sedative (diazepam or lorazepam), and atropine are given as premedication. Sometimes the anesthesiologist may dispense with premedication if the patient is deeply comatose. Cimetidine or ranitidine, histamine antagonists, may be given to suppress gastric secretion and raise gastric pH.

Induction

The goals at induction are to avoid elevation of intracranial pressure (ICP) or reduction in CBF. Hypertension or hypotension, hypoxia, hypercapnia, and coughing should be avoided. When the patient arrives in the operating room, place intravenous lines and monitoring equipment. Preoxygenate the patient and induce anesthesia. Frequently thiopental, a muscle relaxant, a narcotic, lidocaine, and an inhalational agent are given.

Narcotics are given to blunt the cardiovascular responses to intubation. *Fentanyl* or *sufentanil* is commonly used. Both cause a decrease in CBF and cerebral metabolic rate for oxygen ($CMRO_2$) [1]. *Lidocaine* may be given at this time, since it causes a brief but marked reduction in ICP. Give inhalational agents in low doses to prevent the hypertension that often attends early surgical stimulation.

After intubation, check the position of the tube and firmly secure it in place. Protect the patient's eyes with lubricating ointment and tape patches over the lids. Insert the oral airway, esophageal stethoscope, and temperature probe appropriately. Apply the ground plate of the cautery at a suitable location (if a hair-bearing area, shave enough for good contact). If the procedure is expected to last more than several hours, or if diuretics or hyperosmolar agents are to be used, insert a Foley catheter. If cerebral spinal fluid (CSF) drainage is required, place the lumbar drainage catheter. After the patient is positioned, reascertain the functional integrity of the drainage system. If spinal traction will be required, now is a good time to apply the apparatus (if not in place preoperatively). Finally, the surgical team positions the patient for the procedure.

Maintenance

There are two main neuroanesthetic techniques: (1) *intravenous* or *balanced anesthesia*, which involves the use of several drugs, including barbiturates (thiopental), narcotics (fentanyl), tranquilizers (diazepam, droperidol), and muscle relaxants (pancuronium, curare); and (2) the *inhalation* technique, which involves using a halogenated agent.

Both techniques may be used with a nitrous oxide–oxygen mixture (50:50). In favor of the former technique is the cerebral protection offered by a reduction in cerebral metabolic rate (CMR) from barbiturates and narcotics; disadvantages include the multiplicity of medications, delayed emergence from anesthesia, and less control of arterial hypertension. The latter technique recommends itself by its ease of application, fewer agents involved, and the patient's rapid emergence, which makes immediate postoperative evaluation easier. Undesirable effects of inhalational agents include the increase in CBF and decrease in cerebral venous return (CVR), which may aggravate cerebral edema and increase ICP. A newer inhalational agent, isoflurane, has overcome some of the difficulties of this technique [2, 3].

The neuroanesthesiologist selects a technique based on the nature of the intracranial pathologic state and personal experience. To facilitate brain relaxation, mannitol, 0.5 to 1.5 gm/kg intravenously, is given before the craniotomy is completed. It may be supplemented with furosemide, 10 to 40 mg intravenously. Hyperventilation to a pCO_2 of 25 to 30 mm Hg augments brain relaxation.

After craniotomy and dural opening, the anesthetic requirement is less because the brain is insensitive to pain. Narcotics are usually withheld toward the end of the procedure to allow for postoperative neurologic examination.

Recovery

In most cases, neurosurgeons prefer that the patient awaken before leaving the operating room unless otherwise indicated. The awakening should be smooth and unattended by coughing or other activity that may increase ICP. If the head must be bandaged, there should be sufficient anesthesia available to allow for this. All necessary equipment is arranged for transfer of the patient to the recovery room or intensive care unit.

Types of Agents and Induced Hypotension

Inhalational Agents

Inhalational agents are begun in low doses during induction. *Halothane, enflurane*, and *isoflurane* all produce cerebral vasodilatation and increase CBF and ICP; with increasing doses, autoregulatory mechanisms become less effective and CBF more pressure-dependent [4]. This increase in ICP may be attenuated by hyperventilation or barbiturates before introducing the inhalational agent. Isoflurane is the most effective of the three agents in reducing CMR and has the least effect on ICP and CBF. It also has the widest margin of safety. Most of the halogenated agents depress $CMRO_2$ in a dose-related fashion; high doses of enflurane may induce seizures and therefore increase $CMRO_2$. Volatile agents cause an increased sensitivity (left-sided shift) in the carbon dioxide–CBF response curve; i.e., hypocapnia still reduces CBF but hypercapnia causes a greater increase in CBF for a particular value of pCO_2.

Nitrous oxide seems to have less well-defined effects on cerebrovascular dynamics and cerebral metabolism. Some animal studies suggest a vasodilator effect with an increase in CBF; the data from human studies are equivocal. Nitrous oxide may contribute to the development of a tension pneumocephalus. At the conclusion of a craniotomy, some air may be trapped inside the skull; nitrous oxide, being 30 times more soluble than nitrogen, diffuses more rapidly into the air space from the blood than nitrogen can diffuse out, leading to an increase in ICP. For this reason, nitrous oxide should be turned off well before dural closure is complete.

Intravenous Anesthetics

Barbiturates are the prototypical intravenous agent; they depress CMR, cause cerebral vasoconstriction, and reduce CBF and ICP. However, barbiturates may cause systemic hypotension, and recovery from barbiturate anesthesia tends to be prolonged. Barbiturates are particularly useful in providing cerebral protection during regional cerebral ischemia, for example, temporary vessel occlusion during cerebral aneurysm surgery or revascularization.

Benzodiazepines decrease CBF and $CMRO_2$ [5, 6]. Diazepam (Valium), the prototype of this group, has little cardiovascular effect but may cause respiratory depression. The central nervous system (CNS) effects of diazepam are more pronounced in the elderly. Its long half-life makes it less desirable in neurosurgical patients. *Midazolam* (Versed) is a short-acting benzodiazepine; it holds some advantage over the barbiturates as an induction agent by not reducing systemic arterial pressure (MAP) or cerebral perfusion pressure (CPP) in patients with brain tumors. Midazolam is more effective in protecting the brain from hypoxia than is diazepam [7]. The neurolept combination of fentanyl-droperidol reduces CBF, $CMRO_2$, and ICP.

Muscle Relaxants

These are usually given for intubation, to provide relaxation of paraspinal muscles during spinal operations, and to prevent patient movement. *Curare* causes histamine release (especially when administered rapidly), which can decrease CPP, causing cerebral vasodilatation and intracranial hypertension [8]. *Succinylcholine* increases CBF and may increase ICP [9]. In patients with nerve or spinal cord injuries and denervated muscle, succinylcholine, if given during the acute phase, may cause potassium release from denervated muscle leading to cardiac arrest [10]. Succinylcholine is also associated with hyperkalemia in patients with subarachnoid hemorrhage (SAH) [11]. It is preferred when rapid onset, short duration neuromuscular blockade is desired.

As a muscle relaxant in neuroanesthesia, *pancuronium bromide* (Pavulon) is almost ideal; it produces little histamine release, has a minimal effect on ICP, and is a rapid and effective relaxant. It may, however, cause tachycardia and systemic hypertension. *Vercuronium bromide* (Norcuron) is more potent than pancuronium and has a shorter duration of action; compared with pancuronium, its hemodynamic effects are clinically insignificant.

Vasoactive Agents

Phenylephrine, epinephrine, and *norepinephrine* may increase CPP, indirectly increasing CBF. *Trimetaphan*, a ganglion blocker, is used to induce hypotension intraoperatively because it does not increase CBF or ICP as much as do the direct vasodilators. However, by causing cycloplegia and mydriasis, it may confound postoperative neurologic evaluation. *Sodium nitroprusside (Nipride)* is a direct cerebral vasodilator. It increases ICP in patients with decreased intracranial compliance and alters cerebral autoregulation [12]. Nitroglycerin is an alternative to sodium nitroprusside for induced hypotension. Like nitroprusside, it increases ICP [13]. Other useful hypotensive agents include labetalol (Normodyne) and the angiotensin converting enzyme (ACE) inhibitor, enalaprilat (Vasotec).

Induced Hypotension

Arterial hypotension is used to facilitate the dissection of intracranial aneurysm and the resection of arteriovenous malformations (AVMs). By reducing intravascular turgor, it lessens the chance of hemorrhage. Many neurosurgeons prefer that induced hypotension begin soon after the aneurysm is visualized and continue until it has been clipped. The MAP may be maintained at a fixed level (50–70 mm Hg) or tailored according to a level when there is slackening of flow through the aneurysm itself, keeping in mind the physiologic restraints of the patient's condition. Occasionally, the surgical management of complex vascular lesions has been aided by the use of complete circulatory arrest with extracorporeal circulation and deep hypothermia.

Cerebral Protection

There are a number of therapeutic strategies designed to moderate the response of neuronal tissue to various insults and conditions. These are collectively known as "cerebral protection" [14, 15]. (See Chaps. 1 and 2, which address the concepts of cerebral protection.) Such interventions may be *prophylactic* (i.e., mitigate anticipated unfavorable events, e.g., administration of barbiturates before temporary vessel occlusion—focal ischemia) or *therapeutic* (i.e., attempts to reverse a situation already in progress, e.g., the use of calcium channel blockers to improve neurologic outcome from ischemia related to aneurysmal subarachnoid hemorrhage). A number of these therapies are yet to make the transition from bench to bedside; some of those with established clinical use will be discussed in this section.

Agents that control ICP have been discussed in detail in Chap. 2.

Augmentation of Cerebral Blood Flow

Induced Hypertension

With impaired autoregulation, CBF may become pressure-dependent; changes in systemic blood pressure result in concomitant changes in CBF. Focal ischemia from a reduction in CBF can be reversed by induced hypertension. *Dopamine* has been used to this effect. Timing is crucial to obtain the maximum benefit with the fewest side effects [16,

17]. The blood-brain barrier must be relatively intact or vasogenic cerebral edema may result.

Hypervolemic Hemodilution

It is possible to increase CBF by reducing blood viscosity. This is achieved by administering crystalloid or colloid solutions (albumin, low-molecular-weight dextran). This therapy can reduce neurologic deficits in some patients with focal ischemia [16, 18, 19].

Reduction in Metabolic Demand

Barbiturates

Barbiturates are known to produce significant reductions in $CMRO_2$, and this effect has been harnessed clinically. Operative strategies in many cerebrovascular procedures (e.g., aneurysms, carotid endarterectomy) involve temporary vessel occlusion. Barbiturates are often used as an anesthetic adjunct during such procedures because of their cerebral protective effect [20–22]. Barbiturate administration before vessel occlusion significantly reduces infarct size [23]. A similar protection is offered if the drug is given within 30 minutes after occlusion [24], and circulation is restored to the ischemic zone [25, 26].

Other effects of barbiturates that may contribute to their cerebral protective effect include reduction of ICP and the rate of edema formation, free radical scavenging, and vasconstriction in normal tissue with shunting of blood to ischemic zones [27].

Lidocaine

Lidocaine suppresses synaptic transmission and inhibits metabolism in normal tissue [28]. It reduces membrane permeability in ischemic brain tissue and membrane leak of sodium in particular, thereby relieving ionic pumps of their energy expenditure. Lidocaine causes a brief reduction in ICP; it may be given before procedures that can be expected to elevate ICP in patients with marginal intracranial compliance.

Calcium Channel Blockers

The central role of calcium in the intracellular cascade resulting in cell death is now well known [29]. Calcium channel blockers, e.g., nimodipine, may retard calcium influx to metabolically threatened ischemic cells and reduce vascular smooth muscle contraction.

Anticonvulsant Agents

Seizure activity may aggravate an ischemic insult by increasing CMR and elevating ICP. Phenytoin sodium, an anticonvulsant, promotes sodium efflux from neurons and prevents the rise in intracellular sodium (depolarization) that may attend hypoxia [30]. Phenytoin decreases $CMRO_2$ and cerebral lactate production, and increases cerebral glucose. CBF is elevated [31]. Phenytoin reduces the extracellular accumulation of potassium, which retards the rate of edema formation by imposing less demand on the Na^+-K^+-ATPase system [32].

Scalp Preparation

The hair may be clipped on the ward, in the holding area, or in the operating room just before surgery. Surgeons differ in the extent of hair removal; some restrict it to the surgical area, and others remove it all. A "prep" tray containing the following should be at hand:

1. Electric clippers
2. Povidone-iodine scrub and sponge
3. Comb
4. Razors
5. 70% alcohol solution
6. Adhesive tape
7. Cotton balls
8. 4-in. × 4-in. gauze sponges
9. Water

The procedure for scalp preparation is as follows:

1. Place the patient's head on a polyethylene bag to catch the hair, which is saved and returned to the patient.
2. Clip hair with the electric clippers. Lather with povidone-iodine scrub. Comb the hair away from the clipped area so that unclipped locks do not constantly fall into the surgical area.
3. Shave the scalp with safety razors. Keep the blade on the scalp at an angle of 45 degrees. Deliver deliberate strokes while providing countertraction with the other hand over a gauze sponge. Shave once with and then once against the grain.
4. Dry with gauze sponges; examine closely for patches of resistance. Go over these areas again and blot with adhesive tape.
5. Degrease the scalp with nonexplosive degreaser or 70% alcohol. Cleanse with a gauze sponge saturated with water and then dry.
6. Place a small cotton ball in the ear to prevent antiseptic solution from reaching the tympanum, which could irritate the patient postoperatively.
7. The scalp can now be prepared with povidone-iodine scrub and then solution.

Patient Positioning

Proper positioning facilitates the smooth execution of any operative procedure; conversely, inattention to details of positioning may encum-

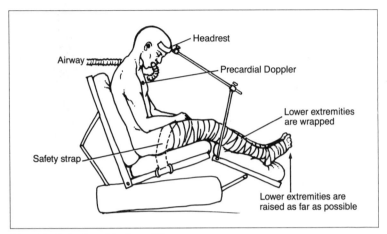

Fig. 6-1. Patient positioning: sitting.

ber the team to no end. The goals are (1) to provide maximum exposure and avoid cardiorespiratory embarrassment, (2) to avoid mechanical distortion of the patient's anatomy, especially the eyes, bony prominences, and peripheral nerves, and (3) to provide an ergonomically optimal arrangement for the surgeon and the operating room team. In many cranial operations the head is immobilized in a three-point pin *head rest* (Mayfield). This is a quadrangular device into which the head is fixed by three sterile pins and a screw that is turned into the skull. Two people are needed to apply the head rest (one supports the patient's head). The pins should be placed at a 90-degree angle and never in a major vessel or nerve or where the bone is very thin. The head can be fixed in virtually any position.

The horseshoe head rest is an incomplete ring upholstered with foam and vinyl covering on which the patient's head rests. It may be used with the patient in the prone position, when rigid fixation is not necessary. Foam doughnuts are used when the patient is in the supine position, and strict fixation is not necessary.

Sitting Position

A number of procedures are carried out within the posterior fossa. These include microvascular decompression of lower cranial nerves, evacuation of cerebellar hematomas and infarcts, resection of tumors and AVMs, and clip ligation of posterior circulation aneurysms. These procedures may be done with the patient in the lateral, prone, or sitting position. The advantages of the sitting position (Fig. 6-1) include the excellent surgical access, improved venous and CSF drainage, and ready access to the head for the anesthesiologist. Potential problems with the sitting position include air embolism, hypotension, tension pneumocephalus, ventilatory difficulties, and pressure injuries [33].

The patient's legs should be wrapped and comfortably flexed at the knees and hips. The legs should be raised to reduce negative venous pressure. The back is supported. The head is flexed onto a head rest (undue flexion impairs venous return). Overzealous head flexion in the patient with cervical spondylosis may precipitate compressive myelopathy. Elbow rests may be provided to support the surgeon's arms.

A recent review of anesthesia and surgery in the seated position reports an overall mortality and morbidity related to the sitting position of 1.0 percent and 0.9 percent, respectively [34].

Venous Air Embolism

In the sitting position the head is higher than the heart; this allows subatmospheric (negative) pressures to develop in the cerebral veins. Because of the large number of diploic veins in the skull and the noncollapsibility of the dural sinuses, air embolism may occur when they are exposed. The physiologic consequences of air embolism can be fatal; therefore, it is best prevented. The neurosurgeon is constantly alert to this possibility; significant venous channels are obliterated. Irrigation of posterior fossa wounds with saline solution and application of bone wax to the edges of the craniectomy also reduce the possibility of air embolism. The period of greatest risk is during muscle and bone dissection. Precordial Doppler ultrasound is a sensitive monitoring parameter [35].

End-tidal carbon dioxide monitoring provides additional vigilance with visual display and an alarm. Some neurosurgeons have questioned the necessity of right atrial catheters in patients undergoing posterior fossa surgery for neurovascular decompressions because it offered no advantages and subjected the patient to the risks of central vein catheterization [36]. If ongoing embolism is suspected, flood the operative field with saline and place the patient head down (this carries a risk of wound contamination); placing the patient in a left-lateral position offers no protection if significant embolism has occurred [33]. Initiate positive end-expiratory pressure (PEEP) ventilation (to raise the central venous pressure [CVP]). Aspirate air through an indwelling right atrial catheter. Nitrous oxide is discontinued.

Postural Hypotension

This is usually of short duration and can be anticipated by wrapping the lower extremities to prevent venous pooling. Maintain anesthesia as lightly as possible and infuse fluids before the patient sits up.

Tension Pneumocephalus

Brain shrinkage during craniotomy may trap extraaxial air. When the patient is sitting, air localizes over the frontal areas as the brain settles with the fluid drainage. If nitrous oxide is continued during dural closure, reexpansion of the brain and diffusion of nitrous oxide into intracranial air pockets may allow tension pneumocephalus to develop [37, 38]. Warming the patient postoperatively fuels the expansion of intracranial air. The syndrome presents as a delay in the resumption of full consciousness or a deterioration in mental status. The differential diagnosis of tension pneumocephalus and the after effects of prolonged anesthesia can be difficult. Diagnosis can be confirmed by computed tomography (CT) scan. To decrease the likelihood of this complication, air is displaced from the subdural space by flushing with saline; hyperventilation is decreased to allow reexpansion of brain. Nitrous oxide is discontinued about 15 minutes before dural closure, although some evidence suggests that this may not be as protective as previously thought [39].

Pressure Injuries

These are prevented by padding risk regions (common peroneal, sciatic, saphenous, and ulnar). Although control of respiration is desirable in the sitting position, some argue that not monitoring the activity of the respiratory center robs the anesthesiologist of a sensitive parameter. A number of centers use brainstem EP as adjunctive monitoring.

Supine Position

The supine position is used for various supratentorial approaches, shunt operations, anterior cervical procedures, many peripheral nerve procedures, and carotid endarterectomy. For craniotomy, the head is either supported on a doughnut or 3-point head rest. The head is usually slightly elevated above the heart to reduce venous engorgement, in such a way that normal brain falls away from the region of interest to minimize retraction. The head may be turned as needed, and the shoulder is buttressed with rolls or sandbags to minimize neck rotation which may cause kinking of the great vessels. Outline the incision before the patient is draped so that all important landmarks are clearly visible. It may also be necessary to mark out key features such as the midline, coronal suture, and mastoid prominence, which may later be referred to for orientation. Some procedures may require accessory incisions, e.g., a burr hole to place an ICP monitor or a stab wound to exit a drain or ventricular catheter. These should be similarly marked out.

Prone Position

The prone position (Fig. 6-2) is used for posterior fossa surgery, posterior cervical approaches, and for thoracic and lumbar laminectomies.

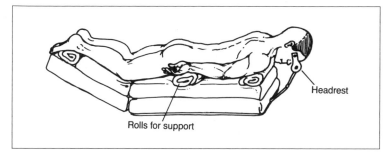

Fig. 6-2. Patient positioning: prone.

Fig. 6-3. Patient positioning: Knee-chest position.

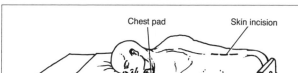

This position may interfere with free costal excursions unless the patient's shoulders are supported away from the table. The shoulders and trunk should be supported on either side and the pelvis from below by padded rolls oriented longitudinally from the chest to the iliac crest. The abdomen is left free to prevent raised CVP. For posterior fossa approaches, the head is flexed and fixed. Exaggerated forward flexion should be avoided to prevent obstruction of venous drainage. When a horseshoe head rest is used, ensure that the orbits are free of pressure to prevent injury to the eye. For lumbar laminectomies, the table can be "broken" (flexed) to bring the spine into a neutral position.

Kneeling on the Andrews Frame

The Andrews frame attaches to the foot section of the operating table. The foot section is flexed 90 degrees and the patient kneels on a horizontal padded support (Fig. 6-3). A chest roll supports the torso. The

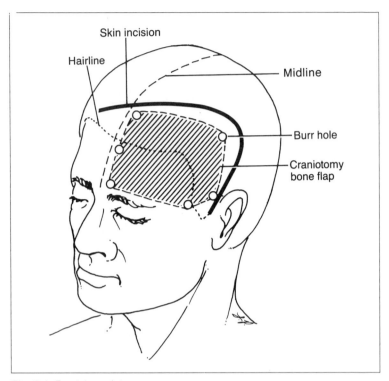

Fig. 6-4. Frontal craniotomy.

abdomen is free to prevent increased venous pressure. The arms rest on padded arm boards and the buttocks and thighs are supported posteriorly and laterally by padded supports. This position is particularly suited for thoracic or lumbar laminectomies. Abdominal decompression is excellent.

Lateral Decubitus Position

This position may be a full or semilateral (also referred to as the "park bench"). The patient is placed on the side. The axilla is supported with a sand bag, and a pillow is placed between the knees (see Fig. 6-11.) If the procedure is an intracranial one (e.g., posterior fossa or subtemporal craniectomy), the head is attached to a three-pin head rest for fixation. For lumbar diskectomy and laminectomies, the head may be supported on a doughnut or soft pillow; the pathologic side is placed uppermost. A suction-activated "bean-bag" or wide strips of tape can be used to stabilize the patient.

Draping

Although each surgeon has a preference, the important features of draping are simplicity and consistency. The main purpose is to isolate the sterile operative field from the surrounding unsterile areas. Drape edges at the craniotomy may be gathered into a kick bucket for drainage. Alternately, many commercially available drapes have a built-in drainage pocket.

Allow for patient access by the anesthesiologist and for movement of the overhead instrument table. The drapes should be waterproof to reduce contamination and may be secured with clips or sutures; many surgeons use a Steri-drape as part of their routine.

After draping, the scrub nurse enters the field with the instrument table and hands off the suction tubing, cautery cords, and energy source for the power drill. These are secured to the drapes and placed in containers.

The surgeon and assistant should have their light sources attached. If a microscope is to be used, it is draped at the appropriate time and positioned safely to avoid contamination.

Antibiotic Prophylaxis

The incidence of neurosurgical infections is low (1 to 2%). The most common organisms causing neurosurgical wound infection are staphylococci; therefore, prophylactic regimens should have excellent anti-staphylococcal coverage. Other things being equal, the least expensive agent should be used. It is unclear whether CSF penetration by the antibiotic is an important factor in preventing wound infection; most infections begin in the soft tissues where the blood-brain barrier is inconsequential. There is as yet no overwhelming reason to select prophylactic antibiotics on the basis of blood-brain permeability. Malis reported a series of 1732 consecutive clean neurosurgical procedures in which prophylactic antibiotics were used without a single postoperative infection [40]. His patients received intraoperative gentamicin or tobramycin and vancomycin. In addition, all wounds were irrigated with streptomycin solution. No adverse effects were noted.

To date, those results have not been duplicated, and the use of prophylactic antibiotics in clean neurosurgical cases remains controversial. There are currently no completed double-blind, randomized, placebo-controlled published trials in clean neurosurgical cases that have not provoked some legitimate criticism, although the weight of current evidence is clearly in favor of the use of prophylactic antibiotics [41]. In a recent literature review of prophylactic antibiotics in clean neurosurgical procedures, Dempsey et al. note that the predominant organisms are gram-positive ones including *Staphylococcus aureus*. They suggest that since the incidence of methicillin and cephalosporin-resistant *S. aureus* in most community hospitals is 0 to 1 percent, the use of a first-generation cephalosporin or antistaphylococcal penicillin as prophylaxis would be appropriate. They recommended cefazolin because of its longer half-life (2 hours); it may be given at the time of premedication on the ward. Cephalothin, oxacillin, and nafcillin have shorter half-lives (under 1 hour) and should be given just before surgery. If the procedure lasts more than 2 or 3 hours, a further dose is needed. For hospitals with a proved incidence of methicillin-resistant *S. aureus* over 10 percent or where methicillin-resistant coagulase-negative staphylococci are associated with postneurosurgical wound infection, the use of one- or two-day perioperative courses of vancomycin appears to be justified. There is no evidence to support continuing prophylaxis postoperatively [41, 42].

Neurosurgical Instrumentation

Cutting Instruments

These vary from the standard scalpel for skin incisions to the microsurgical arachnoid knife for dividing the leptomeninges. *Scissors* are fine to heavy and come in varying lengths, curved and angled. Metzenbaum scissors are dissecting scissors, Mayo scissors are heavy for dividing tough tissue, Frazier and Taylor dura scissors have a guarded point that separates planes and then divides, and Potts scissors have delicate angled blades. Wire scissors are stout with serrated margins. Microsurgical scissors are proportionately smaller with long bayonet shanks; some have a gentle spring action with lock for better control. Cautery pencils may be straight blade (for cutting muscle and fascia) or loops (used to remove meningiomas).

Grasping Instruments

Tissue forceps may be smooth or toothed, straight or bayoneted, and fine to heavy. Adson tissue forceps are fine, with a diamond jaw for gentle pincer action. Cushing tissue forceps are heavier and longer. Penfield tissue and needle pulling forceps have a guard on one shank for a more determined grasp. *Biopsy forceps* may have ring, cup, or hinged jaws. They are frequently long and bayoneted with serrated shanks.

Hooks are used for grasping, retracting, and elevating. Dural hooks have a curved pointed end that penetrates and seats in the dura. Nerve hooks (retractor) are used for retracting nerve roots and trunks, usually during lumbar or cervical laminectomies. Examples include the Dandy, Love, and Krayenbuhl.

Spinal retractors are used for retracting bulky paravertebral muscles and tissues during laminectomy. Examples include the Weitlander, Scoville, Taylor, Adson-Beckman, and Cloward (for anterior cervical procedures).

Bone Instruments

Rongeurs are bone-biting instruments. They may be single or double action and come in different jaw configurations (straight, curved, and angled) and sizes (wide to narrow). The double-action rongeurs have two fulcrum points, which lessen the pressure needed for cutting and give the surgeon better control. Furthermore, the smaller opening action and handle spread permit the double-action rongeur to be inserted further into the operative site than the single-action rongeur. Examples include the Leksell (double action), Stille (double action), and Adson (single action).

Bone punches have a long slender shaft with trigger handles. They are commonly used in laminectomies and for a variety of bone work. The tips are referred to as up and down biting, straight, or angled. Bite size varies from small to large, as does shaft length. Common examples include the Kerrison, Spurling, Schlesinger, and Raney.

Operating Microscope

Microsurgical techniques revolutionized neurosurgery by providing detailed vision and illumination. Delicate structures can be identified and preserved; less retraction and smaller exposures are required. There are many magnification ranges with a varying combination of objective lenses, eyepieces, and body tubes. Microscope angulation and position may be altered to cope with virtually any procedure. The microscope can accommodate several accessories for still or video photography, audio, and laser surgery. The microscope may be a ceiling-mounted or a floor model. It should be "balanced" and draped before use.

Cavitron Ultrasonic Surgical Aspirator

The Cavitron Ultrasonic Surgical Aspirator (CUSA) consists of a handpiece (straight or curved), foot switch, and control console. The console provides variable suction and irrigation to the handpiece. The surgeon activates a longitudinally vibrating tip by depressing the footswitch; this vibration fragments and emulsifies tissue, which is aspirated by suction through the hollow tip and into a reservoir.

One advantage of the CUSA is that tumors may be removed with little movement of adjacent neural and vascular structures; consequently, tumors adjacent to vital structures may be extirpated with minimal risk [43]. The tumor is usually debulked centrifugally (internal decompression) and then its capsule is dissected free. Tumors amenable to the CUSA include meningioma, acoustic neuroma, glioma, and intramedullary spinal neoplasm (ependymoma and astrocytoma). The CUSA is not hemostatic, and the surgeon will pause frequently to secure hemostasis. It is of little value in removing densely calcified or fibrous tissue.

Intraoperative Ultrasound

Real-time intraoperative ultrasound imaging (IUS) has become a useful tool. It helps in localizing lesions not readily visible on the surface of the brain or spinal cord. The concept of real-time imaging means that the image on the screen represents the exact situation at the moment the image is obtained [44, 45].

To obtain an image, a bone "window" is required; this may be a burr hole or craniotomy flap in the head or a laminectomy in the spine. Acoustic coupling, needed between the transducer and the target, is provided by fluid (saline) on the operative surface.

IUS locates the pathologic site and differentiates between the solid and cystic components of lesions. This information minimizes the need for extensive tissue dissection and aids in determining if surgical treatment is adequate. Because the images are real-time images, technical adjustments can be made and the efficacy of those alterations can be assessed by obtaining further images [46–48].

IUS has also been useful for placing ventricular shunt catheters and Ommaya reservoirs. Systems for IUS-guided biopsy have been developed. These ensure accurate needle and probe placement [49].

Neurosurgical Lasers

LASER is the acronym for light amplification by the stimulated emission of radiation [50, 51]. Laser light is electromagnetic energy and has three unique and desirable qualities compared with ambient light: monochromaticity (i.e., composed of a single wave length), coherence (i.e., in phase temporally and spatially, and collimation (i.e., travels as parallel beams over long distances). A laser system requires an active medium (solid, liquid, or gas) that, when stimulated, emits photons to generate the laser beam; examples in neurosurgical use are the carbon dioxide and argon lasers (gas) and the neodymium:YAG laser (solid state).

The laser beam incises, coagulates, or vaporizes depending on the quantity and distribution of power within it. Where the laser beam strikes the tissue surface, a cross-sectional energy profile (laser spot) may be described. The spot size may be varied from finely focused, small diameter (for incision and fine vaporization) to defocused, larger diameter (to coagulate or vaporize more superficial volumes of tissue over a wide area).

Lasers may be used to vaporize tumors in hard-to-reach or critical areas: skull base, brainstem, and spinal cord. Vaporization is a no-touch technique that minimizes manipulation and displacement of surrounding vital structures. However, this loss of proprioceptive information from the tissue may be disadvantageous.

Lasers may find clinical use in the photoradiation therapy (PRT) of gliomas. In this treatment, tissue color is altered by staining with vital dyes, which then enhances the absorption of laser energy by those tissues. One photosensitizing agent (hematoporphyrin derivative [HPD]) has been applied in this fashion [52]. Lasers are also being used in reconstructive vascular procedures to weld anastomoses.

A computer-assisted stereotactic microlaser technique for the precise removal of deep seated intraaxial cranial lesions (gliomas and AVMs) has been developed. This permits the surgeon to maintain accurate three-dimensional orientation during vaporization. The technique may be particularly useful for invasive tumors with indistinct margins [53].

Carbon Dioxide Laser

This is currently the most widely used laser in neurosurgery. Because it is invisible, it must be guided by a coaxial pilot beam. The carbon dioxide laser seals capillaries and small vessels (0.5–1.0 mm) but may incise larger vessels, causing bleeding. Carbon dioxide laser energy can penetrate through a tumor capsule, injuring underlying structures. Reflection of the beam from shiny surfaces (e.g., retractors) and metallic instruments may damage exposed structures; therefore all exposed or underlying tissue is protected by moistened cottonoids. Suction catheters are placed in the field to remove the laser plume that forms during vaporization.

Neodymium:YAG Laser

The neodymium:YAG laser (Nd:YAG, neodymium:yttrium-aluminium-garnet) is selectively absorbed by hemoglobin, making it potentially useful for the surgical removal of vascular lesions. It coagulates small-caliber vessels but is not effective against bleeding from high-flow large vessels because rapid blood flow reduces its heating effect. The neodymium:YAG laser has been useful for excision of AVMs and vascular meningiomas, with significant reduction in blood loss [54, 55].

Argon Laser

The argon laser emits energy in the green part of the spectrum; it is absorbed by pigmented tissue, making it potentially useful in the surgical treatment of AVMs and vascular tumors. Because of its relatively short wavelength, it can be transmitted through fiberoptic systems with little loss of power. The fiberoptic delivery system and a micromanipulator provide accurate localization and movement of the beam to within millimeters, which is ideally suited for microsurgical applications. The argon laser's ability to transmit energy fiberoptically lends it to endoscopic neurosurgical procedures. Its major limitation is low power output.

Laser Safety

When lasers are in use, all operating room personnel should wear eye protection and the patient's eyes are covered with moistened eye pads. For the argon or neodymium:YAG laser, colored protective eyewear is required. Retractors and other shiny surfaces in the operative field are covered with moist sponges, since the laser beam can be reflected off such surfaces. The operating room is appropriately tagged, and entry is restricted.

Hemostasis in Neurosurgery

One of the distinguishing features of neurosurgical technique is the control of hemorrhage without much use of ligature. The delicate consistency of neural tissue, the narrow avenues of approach, and the depth at which most work is done all conspire to make ligature an impractical technique. Electrical methods are not suitable for diffuse topical bleeding from dura and brain. Neurosurgery has few opportunities for pressure packing. Therefore, other means of securing hemostasis have developed including:

1. Horsley's bone wax
2. Clips
3. Electrocautery
4. Chemical agents

Bone wax controls bone bleeding by sealing off diploic channels. It is used slightly softened in small pieces and may be applied with a finger or an instrument. It tends to retard bone fusion.

Clips have long been used in neurosurgery to control bleeding from blood vessels. Cushing used a malleable silver clip; this has been largely abandoned in favor of the Weck hemoclip and the Ethicon ligaclip, both made of tantalum. Vascular clips made of polyglactic acid (Vicryl) are absorbable and can control bleeding from small vessels. Spring-loaded clips were developed for aneurysm surgery, and there are many varieties. Many surgeons consider implanting nonferromagnetic clips because of the increasing use of MRI.

Electrocautery may be unipolar (coagulating and cutting) or bipolar (coagulating). The cutting current is actually a mixed current containing some degree of coagulation. The cutting current will often stop bone bleeding. It may be used with loop tips for resecting meningiomas. Bipolar coagulation provides a minimal, precise current that travels from point to point on a forceps rather than through the patient; consequently, a grounding pad is not necessary. It provides hemostasis without stimulation or current spread to adjacent structures.

Several *chemical agents* in use are discussed below.

1. *Gelatin sponge (Gelfoam)*. The hemostatic effect is partly due to its porousness. Gelfoam absorbs up to 45 times its weight in blood, providing a tamponade effect. Adhesion is preserved by the platelet glue between the sponge and the wound surface. Its activity is enhanced by presoaking in thrombin. Gelfoam is absorbable [56]. It may predispose to infection when used in contaminated wounds [57]. Gelfoam is effective in controling hemorrhage from cancellous bone, as occurs in spinal fusions [58].
2. *Oxidized cellulose (Oxycel) and oxidized regenerated cellulose (Surgicel)*. Both are chemically altered forms of cellulose. They react with blood to form an acid hematin, gelatinous mass that functions as an artificial clot [59]. Both are absorbable. Surgicel has superior handling qualities and does not interfere with epithelialization, as may Oxycel. A major advantage of oxidized cellulose is its activity against a wide variety of pathogenic organisms. Surgicel is thought to be bactericidal in vivo against over 20 pathogenic organisms [60–62]. These agents may retard bone growth. There have been reports of compressive neuropathies and narrowing of blood vessels associated with leaving these agents in confined spaces because they tend to swell. They should be removed when used in laminectomies and around vascular anastomoses if compression is likely [63, 64].
3. Microfibrillar collagen (Avitene, Instat).
   Microfibrillar collagen is thought to react with platelets, increasing their aggregation and accelerating blood coagulation. Avitene is available in powder form or as patties. It must be used dry because moisture impairs its activity. However, Instat works well even wet. It is absorbable and does not appear to retard bone healing [65].
4. Thrombin (Thrombogen, Thrombostat). Thrombin is an integral part of the coagulation cascade and converts fibrinogen to fibrin. It is made commercially from bovine materials and it provides "instant" coagulation when sprayed onto oozing surfaces or adsorbed on cotton pledgets or Gelfoam.

Neurosurgical Approaches and Techniques

This section will familiarize the young trainee with terms and operations in contemporary neurosurgery. Only the more common operations are touched upon. The advanced trainee should consult specialized works on operative neurosurgery (see Suggested Reading).

Craniotomy

Opening

In craniotomy, the skull is opened by making a bone flap, which is replaced after the operation and fixed to adjacent bony margins. (In craniectomy, however, the bone removed from the skull is not returned.

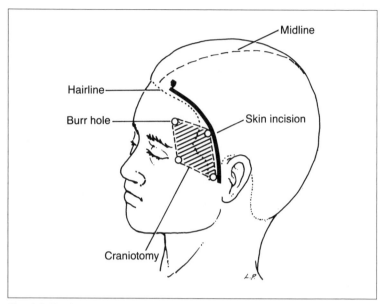

Fig. 6-5. Pterional craniotomy.

This is the method of choice for exposing the posterior fossa, which is discussed on pp. 256–257.) Figures 6-5 to 6-10 illustrate the various approaches for craniotomy.

To obtain adequate exposure, the craniotomy is centered over the lesion. The opening should be large enough to handle untoward complications. In cranial operations, standard reference points of craniocerebral topography are plotted (mentally or graphically) against the location of the lesion on the radiographic studies.

Scalp vascularization is so profuse that it is difficult to render it truly ischemic; however, the principle of preservation of the frontal, temporal, and occipital arteriovenous pedicles applies in the design of standard neurosurgical approaches. A second principle is to place the incision behind the hairline (as far as feasible) so that it remains hidden as hair grows.

Some cranial flaps are described below.
Osteoplastic Flap. In an *osteoplastic* flap, the bone is not separated from the muscle and periosteum, with the theoretical purpose of keeping flap vascularization intact. This technique, pioneered by Cushing, has been largely given up with better knowledge of the flap's blood supply.
Free Flap. A *free* flap implies complete detachment of bone from the muscle, periosteum, and scalp.
Frontal Craniotomy. The unilateral frontal flap exposes the frontal re-

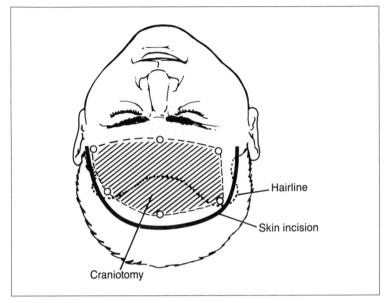

Fig. 6-6. Bifrontal craniotomy.

Fig. 6-7. Subtemporal craniotomy.

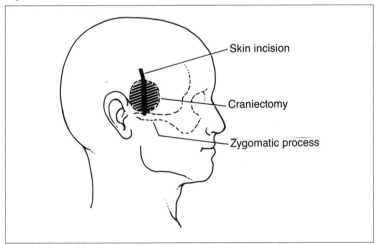

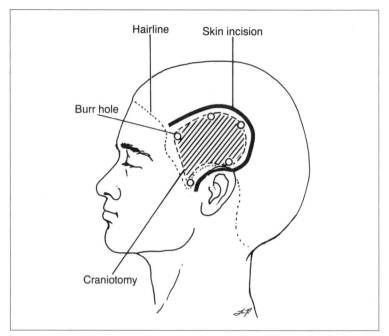

Fig. 6-8. Temporal craniotomy.

gion (see Fig. 6-4). One must preserve the frontalis branch of the facial nerve that supplies the frontalis muscle. In bald patients it is not possible to hide the incision in hair-bearing scalp. Burr holes are placed in the anterior and posterior temporal regions and in the frontal anterior (medial) and posterior (sagittal) regions. Tumors of the frontal region and anterior circulation aneurysms may be approached from this vantage.

Pterional Craniotomy. The pterion is the region of the skull formed by the junction of the frontal, parietal, temporal, and zygomatic bones with the greater wing of the sphenoid bone. Thus, the pterional approach describes a cranial flap centered about this landmark (see Fig. 6-5). The pterional approach is used for the surgical treatment of lesions about the skull base, particularly aneurysms of the anterior cerebral circulation.

The critical burr hole is located at the junction of the temporal line, the zygomatic process of the frontal bone, and the orbital ridge, the so-called "keyhole." Following the development of microneurosurgery, a smaller, more basal exposure has been used. This is accomplished by drilling the sphenoid bone, more anterior placement of the posterior temporal burr holes, and a wider opening of the sylvian fissure.

Bifrontal (Coronal) Craniotomy. This incision is used to gain approach

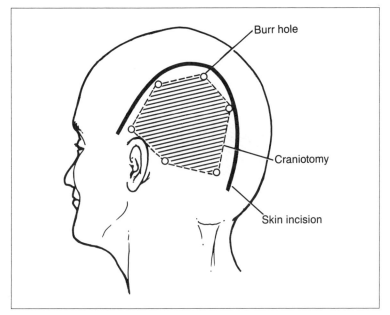

Fig. 6-9. Occipital craniotomy.

to the frontal and frontobasal regions (see Fig. 6-7). It reaches from the ear on one side to the other, somewhat overlying the coronal suture. The bone flap may be single (hinged on one side) or bivalved (separated in the midline and hinged on both sides). It may be used to approach frontobasal tumors and anterior communicating artery aneurysms and to repair CSF rhinorrhea.

Subtemporal Craniectomy. This approach was introduced by Cushing for the palliative treatment of idiopathic intracranial hypertension (see Fig. 6-7). A vertical incision is made in the temporal region (some surgeons add a gentle curve). The approach is now rarely performed for decompression; more commonly it is used to approach aneurysms of the basilar artery and skull base lesions.

Temporal Craniotomy. The questionmark or reverse questionmark incision may be used (see Fig. 6-9). Anterior and posterior temporal burr holes are made as close as possible to the skull base to maximize exposure. Three to four peripheral holes are made to delimit the height of the flap. This approach is used frequently in epilepsy surgery for placing electrodes and for cortical resections of epileptogenic foci; tumors of the temporal region can also be removed from this approach. A large temporal flap is used for traumatic intracranial hematoma. It is commonly referred to as a "trauma flap."

Occipital and Parietal Craniotomy. These are regional craniotomy flaps based on the principles previously outlined (see Fig. 6-9). Lesions

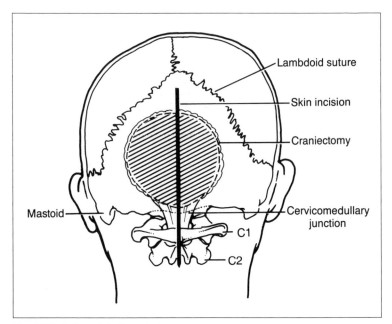

Fig. 6-10. Suboccipital craniectomy.

that may be approached by these exposures include parenchymal tumors (gliomas), intracerebral hemorrhages, and AVMs.

Procedure. The procedure for craniotomy is generally as follows:

1. Outline the incision (usually by a superficial scratch with a needle or a marking pen) before the operative area is draped so that no land marks are obscured. Many surgeons mark out the sagittal midline or other bony landmarks for orientation. Make cross-hatches if necessary to aid reapproximation at closure. Inject local anesthetic (1% lidocaine with 1:100,000 epinephrine solution) between the galea and periosteum to loosen the tissue planes and reduce bleeding.

2. Make the scalp incision with a standard scalpel. The assistant's fingers apply pressure and traction against either side of the skin incision, which helps control bleeding. To further control bleeding, use Raney clips or Dandy hemostats; clips compress the scalp edges and galea, whereas hemostats placed on the galea pull that layer out and back, shutting off the scalp vessels. If the scalp is thin or its blood supply is compromised (e.g., after irradiation), one should be particularly careful or ischemia may result. Obtain additional hemostasis by cautery if needed. Proper scalp hemostasis may make the difference in avoiding transfusion in children.

3. Reflect the scalp flap with the periosteum and check for further

bleeding. Use saline-soaked sponges or Telfa to keep it moist. Protect the pedicle from excessive angulation (which can cut off blood supply) by placing a gauze roll beneath the flap. Apply traction to the scalp with stitches to obtain further exposure and hemostasis.

4. Place burr holes with the power drill or hand-held brace. Irrigation during drilling cools drill friction and flushes bone dust. Remove residual bone fragments of the inner table within the burr hole with a curet to expose the dura fully. Bone dust may or may not be saved. Wax holes with Horsley's bone wax to secure hemostasis.

5. Separate dura from bone with an elevator around the circumference of the burr holes; this maneuver helps prevent dural tears when using the craniotome or Gigli saw. Turn the bone flap with the air-driven craniotome (the craniotome consists of a cranial blade and dura guard) or Gigli saw. In suboccipital craniectomy, bone is removed piecemeal with rongeurs. Irrigate the blade as the flap is being turned; the flap and muscle is retracted away from the drill with Cushing retractors or rakes.

6. Free the bone from underlying dura with an elevator, fracture any bridges, and remove the bone flap; the assistant irrigates to flush away fragments and dust. Place the bone flap in a basin of Betadine or antibiotic solution and return it to the scrub nurse for safekeeping.

7. With an osteoplastic flap, a portion of muscle is left attached to the bone flap; therefore, the bone is never completely removed. Remove rough, fractured edges with a rongeur.

8. In preparation for replacement at closure, drill small holes (wire pass holes) in the bone flap with corresponding holes in the skull; this may be done with a wire pass drill bit or Cone bone punch. These are sites where wires or sutures are placed to anchor the bone flap at closure.

9. Lift dura with a stitch, hook, or screw; it is incised with a blade, and the dural flap is completed with scissors. Moist cottonoids may be inserted beneath the dura to separate it from brain. Place dural tack up sutures to limit epidural bleeding. Surgical or Gelfoam strips and cottonoids may be arranged circumferentially for hemostasis.

10. Keep exposed brain constantly moist with irrigating solution. In many neurosurgical operations, brain retraction provides exposure. Every neurosurgeon knows from training and experience the safe limits of retraction pressure. Retraction pressure monitoring may provide the surgeon with early warning of excessive tissue pressure [88]. Direct retraction against tissue to be removed (e.g., brain tumor) rather than against normal brain tissue. Brain tissue retraction pressure may reach 25 mm Hg compromising and promoting ischemia. Self-retaining retractor systems include the Leyla, Budde, Janetta, and Greenberg.

The conduct of the case from here on depends on the nature of the lesion. For example, aneurysms are usually secured by microsurgical dissection and clip ligation. Tumors are dissected from the brain and

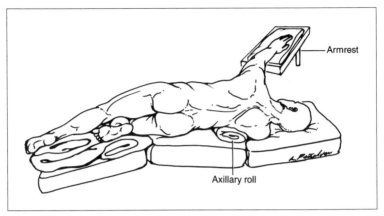

Fig. 6-11. Lateral decubitus ("park bench") position.

resected with the CUSA, laser, or cautery loops. (See procedure descriptions below.)

Closure

The bone flap is retrieved and cleaned; it is replaced within the bony opening and anchored with wire or sutures. If there is infection or a need for decompression, the bone flap may be left out. Muscle is closed separately. The galea is closed with buried stitches (some prefer to close the galea and skin in one layer). Except for a few instances, the dura is closed. This may be a primary closure or, if a defect exists, a secondary closure with artificial substitute or a periosteal graft. Avoiding dural coagulation during opening and keeping it moist prevents shrinkage that makes closure difficult. Small gaps in the edges of a dural closure may be sealed with a piece of Gelfoam; combined with good galeal closure this usually suffices to avoid CSF leak in most cases where there is no obstruction to CSF absorption.

The skin is approximated so that the edges are everted. Subgaleal drainage is occasionally advisable, especially with large flaps; indeed, some neurosurgeons use it routinely. Finally, dressings are applied.

Posterior Fossa Craniectomy

The choice of incision in posterior fossa craniectomy depends on location of the lesion and the surgeon's preference. A midline approach may be used for lesions situated close to the midline or for lesions around the foramen magnum and upper cervical junction (Fig. 6-10). The patient may be sitting (see Fig. 6-1), prone (see Fig. 6-2), or lateral decubitus (park bench) (see Fig. 6-4).

A unilateral approach will secure lesions asymmetrically located in one or the other hemisphere and tumors located in the cerebellopontine angle (e.g., acoustic neuromas and meningiomas) and vascular decompressions for tic douloureux (Fig. 6-12). For cerebellopontine angle approaches, the patient's head is rotated to bring the posterior face of the petrous bone into the anterior-posterior plane. This facilitates exploration of the angle. The incision is a long curvilinear one, 1 to 2 cm medial to the posterior edge of the mastoid process.

A cross-bow incision (combination of a midline occipital with a transverse incision above the external occipital protuberance curving to either side), proffered by Cushing, provides wide exposure to this region.

Combined supratentorial and infratentorial approaches are used for large tumors occupying both compartments or those involving the tentorial hiatus. With coexisting hydrocephalus, intracranial hypertension may be controlled by the placement of an occipital burr hole for tapping the ventricle. A ventricular catheter may be inserted through the burr hole if the patient later develops symptoms of raised ICP.

Burr holes are placed in the occipital squama, avoiding the midline and transverse sinuses; mastoid cells are sealed off with bone wax if they are entered. Burr holes are connected to fashion the craniectomy using rongeurs and bone punches. If dural tension is unacceptably high, the ventricle may be tapped through an already established burr hole after the dura is opened. Dural flaps are retracted with stitches. The intradural procedure is carried out. At the close of the procedure, the dura flaps are approximated. If necessary, artificial dura or periosteal graft is interposed to ensure a tight seal to prevent the development of CSF leak. With hydrocephalus controlled, and a meticulous multilayer closure of muscle fascia, subcutaneous tissue, and skin, CSF leak is seldom a problem even though dural closure is not watertight. The retractors are removed, and the rest of the wound is closed in layers. Figure 6-12 shows a lateral suboccipital craniectomy.

Skull Flaps in Children

In children under 6 months of age, the bone is very thin and the burr holes may even be connected with scissors. Dura and bone adhere closely at suture sites, especially at the fontanelle. Bone regeneration fills in the gaps left by burr holes or a craniotome. The thinness of the skull sometimes makes it difficult to replace the flap in its proper position. Closure of the skin may also be more difficult because the scalp is overstretched.

Flap Reopening

Occasionally it is necessary to reenter an operative site, either to treat some misadventure or to revisit an uncompleted task. It is usually pos-

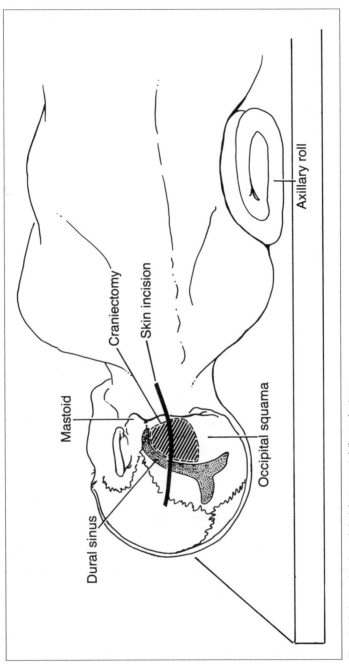

Fig. 6-12. Lateral suboccipital (retromastoid) craniectomy.

sible in the first 2 years after a major craniotomy to reelevate a flap in adults without drilling new burr holes. Adhesions may prevent the easy separation of tissue planes. In children, the healing process is more rapid; usually a new flap is necessary after 1 year has elapsed.

Intracranial Aneurysm

The goal of surgery is to exclude the aneurysm from the circulation, maintain patency, and avoid injury to the parent vessel and its branches. After opening the dura, the approach is usually by subarachnoid dissection. This allows release of CSF, providing further brain relaxation and exposure. The parent vessels are exposed so that proximal and distal control is secured; then the neck of the aneurysm is approached and developed. Microsurgical technique and illumination together with improved neuroanesthesia have made cerebral aneurysm surgery much safer.

Induced hypotension is sometimes necessary during the dissection and clipping of the aneurysm.

Recently, the availability of intraoperative angiography has made it feasible to confirm satisfactory clip placement and to visualize vessels around the neck of the aneurysm.

Most aneurysms of the internal carotid artery, middle cerebral artery, anterior cerebral artery complex, and upper basilar bifurcation can be treated by pterional craniotomy. Posterior fossa aneurysms may be approached by subtemporal or suboccipital craniotomy.

Arteriovenous Malformations

AVMs are exposed by regional craniotomy. The dura is carefully reflected to avoid injury to any underlying vessels that may arise from the malformation. The AVM is traced by following cortical cues such as a red vein. Surgical strategy is guided by study of the preoperative angiogram. Initial dissection begins in the gliotic plane between the AVM and normal brain. Feeding vessels are progressively taken, and finally the draining vein and the malformation are delivered. Induced hypotension may help to reduce intravascular turgor during stages of the dissection.

Attention is given to hemostasis because of the risk of postoperative hemorrhage. The use of intraoperative angiography may improve the safety of the resection by better defining the exact destination of dubious vessels. Intraoperative embolization of major feeding vessels may be used in the early intraoperative stages of AVM resection [66, 67].

Surgery for Epilepsy

Operations for epilepsy are performed under general or local anesthesia. For local anesthesia, a long-acting solution is injected into the scalp at relevant sites and into the dura mater adjacent to meningeal vessels. Intravenous fentanyl and droperidol may be added during the craniotomy. Motor, sensory, and speech areas can be mapped using electrical stimulation (functional mapping) or an EP electrocorticogram (EcoG); depth-electrode recording may also be obtained intraoperatively. Stimulation may produce auras or seizures. Some neurosurgeons use the data from functional mapping and intraoperative EcoG to determine the extent of safe resection for maximal therapeutic benefit [68, 69]. Others rely on the preoperative workup and perform anatomically standardized temporal lobe resections [70, 71].

Corpus callosotomy (callosal section) is performed to treat patients with generalized major motor seizures; it is also of value in patients with partial seizures characterized by loss of postural tone. The extent of section (complete or partial anterior section only) necessary for full therapeutic benefit is not well established. Although callostomy is a relatively benign procedure, some patients experience a muted form of akinetic mutism that is usually transient [72–74]. Damage to the fornix or other deep midline transmission bundles may cause a memory deficit.

Carotid Endarterectomy

Carotid endarterectomy may be performed under local or general anesthesia. Many patients with cerebrovascular insufficiency have coexistent ischemic cardiac disease and an enhanced risk of neurologic deficit from intraoperative hypotension. All cardiac and antihypertension medications are usually continued up to the time of surgery. Because of the high risk of hypertension and tachycardia in these patients, premedication should be sufficient enough to blunt this response while inserting vascular catheters. Local anesthesia allows for clinical assessment of cerebrovascular insufficiency and is associated with a lower risk of myocardial infarction [75].

Hypotension may be avoided by preoperative volume loading and intraoperative use of vasoconstrictors. During carotid artery clamping, hypotension may be deleterious, especially if collateral blood flow is inadequate. For this reason many surgeons place a temporary shunt during this phase of the procedure. The need for shunts has been variously determined by carotid stump pressure, clinical monitoring, CBF, EEG, and somatosensory EP monitoring [76, 77].

The patient is positioned supine, with the head slightly extended and turned away from the side to be operated on. An oblique linear incision is made along the anterior border of the sternocleidomastoid muscle. Blunt dissection is continued in this plane until the carotid sheath is exposed. The carotid artery is secured. A small amount of lidocaine is injected into the region of the bifurcation to prevent reflex bradycardia and hypotension from manipulation of the vessel. The patient is heparinized, and the external, common, and internal carotid arteries are clamped. Some neurosurgeons give barbiturates at this point for their cerebral protectant effect in focal ischemia. Monitoring is by EEG or CBF. If local anesthesia is preferred, monitor the patient clinically for neurologic deficit. The arteriotomy is made in the carotid artery, and the endarterectomy is completed. The arteriotomy is closed (a patch graft may be necessary if the arterial lumen is small) and the clamps are removed. The wound is closed in the standard fashion with or without a drain.

Transsphenoidal Adenomectomy

The patient is positioned supine. The head, held by pin fixation, is turned to face the surgeon, who stands to the right. The left arm is abducted at 90 degrees to the torso. A lumbar drain may be used if the tumor is large [78]. The face, nares, and upper gingival and nasal mucosa are cleansed with antiseptic solution. A separate field is prepared in the left lower quadrant of the abdomen to harvest a fat graft. The initial part of the procedure is performed with low-power loupes. A sublabial incision is made and dissection continues posteriorly in a submucosal plane along the nasal floor and septum (unilateral septal) [79]. The septum is cracked from left to right and a Hardy speculum is placed for exposure. The sphenoid sinus is entered and the operating microscope is brought into the field. The sellar floor is removed and the dura is incised and opened to expose the pituitary gland. The tumor is identified and gently removed under direct vision. Pituitary adenomas have a predilection for different sites within the gland according to histologic subtype; this is important for localizing small tumors. Intraoperative problems occasionally encountered include bleeding in and around the sella, CSF leak, and failure to identify an adenoma. The sublabial incision is closed with catgut suture, and nasal airways are placed in both nares with anchoring silk stitch.

Stereotactic Neurosurgery

There are currently a number of CT-guided stereotactic systems for use in neurosurgery (Brown-Roberts-Wells [BRW], Leksell, Reichert-Mundinger,) (Fig. 6-13). These systems may be used for biopsy of intraparenchymal lesions and functional neurosurgical procedures [80, 81]. The basic concept involves a reformation of the two-dimensional coordinates of a CT or MRI image to a three-dimensional point in real space. In the BRW system, for example, the components of the system include the following:

1. Head ring
2. Localizing rods
3. Arc guidance system
4. Phantom base ring and dummy point

The conduct of the procedure is generally as follows.

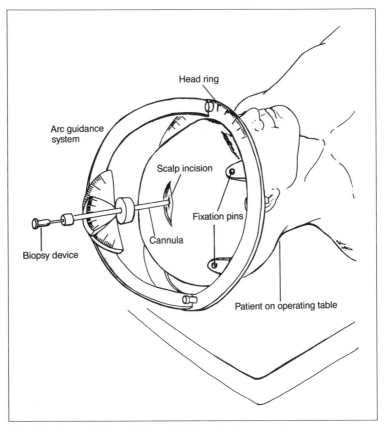

Fig. 6-13. Brown-Roberts-Wells (BRW) stereotactic apparatus.

The head ring is fixed to the skull to provide the reference plane. The localizing system is attached to the base ring; then the patient undergoes scanning. The anteroposterior and lateral coordinates of the nine localizing rods and selected target points are read from the scanner console and entered into the computer for processing. Meanwhile, the patient is transported into the operating room. The Mayfield head rest adaptor is attached to the head ring. The computer program calculates the anteroposterior, lateral, and vertical coordinates of the target, the arc settings (alpha, beta, gamma, and delta), and the distance from a reference point on the arc sleeve to the target. The settings are checked on the phantom simulator. The arc is returned to the head ring on the patient. The entry point is marked on the scalp, which is shaved and prepared. A twist drill hole is made and the biopsy is taken.

Tic Douloureux

Procedures for treatment of tic douloureux are described below.

Percutaneous Trigeminal Radiofrequency Rhizotomy

This is an ablative procedure. Under local anesthesia, a probe (insulated needle) is inserted through the cheek into the foramen ovale, free hand, under radiographic guidance (Härtel technique). By a weak electrical current (generally a nonpainful stimulus), the appropriate site can be correctly localized before lesion making. A short-acting intravenous anesthetic (usually methohexital) and nitrous oxide–oxygen (by mask) are given so that the patient can awaken rapidly for sensory testing during the operation. A selective radiofrequency (RF) lesion(s) with precise temperature control is made in the gasserian ganglion or sensory root [82–84].

Percutaneous Retrogasserian Glycerol Rhizotomy

This is similar to the RF technique. Instead of making an RF lesion, a needle is introduced in the same fashion into the arachnoid cistern of the gasserian ganglion, and a small volume of anhydrous glycerol is injected. The patient is kept sitting in bed with the head flexed for at least an hour following the procedure to keep the glycerol within the trigeminal cistern [85, 86].

Posterior Fossa (Retromastoid) Craniectomy for Microvascular Decompression of the Trigeminal Nerve (Jannetta Procedure)

The Janetta procedure is a microvascular compression. It is performed through a small, lateral posterior fossa craniectomy. The cerebellum is retracted medially and inferiorly to expose the trigeminal nerve as it enters the pons. Then, a microsurgical exploration of the root entry zone for a loop of artery is undertaken. The arterial loop is separated from the nerve. A sponge (Ivalon or Teflon felt) is inserted to maintain separation of the vessel from the nerve. If a vein is found, it is coagulated and divided. About 90 percent of patients will have clear-cut impingement by an artery or vein. The usual finding is an ectatic superior cerebellar artery that abuts on the nerve [87].

Spinal Surgery

In spinal surgery one is guided by palpation of the spinous processes and other bony landmarks. Skin marks made during myelography are sometimes helpful. The appropriate level may be verified by intraoperative x-ray film.

Lumbar Disk In lumbar disk surgery, the patient may be prone, lateral, or kneeling on the Andrews frame (see Fig. 6-3). A midline incision is made in the lumbosacral region. The paravertebral muscles are stripped laterally by periosteal elevators to skeletonize the posterior elements. A laminectomy retractor (Scoville, Taylor, or Weitlander) is placed in the wound for exposure. Spinous processes may or may not be removed. The laminectomy or laminotomy is performed on the side of the lesion; it may be accomplished with rongeurs, bone punches, or a high-speed drill. The ligamentum flavum is incised and removed by sharp dissection or bone punches to expose the epidural space. The nerve root is retracted. The annulus is incised and the disk is removed.

Lumbar Stenosis

This approach is similar to that for lumbar disk surgery. Generally, wide multiple-level laminectomies and foraminotomies are required for adequate decompression of the neural elements.

Intramedullary Tumors and Syrinx

The same midline approach is used. The dura is opened in the midline. Microsurgical technique is used for the intradural portion. Intraoperative ultrasound may be needed for precise localization of the lesion. The laser or CUSA may be used depending on the type of tumor.

References

1. Carlsson C., Smith D. S., Keykhah M. M., et al. The effects of high-dose fentanyl in cerebral circulation and metabolism in rats. *Anesthesiology* 57:375, 1982.
2. Adams R. W., Cucchiara R. F., Gronert G. A., et al. Isoflurane and cerebrospinal fluid pressure in neurosurgical patients. *Anesthesiology* 54:97, 1981.
3. Newberg L. A., Michenfelder J. D. Cerebral protection by isoflurane during hypoxemia or ischemia. *Anesthesiology* 59:29, 1983.
4. Jennett W. B., Barker J., Fitch W., et al. Effect of anesthesia on intracranial pressure in patients with space-occupying lesions. *Lancet* 1:61, 1969.
5. Carlsson C., Chapman A. G. The effects of diazepam on the cerebral metabolic rate in rats and its interaction with nitrous oxide. *Anesthesiology* 54:488, 1981.
6. Forester A., Juge O., Morel D. Effects of midazolam on cerebral blood flow in human volunteers. *Anesthesiology* 56:453, 1982.
7. Giffin J. P., Cottrell J. E., Shwiry B., et al. Intracranial pressure, mean arterial pressure, and heart rate following midazolam or thiopental in humans with brain tumors. *Anesthesiology* 60:491, 1984.
8. Tarkkanen L., Laitnen L., Johansson G. Effects of d-tubocurarine on intracranial pressure and thalamic electrical impedance. *Anesthesiology* 40:247, 1974.
9. Cottrell J. E., Hartung J., Giffin J. P., et al. Intracranial and hemodynamic changes after succinylcholine administration in cats. *Anesth. Analg.* 62:1006, 1983.
10. Gronert G. A., Theye R. A. Pathophysiology of hyperkalemia induced by succinylcholine. *Anesthesiology* 43:89, 1975.

11. Iwatsuki N., Kuroda N., Amaha K., et al. Succinylcholine induced hyperkalemia in patients with ruptured cerebral aneurysms. *Anethesiology* 53:64, 1980.
12. Weiss M. H., Spence J., Apuzzo M. J., et al. Influence of nitroprusside on cerebral pressure autoregulation. *Neurosurgery* 4:56, 1979.
13. Rogers M. C., Hamburger C., Owen K., et al. Intracranial pressure in the cat during nitroglycerin-induced hypotension. *Anesthesiology* 51:227, 1979.
14. Frost E. A. M. Some inquiries in neuroanesthesia and neurological supportive care. *J. Neurosurg.* 60:673, 1984.
15. Hoff J. T. Cerebral protection. *J. Neurosurg.* 65:579, 1986.
16. Kassell N. F., Peerless S. J., Durward Q. J. Treatment of ischemic deficits from vasospasm with intravascular volume expansion and induced arterial hypertension. *Neurosurgery* 11:337, 1982.
17. Montgomery E. B. Jr., Grubb R. L., Raichle M. E. Cerebral hemodynamics and metabolism in postoperative cerebral vasospasm and treatment with hypertensive therapy. *Ann. Neurol.* 9:502, 1981.
18. Aberg E., Adielson G., Almqvist A., et al. Multicenter trial of hemodilution in ischemic stroke—background and study protocol. *Stroke* 16:885, 1985.
19. Grotta J. C., Pettigrew L. C., Allen S., et al. Baseline hemodynamic state and response to hemodilution in patients with acute cerebral ischemia. *Stroke* 16:790, 1985.
20. Bendtsen A. O., Cold G. E., Astrup, et al. Thiopental loading during controlled hypotension for intracranial aneurysm surgery. *Acta Anesthesiol. Scand.* 28:473, 1984.
21. Markowitz I. P., Adinolfi M. F., Kerstein M. D. Barbiturate therapy in the postoperative endarterectomy patient with a neurologic deficit. *Am. J. Surg.* 148;221, 1984.
22. Shapiro H. M. Barbiturates in brain ischemia. *Br. J. Anaesth.* 57:82, 1985.
23. Smith A. L., Hoff J. T., Nielsen S. L., et al. Barbiturate protection in acute focal cerebral ischemia. *Stroke* 5:1, 1974.
24. Black K. L., Weidler D. J., Jallad N. S., et al. Delayed pentobarbital therapy of acute focal cerebral ischemia. *Stroke* 9:245, 1978.
25. Selman W. R., Spetzler R. F., Roessmann U. R., et al. Barbiturate-induced coma therapy for focal cerebral ischemia. Effect after temporary and permanent occlusion. *J. Neurosurg.* 55:220, 1981.
26. Hoff J. T., Pitts L. H., Spetzler R. F., et al. Barbiturates for protection from cerebral ischemia in aneurysm surgery. *Acta Neurol. Scand.* 56 (Suppl. 64):158, 1977.
27. Hoff J. T., Marshall L. Barbiturates in neurosurgery. *Clin. Neurosurg.* 26:245, 1979.
28. Astrup J., Sørensen P. M., Sørensen H. R. Inhibition of cerebral oxygen and glucose consumption in the dog by hypothermia, pentobarbital, and lidocaine. *Anesthesiology* 55:263, 1981.
29. Schwanne F. A. X., Kane A. B., Young E. E., et al. Calcium dependence of toxic cell death: A final common pathway. *Science* 206:700, 1979.
30. Pincus J. H., Grove I., Marino B. B., et al. Studies on the mechanism of action of diphenylhydantoin. *Arch. Neurol.* 22:566, 1970.
31. Cullen J. P., Aldrete J. A., Jankovsky L., et al. Protective effect of phenytoin in cerebral ischemia. *Anesth. Analog.* 58:165, 1979.
32. Artu A., Michenfelder J. D. Anoxic cerebral potassium accumulation reduced by phenytoin: Mechanism of cerebral protection? *Anesth. Analg.* 60:41, 1981.
33. Albin M. S., Babinski M., Maroon J. C., et al. Anesthetic management of posterior fossa surgery in the sitting position. *Acta Anaesthesiol. Scand.* 20:117, 1976.

34. Matjasko J., Patrozza P., Cohen M., et al. Anesthesia and surgery in the seated position: analysis of 554 cases. *Neurosurgery* 17:695, 1985.
35. English J. B., Westenskow D., Hodges M. R., et al. Comparison of venous air embolism monitoring methods in supine dogs. *Anesthesiology* 48:425, 1978.
36. Mogos B. L., Phillips P. L., Apfelbaum R. I., et al. Is right atrial catheterization always indicated for anesthesia in the sitting position? *Anesth. Analg.* 61:205, 1982.
37. Kitahata L. M., Katz J. D. Tension pneumocephalus after posterior-fossa craniectomy, a complication of the sitting position. *Anesthesiology* 44:448, 1976.
38. Lunsford L. D., Maroon J. C., Sheptak P. E., et al. Subdural tension pneumocephalus. Report of two cases. *J. Neurosurg.* 50:525, 1979.
39. Friedman G. A., Norfleet E. A., Bedford R. F. Discontinuation of nitrous oxide does not prevent tension pneumocephalus. *Anesth. Analg* 60:57, 1981.
40. Malis L. I. Prevention of neurosurgical infection by intraoperative antibiotics. *Neurosurgery* 5:339, 1979.
41. Dempsey R., Rapp R. P., Young B., et al. Prophylactic antibiotics in clean neurosurgical procedures: a review. *J Neurosurg.* 69:52, 1988.
42. Haines S. J. Efficacy of antibiotic prophylaxis in clean neurosurgical operations. *Neurosurgery* 24:401, 1989.
43. Flamm E. S., Ransohoff J., Wachinich D., et al. Preliminary experience with ultrasonic aspiration in neurosurgery. *Neurosurgery* 2:240, 1978.
44. Rubin J. M., Mirfakbraee M., Duda E. E., et al. Intraoperative ultrasound examination of the brain. *Radiology* 137:831, 1980.
45. Rubin J. M., Dohrmann G. J. Use of ultrasonically guided probes and catheters in neurosurgery. *Surg. Neurol.* 18:143, 1982.
46. Chandler W. F., Knake J. E., McGillicudy J. E., et al. Intraoperative use of real-time ultrasonography in neurosurgery. *J. Neurosurg.* 57:157, 1982.
47. Gooding G. A., Boggan E. E., Powers S. K., et al. Neurosurgical sonography: Intraoperative and postoperative imaging of the brain. *A.J.N.R.* 5:521, 1984.
48. Rubin J. M., Dohrmann G. J. The spine and spinal cord during neurosurgical operations: Real-time ultrasonography. *Radiology* 155:197, 1985.
49. Knake J. E., Bowerman R. A., Silver T. M., et al. Neurosurgical applications of intraoperative ultrasound. *Radiol. Clin. North. Am.* 23:73, 1985.
50. Saunders M. L., Young H. F., Becker D. P., et al. The use of the laser in neurological surgery. *Surg. Neurol.* 14:1, 1980.
51. Edwards M. S. B., Boggan J. E., Fuller T. A. The laser in neurological surgery. *J. Neurosurg.* 59:555, 1983.
52. Laws E. R., Jr., Cortese D. A., Kinsey J. H., et al. Photoradiation therapy in the treatment of malignant brain tumors: A phase I (feasibility) study. *J. Neurosurg.* 9:672, 1981.
53. Kelly P. J., Alker G. J., Goerss S. Computer assisted stereotactic laser microsurgery for the treatment of intracranial neoplasms. *Neurosurgery* 10:324, 1981.
54. Takeuchi J., Handa H., Taki W., et al. The Nd:Yag laser in neurological surgery. *Surg. Neurol.* 18:140, 1982.
55. Beck O. J. The use of the Nd-Yag and the CO_2 laser in neurosurgery. *Neurosurg. Rev.* 3:261, 1980.
56. Ulin A. W., Gollub S. S. *Surgical Bleeding: A Handbook for Medicine, Surgery and Specialties.* New York: McGraw-Hill, 1966. Pp. 427–431.
57. Lindstrom P. A. Complications from the use of absorbable hemostatic sponges. *Arch. Surg.* 73:133, 1956.

58. Cobden R. H., Trasher E. L., Harris W. H. Topical hemostatic agents to reduce bleeding from cancellous bone. *J. Bone Joint Surg.* 58A:70, 1976.
59. Ulin A. W., Gollub S. S. *Surgical Bleeding: A Handbook for Medicine, Surgery and Specialities.* New York: McGraw-Hill, 1966. Pp. 404–408.
60. Dineen P. Antibacterial effect of oxidized regenerated cellulose. *Surg. Gynecol. Obstet.* 142:481, 1976.
61. Scher K. S., Coil J. A. Jr. Effects of oxidized cellulose and microfibrillar collagen on infection. *Surgery* 91:301, 1982.
62. Arand A. G., Sawaya R. Intraoperative chemical hemostasis in neurosurgery. *Neurosurgery* 18:223, 1986.
63. Sugar O. Oxidized cellulose hemostat (Surgicel) (editorial). *Surg. Neurol.* 21:521, 1984.
64. Abbott W. M., Austen W. G. Microcrystalline collagen as a topical hemostatic agent for vascular surgery. *Surgery* 75:925, 1974.
65. Abbott W. M., Austen W. G. The effectiveness and mechanism of collagen-induced topical hemostasis. *Surgery* 78:723, 1975.
66. Stein B. M. General techniques for the surgical removal of arteriovenous malformations. In Wilson C. B., Stein B. M. (eds.). *Current Neurosurgical Practice: Intracranial Arteriovenous Malformations.* Baltimore: Williams & Wilkins, 1984. Pp. 156–183.
67. Drake C. G., Friedman A. H., Peerless S. J. Posterior fossa arteriovenous malformations. *J. Neurosurg.* 64:1, 1986.
68. Lüders H. Lesser R. P., Hahn J., et al. Basal temporal language area demonstrated by electrical stimulation. *Neurology* 36:505, 1986.
69. Ojemann G. A. Individual variability in cortical localization of language. J. Neurosurg. 50:164, 1979.
70. Engel J. Jr., Crandall P. H., Rausch R. The partial epilepsies. In Rosenberg R., Grossman R (eds.). *The Clinical Neurosciences, Vol. II. Neurosurgery.* New York: Churchill Livingstone, 1983. Pp. 1149–1380.
71. Falconer M. Anterior temporal lobectomy for epilepsy. In Logue V (ed.): *Neurosurgery*, ed 2; *Operative Surgery,* vol. 14. London: Butterworths, 1971. Pp. 142–149.
72. Gates J. R., Leppik I. E., Yap J., et al. Corpus callosotomy: Clinical and electroencephalographic effects. *Epilepsia* 25:308, 1984.
73. Marino R. Jr., Ragazzo P. C. Selective criteria and results of selective partial callosotomy. In Reeves A. G. (ed.). *Epilepsy and the Corpus Callosum.* New York: Plenum Press, 1985. Pp. 281–302.
74. Ferguson S. M., Rayport M., Corrie W. S. Neuropsychiatric observations on behavioral consequences of corpus callosum for seizure control. In Reeves A. G. (ed.): *Epilepsy and the Corpus Callosum.* New York: Plenum Press, 1985. Pp. 501–504.
75. Prough D. S., Scuderi P. E., Shuttken E., et al. Myocardial infarction following regional anesthesia for carotid endarterectomy. *Can. Anesth. Soc. J.* 31:192, 1984.
76. Hays R. J., Levinson S. A., Wylie E. J. Intraoperative assessment of carotid back pressure as a guide to operative management for carotid endarterectomy. *Surgery* 72:853, 1972.
77. Sharbrough F. W., Messick J. M., Sundt T. M. Correlation of continuous electroencephalograms with cerebral blood flow measurements during carotid endarterectomy. *Stroke* 4:674, 1973.
78. Sung Y. F. Anesthetic considerations for patients undergoing transphenoidal surgery. In Tindall G. T., Collins W. F. (eds.): *Clinical Management of Pituitary Disorders.* New York: Raven Press, 1979. Pp. 413–424.
79. Tindall G. T., Collins W. F. Jr., Kirchner J. A. Unilateral septal technique for

transphenoidal microsurgical approach to the sella turcica: Technical note. *J. Neurosurg.* 49:138, 1978.

80. Heilbrun M. P. Computed tomography-guided stereotactic systems. *Clin. Neurosurg.* 31:564, 1983.
81. Heilbrun M. P., Roberts T. S., Apuzzo M. L. J., et al. Preliminary experience with Brown-Roberts-Wells computerized tomography stereotaxic guidance system. *J. Neurosurg.* 59:217, 1983.
82. Sweet W. H., Wepsic S. G. Controlled thermocoagulation of trigeminal ganglion and results for differential destruction of pain fibers. *J. Neurosurg.* 39:143, 1969.
83. Tew J. M., Keller J. T. The treatment of trigeminal neuralgia by percutaneous radiofrequency technique. *Clin. Neurosurg.* 24:557, 1976.
84. Nugent G. R. Technique and results of 800 percutaneous radiofrequency themocoagulations for trigeminal neuralgia. *Appl. Neurophysiol.* 45:504, 1982.
85. Häkanson S. Trigeminal neuralgia treated by the injection of glycerol into the trigeminal cistern. *Neurosurgery* 9:639, 1981.
86. Lunsford L. D. Treatment of tic douloureux by percutaneous retrogasserian glycerol injection. *J.A.M.A.* 45:504, 1982.
87. Jannetta P. J. Microsurgical approach to the trigeminal nerve for tic douloureux. *Prog. Neurol. Surg.* 7:180, 1976.
88. Hongo K., Kobayashi S., Yokoh A., et al. Monitoring retraction pressure on the brain: An experimental and clinical study. *J. Neurosurg.* 66:270, 1987.

Suggested Reading

Cottrell J. E., Turndorf H. *Anesthesia and Neurosurgery,* 2nd. ed. St. Louis; Mosby, 1986.

Kempe L. G. *Operative Neurosurgery,* Vol. 1. Berlin: Springer-Verlag, 1968.

Kempe L. G. *Operative Neurosurgery,* Vol. 2. Berlin: Springer-Verlag, 1970.

Long D. M. *Atlas of Operative Neurosurgical Technique, Vol. 1. Cranial Operations.* Baltimore: Williams & Wilkins, 1988.

McLaurin R. L., Schut L., Venes J. Epstein F. (eds). *Pediatric Neurosurgery: Surgery of the Developing Nervous System,* 2nd ed. Philadelphia: Saunders, 1989.

Schmidek H. H., Sweet W. H. (eds). *Operative Neurosurgical Techniques: Indications, Methods, and Results,* 2nd ed. Philadelphia: Saunders, 1988.

Symon L., Thomas D. G. T., Clark K. (eds). *Rob & Smith's Operative Surgery—Neurosurgery,* 4th ed. London: Butterworths, 1989.

7. Postoperative Care

The principles of postoperative care following most intracranial procedures are quite similar. Careful clinical observation repeated at frequent intervals by trained nursing personnel and neurosurgical housestaff will generally identify potential problems and significant trends. Nurses in the recovery room or intensive care unit (ICU) may not have met the patient before surgery. Therefore, they should be apprised of the preoperative neurologic status or existing medical problems. The surgeon should give some indication about short-term prognosis. A general scheme for postoperative management is described, followed by specific issues for different conditions.

Craniotomy

Postoperative care for the craniotomy patient is described below.

General Orders

1. Perform vital signs and neurologic checks according to the post-anesthesia care routine; then, at least every hour in the neurosurgical ICU for the first 24 hours and every 2 hours if the patient is stable. Findings should be reported in a standard fashion so that different examiners can compare results. The examination of patients in altered states of consciousness is an essential clinical skill (see Plum and Posner [1]). Briefly, one needs to determine the level of consciousness and assess cranial nerve integrity and sensorimotor function.

   Subtle changes in a patient's condition may go unnoticed, especially in patients who are intubated or aphasic. Postoperative systemic hypertension may be secondary to pain or elevated intracranial pressure (ICP). Hypertension may precipitate postoperative hemorrhage, especially following evacuation of an intraparenchymal hematoma or resection of an arteriovenous malformation (AVM); therefore, control of blood pressure in these situations is important.
2. Do not give anything orally until the patient is fully awake and alert; then try clear liquids and advance diet as tolerated. Tube feeding may be necessary in patients who cannot tolerate conventional oral diets. These include comatose patients, those with impaired deglutition, or those requiring prolonged intubation. Some patients may need a gastrostomy or other enterostomy if tube feedings are to continue indefinitely.
3. Elevate the head of the bed to 30 degrees. This improves cerebral venous drainage and reduces ICP in most instances. Allow activity as tolerated. Endeavor to get the patient out of bed on the first or second postoperative day.

4. A Foley catheter is placed during most craniotomies. This should be removed as soon as possible. In the initial postoperative period, follow intake and output hourly. Check urine specific gravity if urine output is over 300 ml/hour or more than 500 ml/2 hours. Polyuria may be secondary to intraoperative volume loading or may be indicative of diabetes insipidus (DI). Check the intraoperative fluid balance sheet to ascertain this and monitor the progress of urine output. Check serum electrolytes and blood counts as indicated.
5. Before fluid orders are written, review intraoperative fluid administration and urine output. Hyperosmolar agents may have been given, resulting in a delayed diuresis; blood loss and transfusions should also be considered. Output from a cerebrospinal fluid (CSF) drain is also relevant. Hypotension during anesthesia for cerebrovascular surgery may reduce renal perfusion and urine output transiently. Restoration of normal arterial pressure results in a brisk diuresis. Determine the patient's daily maintenance of fluid and electrolytes based on age and weight. Other losses from fever, respiration, and, in multiple system trauma, third space loss must be considered. The usual plan is to write tentative orders based on the best estimate of potential needs and the vital signs. Revise the fluid orders based on clinical and laboratory assessment. Although general surgeons have generally been "volume-oriented" and "perfusion-oriented," neurosurgeons have tended to "keep their patients dry."

Water intoxication is an undesirable complication; it is not frequent in the usual postoperative neurosurgical patient but may be seen with large sudden fluid shifts between fluid spaces after substantial volume replacement in patients with multiple trauma or as an iatrogenic complication when correcting hypernatremia.

Although it is important to avoid overexpansion of the intravascular space because systemic hypertension and elevated hydrostatic pressure may promote the spread of vasogenic cerebral edema, it is equally true that autoregulation of cerebral blood flow (CBF) is regionally defective in many diseases as well as during general anesthesia; indeed CBF may be pressure passive, making an adequate cerebral perfusion pressure (CPP) even more crucial. Typical initial intravenous fluid orders for an adult patient are as follows:

5% dextrose and 0.5 normal saline

+ 20 mEq KCl/L at a rate to maintain euvolemia

Where cerebral ischemia is present, the addition of glucose to the infusate may be deleterious (see Chap. 1 for a discussion on cerebral metabolism). Under these circumstances, normal saline is an acceptable option.
6. If an arterial line has been placed, connect it to a continuous monitor; set parameters for which to implement necessary interventions.
7. Provide humidified oxygen (FiO$_2$ 40%) by face mask. If the patient

is comatose or has a poor cough, chest physiotherapy every 2 hours and aerosolized bronchodilators as necessary may help in clearing pulmonary secretions. The awake patient may also benefit from incentive spirometry. Most postoperative pulmonary problems are accentuated in smokers and patients with chronic lung disease.

If the patient is to remain intubated, orders for ventilatory support (tidal volume, respiratory rate, inspired oxygen concentration, and positive pressure) are written. Patients who remain comatose and intubated for a significant period may require tracheotomy in order to maintain the airway.

8. Provide thigh-high antiembolism stockings or pneumatic compression stockings if indicated.

9. Give an analgesic (e.g., acetaminophen [Tylenol] 650 mg with codeine phosphate 60 mg orally or codeine phosphate 60 mg intramuscularly every 4 hours) as needed for pain. This regimen does not significantly depress respiration or alter pupillary responses. A certain amount of cephalalgia can be expected after craniotomy. Most of the pain originates from nerves in the scalp. The head dressing should not be applied too tightly as this may be uncomfortable.

10. Give acetaminophen 650 mg orally every 4 hours as needed for temperature over 101.5°F. Some fever can be expected soon after craniotomy, especially if blood has been spilled in the subarachnoid space or if cranioplasty has been performed with prosthetic materials. Occasionally, hyperpyrexia may follow surgery around the hypothalamus. Embark on a fever workup if other considerations warrant it. Hypothermia in the early postoperative period may occur after lengthy procedures.

11. Nausea or vomiting are not infrequent in the early postoperative period. Vomiting should be discouraged as it may elevate ICP at least transiently. Conversely, raised ICP may result in vomiting. More often nausea and vomiting are side effects of general anesthesia rather than intracranial hypertension, although this must be considered. For symptomatic relief, prochlorperazine maleate (Compazine) 10 mg intramuscularly or rectally every 6 hours as needed may be given for nausea. Note that phenothiazine derivatives are contraindicated in some neurosurgical patients.

12. Steroids are sometimes used in the perioperative period, especially with intracranial tumors. The rationale is that steroids reduce peritumoral edema. Generally, the regimen is maintained through the expected peak of cerebral edema, which commonly occurs 48 to 72 hours after operation. Dexamethasone sodium (Decadron) 10 mg orally or intravenously every 6 hours and then in tapering doses is an acceptable regimen. The oral route is preferable when possible. The intravenous route is less effective for maintaining steady blood levels. Assume some suppression of the adrenal cortex whenever corticosteroids are administered in pharmacologic doses for a significant duration. Unless a complication such as gastrointestinal hemorrhage intervenes, gradually taper the dose of steroids. This

reduces the likelihood of an iatrogenic addisonian crisis or a recrudescence of cerebral edema. The patient's clinical condition is the best indicator of when steroids may be withdrawn.

13. Give an antacid (e.g., Maalox 30 ml orally every 4 hours) or a histamine (H_2-receptor) blocker (e.g., ranitidine [Zantac] 50 mg intravenously every 8 hours or 150 mg orally 2 times a day) for stress ulcer prophylaxis. This is particularly necessary if the patient is on steroids; therapy should ordinarily be continued through the period when the patient is taking steroids.

14. Anticonvulsant therapy with phenytoin sodium (Dilantin) or other agents may be necessary for some intracranial lesions. Many cerebral lesions present with seizures (e.g., tumors and AVMs); furthermore, surgery is traumatic to neural tissue and may lead to an irritative focus. The usual adult maintenance dose of phenytoin sodium is 300 to 500 mg orally or intravenously daily in divided doses after an initial loading dose of 1 gm (see Chap. 4 for a discussion on prophylactic convulsants in neurosurgery).

15. Routine laboratory assessment includes a complete blood count (CBC), serum electrolytes, and arterial blood gases (ABGs). These should be monitored as frequently as is clinically warranted.

16. *Wound management.* The craniotomy dressing is left in place for 24 to 48 hours and then removed, leaving the incision open. It is not unusual to precipitate a slight superficial ooze when the dressings are removed; this is almost never significant. Inspect the wound daily. Remove the sutures or staples between the tenth and fourteenth postoperative day. The rate of wound infection following clean neurosurgical cases is between 1 and 2 percent.

Postoperative Care in Specific Conditions

Intracranial Aneurysm

Cerebral Perfusion

Maintaining an adequate CBF and reducing morbidity from vasospasm are important goals in the postoperative care of the patient with a ruptured cerebral aneurysm.

Volume expansion with crystalloid or colloid solutions is one method of achieving an adequate CBF. Monitoring intravascular volume by central line or Swan-Ganz catheter is necessary to tailor therapy appropriately. In some patients with symptomatic vasospasm, a pressor agent (e.g., dopamine) may be required to elevate blood pressure and further augment CBF, providing the aneurysm has been excluded from the circulation.

Calcium Channel Blockers

The calcium channel blocker nimodipine may be given to reduce the severity of ischemic neurologic deficits associated with vasospasm.

The usual dose is 60 mg orally every 4 hours beginning within 96 hours of the event and continuing for 21 consecutive days following subarachnoid hemorrhage (SAH) (see Chap. 4).

Postoperative Angiogram

Although some neurosurgeons are able to confirm satisfactory treatment of the aneurysm intraoperatively, others prefer a postoperative angiogram. Incomplete clipping of the aneurysm with continued filling of the aneurysm may occur in up to 5 percent of patients; this constitutes a valid reason for reoperation since the residual neck may expand into another sac. An angiogram may also be indicated for the differential diagnosis of vasospasm from other postoperative complications of aneurysm surgery that have a similar clinical presentation.

Complications

Complications of intracranial aneurysms include cerebral infarction, hydrocephalus, and cerebral edema.

1. *Infarction.* Even after a technically successful operation, some patients may fail to awaken from anesthesia; others awaken with a new neurologic deficit. Some may deteriorate a few days after surgery.

   Some of these problems are due to systemic factors (metabolic, hypotension); others are the result of a major vessel occlusion, cerebral vasospasm, or hydrocephalus [2, 3]. Vessel occlusion may be from malpositioning of an aneurysm clip. A misplaced clip, if discovered early, should prompt a return to the operating room for clip repositioning. Intraoperative angiography may reduce the incidence of such mishaps [4].

   Surgery in the proximity of striatal or brainstem perforators may disrupt these fragile channels, resulting in significant morbidity.

   Intraoperative induced hypotension may precipitate "watershed infarcts" if collateral circulation is poor.
2. *Recurrent SAH.* Likely causes include inadequate clipping [5], rupture of an untreated lesion in a patient with multiple aneurysm [6], or the "slipped clip" [7, 8].
3. *Hydrocephalus* following SAH may be acute, obstructive (noncommunicating) from intraventricular hemorrhage [9], or delayed (secondary [communicating]) due to basal adhesions.

Arteriovenous Malformation

Postoperative considerations include the following:

1. *Hemorrhage.* This may be the result of poor hemostasis, hypertension in the immediate postoperative period, or the normal perfusion-pressure breakthrough phenomenon. Blood pressure must therefore be

carefully controlled, and extremes of hypotension or hypertension must be evaluated and treated appropriately.

2. *Cerebral edema* may be from excessive brain retraction, normal perfusion breakthrough, or other forms of altered cerebral autoregulation. Steroids may be helpful in the treatment of cerebral edema.

3. Postoperative angiography is necessary to confirm completeness of the AVM resection. Residual lesions may require reoperation or, in some cases, radiotherapy.

4. *Seizure.* Seizures are common with supratentorial AVMs. They may worsen cerebral edema or precipitate a hemorrhage; therefore, prompt effective management is necessary.

5. Postoperative *neurologic deficit* may be transient or permanent. Transient ischemic deficits may be due to cerebral edema or disordered autoregulation as the cerebral circulation adjusts to the removal of the AVM. Permanent deficits may be the result of an en passant vessel sacrificed during the resection.

Epilepsy Surgery

Anticonvulsants should generally be continued at preoperative levels. Serum drug levels are checked to ensure that dosing is within therapeutic range. Patients continue to take anticonvulsants for the first year after surgery. If they have no seizures, the anticonvulsant is gradually tapered.

If the ventricle was entered at surgery, some patients may experience an aseptic meningitis syndrome with lethargy, nausea, and fever. This is a reaction to breakdown products of blood in the CSF. Spinal fluid cultures are negative, and cytologic findings show chronic inflammatory cells.

Complications of epilepsy surgery include the following:

1. *Hemiparesis.* Sacrifice of a vessel (e.g., the anterior choroidal artery) during anterior temporal lobectomy may lead to infarction of the adjacent internal capsule and globus pallidus.

2. *Visual field defect* (e.g., superior quadrantanopsia).

3. Subtle deficits of recent *memory.*

Carotid Endarterectomy

Blood pressure fluctuations are not infrequent in the early postoperative period and may be due to baroreceptor dysfunction [10]. The patient should be cautiously ambulated to prevent postural hypotension. Postoperative *hypertension* correlates with postoperative complications. Control of hypertension diminishes the risk of *myocardial ischemia* and *intraparenchymal hemorrhage* [11]. *Cardiac arrhythmias* are common in the postoperative period because of associated coronary artery disease in these patients.

The wound should be inspected for development of hematoma. Airway obstruction from hematoma is an indication for reexploration. If a drain is used, it is removed by the second postoperative day.

Most patients are ready for discharge within a week of surgery. The main complications are perioperative myocardial infarction, stroke, and neck hematoma. Continued risk reduction of atherosclerotic cerebrovascular disease by diet modification and an antiplatelet drug regimen is advised.

Pituitary Adenomectomy

Most pituitary adenomas are removed by the transsphenoidal route. The primary considerations in the postoperative period are those of fluid balance and corticosteroid coverage. Typical postoperative orders include:

1. The patient should avoid blowing the nose. Dab dry any rhinorrhea.
2. Remove nasal airways on the first postoperative day.
3. Hydrocortisone 100 mg orally or intravenously every 8 hours is continued after surgery. This dose is tapered over 72 hours to maintenance levels. Check serum cortisol at 6 A.M. after holding the P.M. dose the previous day to determine possible corticotropin deficiency and the need for hydrocortisone maintenance at discharge [12]. Seven to ten days following surgery, the patient undergoes endocrinologic testing (T_4, LH, FSH, testosterone [in male patients], and estradiol [in female patients]) to assess residual pituitary function. Replacement thyroid medication may be required. If prolactin was elevated preoperatively, a postoperative level is obtained at this time.
4. Monitor fluid intake-output and urine specific gravity for DI. Most cases of DI following transsphenoidal surgery are transient and resolve spontaneously. Most patients will have an adequate oral intake in response to thirst. If the patient is not alert or oral intake is insufficient, intravenous fluids may be required (this is unusual).

Fortunately, there is enough circulating antidiuretic hormone (ADH); therefore, DI rarely occurs within the first 24 to 36 hours. Early polyuria may be an appropriate response from intraoperative fluid loading. If urine output exceeds 500 ml/2 hours or 300 ml/hour and urine specific gravity is less than 1.005 or urine osmolality is between 50 and 150 mOsm/kg, obtain a serum sodium level. If fluid replacement is not effective and serum sodium exceeds 150 mEq/L, give aqueous vasopressin (Pitressin) 5 units intramuscularly or subcutaneously. Alternately, desmopressin acetate (DDAVP) 0.5 to 1.0 ml (2.0–4.0 μg) intravenously or subcutaneously may be given in two divided doses over 24 hours.

Complications of Transsphenoidal Adenomectomy

1. *Diabetes insipidus.*
2. Varying degrees of *anterior lobe dysfunction* (hypopituitarism). In experienced hands, the incidence of permanent difficulties is low [13].

3. Injury to the *visual apparatus*. Damage is likely when the tumor capsule is firmly attached to the visual apparatus. Dissection may interfere with the blood supply of the optic chiasm, resulting in ischemia.
4. *CSF rhinorrhea* is infrequent and usually transient. If sustained, it may lead to meningitis. Persistent CSF leak may require continuous lumbar drainage or operative repair for control.
5. *Nasal congestion or sinusitis* is usually transient; pseudoephedrine hydrocholoride (Actifed) 60 mg orally every 6 hours offers symptomatic relief.

Brain Tumor (Glioma)

Gliomas are the most common variety of brain tumor. Craniotomy for resection or biopsy for diagnosis are the usual procedures performed.

Postoperatively, steroids are generally continued and tapered as clinically indicated. Patients with preoperative seizure should have their anticonvulsants continued. If craniotomy was performed for recurrent tumor in a patient who has had previous radiation, the wound must be carefully watched; sutures may need to be kept in slightly longer because of delayed healing.

Alterations in neurologic status may be due to postoperative hemorrhage or cerebral edema. A nonenhanced computed tomography (CT) scan can differentiate between these entities. Residual tumor may be determined by contrast-enhanced CT or MRI. Posterior fossa craniectomies may be complicated by aseptic meningitis, CSF leak, or hydrocephalus.

Chemotherapy

At present, the use of chemotherapy for malignant gliomas is *adjunctive*. The nitrosoureas are the best-known chemotherapeutic agents for brain tumor therapy. They are highly *lipid soluble* and readily *cross* the blood-brain barrier. The most effective agent is carmustine (BCNU) [14]. Improved median survival times with BCNU therapy after surgery and radiotherapy has been demonstrated in several studies. BCNU may cause bone marrow toxicity, liver dysfunction, and pulmonary fibrosis if the cumulative dose exceeds 1400 mg. Still at issue is the optimal timing of chemotherapy [15–17]. The intracarotid route of delivery may reduce systemic toxicity while enhancing delivery to the tumor.

Many chemotherapeutic agents are under phase I and II trials, and varying clinical protocols are being explored [18].

Immunotherapy

This modality takes its cue from the observation that patients with brain tumors demonstrate impaired humoral and cellular immunity. Promising lines of investigation include (1) active immunization of patients with irradiated autologous tumor cells or with human glioma cell lines, (2) interferon therapy, and (3) passive immunotherapy with monoclonal antibodies tagged to radioisotopes and biological toxins [19].

Radiotherapy

Radiotherapy is currently the most effective and widely used form of adjunctive therapy for malignant gliomas. Conventional radiotherapy is usually given in the range of 5500 to 6000 rad delivered in 30 to 35 fractions, five treatments each week. Adjuvant radiotherapy for brain tumors shows a linear dose relationship between 4500 and 6000 rad. Lower doses are less likely to be effective. Doses above 6000 rad present an increased risk of radionecrosis. Whether postoperative adjuvant radiation therapy in cerebral astrocytoma (grades I and II astrocytomas of the Kernohan classification) is more beneficial than harmful is not fully resolved [20, 21].

Other forms of delivering radiation include *brachytherapy, hyperfractionation,* and *heavy particle radiotherapy.*
Brachytherapy. Interstitial radiotherapy or brachytherapy, which literally means "short therapy," is achieved by placing a source (usually iodine 125 [^{125}I] or iridium 192 [^{192}Ir]) at or near the center of the tumor. The appeal of brachytherapy is that more radiation can be delivered to a focal area, thus obviating the main drawback of teletherapy (external beam radiation), i.e., unnecessary radiation spill to surrounding normal brain tissue. The main dose of radiation (10,000 rad or more) is directed at the tumor with an exponential decline in radiation from the center of the lesion. The surrounding brain tissue is therefore unlikely to receive lethal doses of radiation. Another advantage of brachytherapy is that radiation is delivered at a considerably lower dose rate compared with conventional radiation; this maximizes the effectiveness of differential cell killing between neoplastic tissue and normal tissue.

Brachytherapy is frequently used in the management of malignant gliomas in combination with teletherapy so that the "booster dose" is given by brachytherapy. Patients with recurrent malignant gliomas who have failed other adjuvant therapy are also potential candidates for brachytherapy. The ideal lesion is small (<5 cm), solitary, and well defined on contrast-enhanced CT scan. Typically, the patient has had debulking surgery or stereotactic biopsy as a primary procedure, and a tissue diagnosis has been made. A CT-guided stereotactic procedure is performed for implantation of one or more removable catheters into the tumor and then the radioactive seeds are loaded into them [22].
POSTOPERATIVE CARE. During treatment there is some risk to health personnel and visitors; therefore, the patient should be relatively isolated. Radiation monitoring protocols should be followed. Lead-lined helmets are necessary for patients with iodine implants; portable lead shields can limit iridium isotopes.

The main risks of brachytherapy are those associated with the stereotactic procedure itself and radiation necrosis [23, 24].

Hyperfractionation. This is a technique designed to increase central nervous system (CNS) tolerance by using a larger number of smaller fractions of radiation. Proliferating glioma cells are more likely to be exposed to radiation during the most sensitive part of their cell cycle if radiation is delivered at frequent intervals during a 24-hour period. Furthermore, normal glial cells are better able to repair the sublethal damage induced at a lower dose of radiation.

Heavy Particle Radiotherapy. Heavy particle radiotherapy refers to treatment with beams of subatomic particles (such as neutrons and protons) rather than photon beams (x-rays or gamma rays).

Heavy particle radiotherapy offers two advantages. Except for neutrons, heavy particle beams give a superior localization of radiation dose to the target, thereby decreasing the dose to surrounding normal tissue. This is a result of the Bragg peak effect—the charged particle penetrates to a definite predetermined distance within tissue and deposits most of the radiation dose at that locus, which is called the Bragg peak. The other advantage is that most heavy particles have biological superiority in terms of tumor cell killing. Several subsets of tumor cells (e.g., hypoxic cells and cells in the S phase of the mitotic cycle) are relatively resistant to x-ray beams; furthermore, recovery of tumor cells by repair of sublethal damage is less likely with some of the heavy particle beams. Neutrons are not charged particles and therefore do not exhibit the Bragg peak effect but do have biological advantages. Protons have a very sharp Bragg peak but little or no biological advantage [20].

Heavy particle beams that have undergone clinical trial include neutrons, protons, and pions.

Neutron therapy is being explored because it is more effective against hypoxic cells (which are relatively radioresistant and are present in significant numbers within tumors) and shows less variation in radiation sensitivity relative to the cell cycle [25].

Radiation-sensitizing drugs (radiosensitizers) are chemotherapeutic agents that modify the effects of radiation therapy. They include misonidazole and the halogenated pyrimidines (5-iodo-2-deoxyuridine [IUdR] and 5-bromodeoxyuridine [BUdR]). They are given to enhance the lethal effect of radiotherapy. None of the agents studied so far has proved to be of significant therapeutic benefit [14].

Hazards of CNS Radiation. Adverse effects of radiation on the CNS limit the amount of radiation that may be delivered in the treatment of brain tumors. *Early reactions* may be due to cerebral edema or breakdown products of the tumor cells. Presenting symptoms are nonspecific: fatigue, malaise, anorexia, or manifestations of raised ICP. Steroid therapy is frequently effective in controlling these early reactions.

Intermediate reactions may occur weeks to a few months after completion of treatment and are probably due to demyelination.

Late reactions are delayed for many months and are usually due to radiation necrosis. These areas of necrosis may present as space-occupying lesions, mimicking the original tumor. It is difficult to assess the incidence of radionecrosis since it is similar in clinical and radiologic appearance to recurrent tumor [26].

Acoustic Neuroma

Most of these tumors are approached through a retromastoid posterior fossa craniectomy. Following *posterior fossa operations,* particular considerations include attention to the status of the lower cranial nerves, respiratory pattern, and the common occurrence of nausea and vomiting from medullary irritation.

Complications

1. *Facial palsy* may result from excessive manipulation of the facial nerve or division of its fibers at surgery. Some patients will need a tarsorrhaphy to protect the cornea. If the facial nerve was grossly intact at the end of the procedure and there is a postoperative facial palsy, it is reasonable to wait a few months to assess the resolution of the deficit. If the nerve was divided at the time of surgery, hypoglossal-facial nerve anastomosis or primary repair of the facial nerve are useful procedures designed to promote regeneration of the nerve.
2. *CSF rhinorrhea* may result from leakage of CSF into exposed mastoid air cells and then into the nasopharynx by way of the middle ear and eustachian tube. It is therefore important to wax exposed air cells adequately. Although many cease spontaneously, others may require a short period of lumbar drainage (see Chap. 3). In persistent cases, the wound may need to be reexplored and the mastoid air cells packed.
3. *Meningitis* may be aseptic or bacterial (the more serious variety). Aseptic meningitis is generally the result of the meningeal reaction from subarachnoid blood spilled during surgery.
4. Other potential complications of lesser frequency include *hydrocephalus, cranial nerve palsies* (fifth, sixth, ninth, tenth), and brainstem infarction.

Cerebrospinal Fluid Shunts

Postoperative Management: Children

The anterior fontanelle should be soft or depressed in a quiet, sitting infant. Most patients who have undergone uncomplicated shunts can be discharged on the second postoperative day. The child is usually seen in the clinic initially at 2 weeks and then at regular intervals. Irritability, failure to thrive, vomiting, and headache may suggest shunt malfunction or infection. CT scans are obtained to monitor ventricular size. The length of shunt tubing is followed by abdominal x-rays (for ventriculoperitoneal shunts) and chest x-rays (for ventriculoatrial shunts).

Shunt Revisions

Revisions may be prophylactic to accommodate normal growth or to treat a shunt malfunction.

Complications of CSF Shunts

1. *Shunt malfunction.* This should be suspected if there is persistent bulging of the anterior fontanelle or increasing head circumference in an infant or signs of increased ICP in the older child.

   Progressive ventricular enlargement on serial CT scans without clinical symptoms is also a sign of malfunction. Sometimes CSF may accumulate along the shunt tract in the neck, chest, or abdomen.

   Commonly there is an obstruction (choroid plexus or blood clot) at the ventricular end of the shunt. The peritoneal end may also cause difficulty from reduced absorption or formation of a pseudocyst. Shunt catheters have also been known to migrate into the most unlikely locations.

2. *Shunt Infections.* One of the major complications of shunts is *infection.* The incidence is less with the more experienced operator and is higher in infants. *Staphylococcus epidermidis* is the commonest organism.

   An *internal shunt infection* is an infection of the shunt hardware, ventriculitis, or meningitis. It may be associated with peritonitis or bacteremia. Skin infection is usually not an important feature. Intermittent low-grade fever in the presence of negative systemic cultures is a suspicious sign. There may be evidence of shunt malfunction. Less frequent signs include anemia, nuchal stiffness, and hepatosplenomegaly.

   An *external shunt infection* is defined as a wound infection or skin breakdown with exposure of the shunt hardware over some length of its course.

   Shunt infections may be treated by removing the shunt system and administering antibiotics according to result of CSF culture and sensitivities. If symptoms of increased ICP are present, an external ventricular drainage system should be employed (see External Ventricular Drainage in Chap. 2, p. 33).

3. Postshunt subdural hematoma. This is especially likely in the patient with markedly dilated ventricles before shunting. Preventive measures include limiting the amount of CSF drained at the time of shunt insertion, coagulating the cortex to the dura, and gradually ambu-

lating or sitting the patient up postoperatively. Treatment may include surgical evacuation through burr holes or craniotomy.
4. Postshunt craniosynostosis. This usually occurs from overshunting in infants with open sutures. Overriding of sutures and premature fusion may result in secondary craniosynostosis.

Spinal Surgery

Spinal Injuries

Most spinal injuries do not require operative treatment. However, in some patients neural decompression may improve function or spinal fusion may be required to secure a reduction. The main goals of postoperative care in these instances are the maintenance of reduction, promotion of healing, and avoidance of further neurologic injury and secondary medical conditions that may arise from prolonged immobilization. Management during this time may include:

1. Log rolling every 2 hours maintains spinal alignment and reduces periods of recumbency. If the patient is immobile, a Kinnair or Clinitron bed is helpful in preventing decubitus ulcers and nerve palsies as well as promoting postural lung drainage. For paraplegic patients, a foot board or hightop sneakers helps prevent contracture with the ankle in extension.
2. Physical and occupational therapy help the patient avoid contractures and atrophy of disuse. Passive range-of-motion exercises help maintain joint mobility. Splinting of the hand in the position of function is useful between periods of manipulation. Rehabilitative efforts should be initiated early. The medical social worker can help marshall local support systems for discharge planning.
3. Chest physiotherapy. Patients with cervical spine injuries may lose intercostal control and tend to breath with the diaphragm and accessory respiratory muscles. Such excursions are shallow and poorly coordinated, and clearance of secretions is impaired. Chest physiotherapy helps promote drainage and aeration of the lung fields.
4. Maximize intravascular volume. During the period of "spinal shock," impaired sympathetic tone results in a dilated vascular bed and hypotension. This may persist for days. Volume support is necessary to maintain critical spinal cord blood flow and perfusion of other organs. As much as 4 or 6 liters/day may be necessary. Watch for the return of vascular tone, which is heralded by a brisk diuresis.
5. Adynamic ileus may follow spinal shock. A bowel regimen with stool softeners and laxatives will maintain bowel function and prevent constipation and fecal impaction. A nasogastric tube may be needed for gastric decompression.
6. Provide for bladder drainage. Following a spinal cord injury, the bladder may be initially flaccid but soon regains its tone and may even become hypertonic or spastic. Early on, an indwelling catheter may

be necessary if the bladder is atonic, a not infrequent condition in many patients with cervical spinal cord injuries. This should be replaced by a regimen of intermittent catheterization as soon as possible to reduce the risk of urinary tract infection and promote bladder retraining. With increasing bladder tone, voiding may be more frequent and one may settle for a condom catheter. If prolonged indwelling catheter drainage must be used, initiate suppressant antibiotic therapy with trimethoprim-sulfamethoxazole (Bactrim) or an equivalent agent.

With cauda equina lesions (e.g., from lumbar spine injuries), the bladder may remain hypotonic. Bethanechol (Urecholine) 10 to 50 mg orally 4 times a day may be used. These patients can be trained to urinate by the Crede maneuver.
7. Cervical traction. With cervical spine injuries, it is often necessary to apply cervical spinal traction to reduce a subluxation or fracture-dislocation. Examples include the Gardner-Wells, University of Virginia, and the Trippi-Wells tongs. These devices are simple to apply. Their application and care of the patient in traction are discussed in Chap. 5.

Benign Spine Lesions

Herniated Lumbar Disk and Lumbar Spinal Stenosis. Most patients with herniated lumbar disk are otherwise healthy. Lumbar stenosis is a disease of older persons with the associated medical problems of aging. The commonest procedure for herniated lumbar disk is a laminotomy and diskectomy. Decompressive lumbar laminectomy (often multiple levels) is the procedure of choice for lumbar stenosis.

Typical postoperative orders include the following:

1. Vital signs and neurologic status checks every 4 hours, with attention to limb movement. Rarely, an epidural hematoma may lead to postoperative deficit.
2. Activity as tolerated. If epidural anesthesia has been used, watch for full return of function before ambulation. The patient should avoid vigorous physical activity involving lifting or bending. Walking should be encouraged as soon as the patient can get out of bed. A prolonged period in bed invites the complications of thrombophlebitis, pulmonary embolism, urinary tract infection, and atelectasis. Defer physical therapy until the patient is free of acute postoperative pain and is willing to devote full effort. Various orthotic devices are available to aid the disabled patient. If a spinal fusion has been performed, further immobilization in a brace may be required. If the neurosurgeon has collaborated with an orthopedic surgeon for spinal fusion, it is well to consult with him or her regarding ambulation, position in bed, and orthotic devices.
3. Postoperative analgesia. Demerol, 50 to 100 mg intramuscularly every 4 hours, or morphine, 10 to 15 mg intramuscularly every 4 hours

with promethazine hydrochloride (Phenergan) or hydroxyzine (Vistaril), 25 mg intramuscularly every 6 hours, for narcotic potentiation is a good regimen. Diazepam may be necessary if muscular spasms are bothersome, especially in a patient with a multiple-level laminectomy.
4. Postoperative radicular symptoms. After lumbar disk surgery, it is not uncommon for the patient to experience a temporary relapse of radicular symptoms on the second or third postoperative day. This has been ascribed to recovery of the nerve from a period of compression or edema from handling at surgery. The condition is frequently a source of anxiety to the patient and, occasionally, to the surgeon as well. Some patients respond to a short course of dexamethasone; others, to a decrease in activity. In any event, the problem is generally self-limited.

Complications of these procedures include the following:

1. *Dural tears.* Dorsal dural tears are easily repaired in the majority of cases. Failure to notice it or to close it firmly may result in a pseudomeningocele. Careful closure of overlying layers (muscle, fascia, and subcutaneous tissue) is required in this situation. Postoperatively, the patient should be kept recumbent for a few days to promote healing.
2. *Root avulsion.* Root avulsion is the result of a technical misadventure. It is not ordinarily amenable to repair but fortunately it is rare.
3. *Wound infection.* Most of these are superficial and can usually be treated with a short course of antibiotics and local wound care. Deep infections (below the lumbodorsal fascia) may require drainage and secondary closure in addition to antibiotic therapy.
4. *Postoperative diskitis.* The incidence of postoperative diskitis is less than 1 percent. It may be caused by bacterial (most commonly *S. epidermidis*) contamination of the disk space, which leads to inflammatory destruction of the cartilaginous end plates and vertebral body [27]. In the acute phase the patient has intense progressive back pain and spasms and prefers immobility. Sudden jolts to the bed are extremely painful. Physical findings are muted, and the wound is usually well healed. In the chronic form the patient presents weeks after successful surgery with severe back pain and a paucity of objective findings. Diagnosis is by history, elevated erythrocyte sedimentation rate (ESR), positive cultures from blood or disk space, and plain spine films; CT scan is often quite specific. Gallium scans are more sensitive. Therapy involves immobilization (4 to 8 weeks), intravenous antibiotics (about 6 weeks), and surgery (to obtain cultures by needle aspiration or open biopsy, to decompress neural elements, or to drain an abscess).
5. Arachnoiditis. The underlying cause is ill-defined; however, contributory factors include previous myelography and multiple spinal procedures. The myelographic appearance is quite typical, with irreg-

ularity of the contrast column, matting of nerve roots, and varying degrees of block. Patients present with recurrent episodes of low back pain and dysesthesia. There is as yet no uniformly satisfactory treatment.

Anterior Cervical Diskectomy with or without Interbody Fusion. Typical postoperative considerations include the following:

1. Obtain a lateral cervical cross-table x-ray film in the recovery room or soon thereafter, to ascertain the position of the graft if a fusion has been performed.
2. Use a cervical collar to avoid extremes of neck motion, which may dislodge the bone plug. When the operation has been done for a fracture-dislocation or other problem in which a great deal of instability is anticipated, it may be necessary to use a halo device.
3. Sore throat, dysphagia, or hoarseness. These are usually from retraction of the trachea and esophagus during surgery. Dysphagia and sore throat are commonly present for a few days postoperatively. Patients with dysphagia may find it easier to swallow a soft diet until the problem is resolved. Humidification of the room air helps liquefy bronchial secretions; giving viscous lidocaine or Chloraseptic lozenges orally every hour provides symptomatic relief. Occasionally the recurrent laryngeal nerve is injured at surgery, resulting in hoarseness.
4. If iliac crest bone was harvested for the bone graft, ambulation may be uncomfortable, if not painful. The patient may require strong analgesic medication.

Complications of anterior cervical diskectomy include the following:

1. *Extrusion of bone graft.* The sudden reappearance of radicular arm pain following the procedure may indicate that the bone graft has slipped out of position, with resultant nerve root compression. Obtain a lateral x-ray film of the cervical spine for diagnosis. The graft may need to be repositioned.
2. Cervical spine deformity. A "swan neck" deformity has been reported after anterior cervical diskectomy without fusion. This may result in recurrent neck pain.

Unlike lumbar disk herniation, cervical disk herniations rarely recur.

Postoperative Complications Following Intracranial Surgery

Postoperative Hematomas

Postoperative intracranial hemorrhage may be a serious and sometimes fatal neurosurgical complication. These clots may be located in the extradural, subdural, or intraparenchymal compartments. The clinical effects result from mechanical compression of adjacent brain tissue and intracranial shifts. Brain shifts may progress to herniation. In the posterior fossa, clinical deterioration from intracranial hematomas is generally quicker than in the supratentorial compartment because of the obvious constraints of space.

In a recent review, a series of 4992 intracranial procedures was evaluated. The overall incidence of postoperative intracranial hemorrhage following intracranial procedures was approximately 0.8 percent. Most (60 percent) were intraparenchymal hematomas. Intracranial tumor was the reason for operation in 56 percent of the patients developing a clot, and meningioma was the most common tumor associated with this complication. Disturbances of coagulation and hypertension were potential precipitating factors [29].

Certainly, it is preferable to prevent a postoperative intracranial hemorrhage than to treat one. Prophylactic measures include evaluation of the patient's preoperative hemostatic status: the platelet count and prothrombin and partial thromboplastin time are good screening tests in addition to a history of bleeding tendency and medications known to interfere with coagulation. If multiple transfusions are required during surgery, one unit of fresh frozen plasma should be given for every four to five units of banked blood. Meticulous hemostasis at surgery is important. Control of postoperative hypertension following certain high risk procedures (resection of an AVM, evacuation of an intraparenchymal hemorrhage, and resection of intraaxial tumors) is also important. Vigorous coughing and gagging are best avoided. In the immediate postoperative period, sudden unexplained neurologic deterioration (lethargy, lateralized neurologic deficit) in a patient who initially appeared to be progressing satisfactorily should raise the question of a postoperative clot. Other conditions (cerebral edema, infarction, acute hydrocephalus, metabolic disturbances, cerebral vasospasm) may all simulate a clot. Whether to reopen a craniotomy depends on the judgment of the neurosurgeon and the particular circumstances of the case. Not all postoperative intracranial hemorrhages need to be evacuated. Even if postoperative hematomas are successfully evacuated, they may leave significant neurologic deficits.

Subgaleal hematomas following large supratentorial flaps may cause local discomfort, threaten the suture line, and even serve as a nidus for subsequent infection since blood is an excellent culture medium. In most cases, these resolve with time. Some surgeons use a subgaleal drain, which exits through a separate stab wound, and a firm circumferential dressing to reduce the likelihood of this occurrence.

Postoperative Cerebral Edema

A certain degree of postoperative edema accompanies many intracranial operations. It is more likely with lesions associated with disruptions of the blood-brain barrier or disordered autoregulation (e.g., brain tumors and AVMs). Intraoperative factors that may contribute include (1) patients with malignant gliomas deep in the white matter in whom only a limited resection is performed, (2) large extraaxial tumors or difficult aneurysms around the base of the brain where prolonged retraction of the brain is required for exposure, and (3) convexity tumors (e.g., meningiomas) that have embedded themselves deep into the surrounding parenchyma.

When postoperative cerebral edema is anticipated, prophylactic measures can be instituted perioperatively, for example, (1) the use of corticosteroids before and after surgery; (2) intraoperative use of mannitol and furosemide (Lasix) to facilitate brain relaxation, reducing the need for brain retraction; and (3) spinal drainage for surgery of cerebral aneurysms and large basal tumors, which provides more exposure, obviating the need for prolonged, vigorous brain retraction.

Unless intraoperative trauma has been severe, postoperative cerebral edema is generally not seen until after the first 6 hours following surgery. Lateralizing signs and a declining level of consciousness may appear in a patient who was initially doing well. The only certain way to distinguish edema from a postoperative hematoma is by CT or magnetic resonance imaging (MRI).

Treatment

Restriction of fluids may reduce intravascular hydrostatic pressure, increase serum osmolality, and retard the progression of cerebral edema, particularly the vasogenic variety.

Steroids may be used (e.g., dexamethasone in a dose of 10 mg intravenously every 6 hours).

ABGs should be checked since hypercarbia and anoxia may exacerbate or even precipitate cerebral edema. If the clinical situation is desperate, it may be necessary to proceed with endotracheal intubation and hyperventilation until the edema and clinical status begin to improve.

Occasionally, insertion of an ICP monitor and vigorous treatment of intracranial hypertension with mannitol, diuretics, or even barbiturates will be necessary.

Generally, if the patient can be satisfactorily treated through the period of maximal swelling (1–3 days) following surgery, edema begins to resolve. The course is followed clinically and by serial CT scans.

A particularly malignant form of postoperative swelling may occur as a result of major vessel occlusion following cerebrovascular surgery or penetrating injuries of the brain. A whole hemisphere may be infarcted. These instances may be completely resistant to medical management. Further surgery to decompress and remove edematous brain tissue may be the only option for this often life-threatening situation.

Postoperative Seizures

Patients with preoperative seizures and those in whom the operative procedure involves a particularly epileptogenic area of the hemisphere (the rolandic regions, temporal lobes) are especially prone to postoperative seizures. One must abort seizures as quickly as possible since continued seizure activity stimulates and may uncouple cerebral metabolism, increases ICP, and may worsen cerebral edema. Intravenous barbiturates, dilantin, or diazepam may be used initially, followed by maintenance oral therapy.

Seizures may be due to metabolic (hyper- or hyponatremia, hypoglycemia, hypoxemia) derangements; therefore, ABGs, serum electrolytes, and blood sugar should be evaluated. A structural cause such as postoperative hematoma or venous or arterial infarction is also likely. A CT scan should be performed to exclude these possibilities.

Postoperative Systemic Complications

Deep Venous Thrombosis and Pulmonary Embolism

Recent reviews suggest that the frequency of postoperative deep venous thrombosis (DVT) in the calf of neurosurgical patients may be up to 29 to 43 percent as measured by the radiolabeled fibrinogen technique [30–32].

Factors that enhance the risk of developing DVT include previous DVT, lengthy surgical procedures, immobilization, advanced age (over 60 years), obesity, limb weakness, heart failure, varicose veins, oral contraceptives, and lower extremity trauma. Clinical diagnosis of venous thrombosis may be augmented by noninvasive screening tests such as fibrinogen-125 scanning, Doppler ultrasonography, and impedance plethysmography. Venography is the definitive test for diagnosing DVT, but it is an invasive method [30–32].

The best therapy for DVT is prevention. Simple methods, such as elevation of the legs and use of elastic stockings, may be employed. Early ambulation is probably the most effective measure when feasible. Prophylactic measures such as external pneumatic compression stockings [33–36] and minidose heparin have decreased the incidence of DVT in neurosurgical patients. Although there is a higher frequency of wound hematomas in patients receiving low-dose heparin, the incidence of major bleeding complications is not increased [36, 37].

Standard management of proximal DVT includes anticoagulation with heparin and warfarin. There has been no evaluation of the safety of full anticoagulation in postoperative neurosurgical patients. There is the possibility of precipitating intracranial or intraspinal hemorrhage in patients with vascular lesions and tumors. Interruption of the inferior vena cava to prevent pulmonary embolism (PE) is an alternative to anticoagulation.

Neurogenic Pulmonary Edema

Neurogenic pulmonary edema (NPE) is pulmonary edema following a CNS insult. It may occur in an *early* or *delayed* form.

The early form develops within minutes to hours of an acute, well-defined CNS condition, most commonly seizures but including intracranial hemorrhage, increased ICP, nonhemorrhagic cerebrovascular accident (CVA), and SAH. There may be a past history of heart failure or breathing problems. Presenting symptoms include dyspnea, tachypnea, and rales. Fever is variable. Hypoxemia, leukocytosis, and bilateral pulmonary infiltrates are classic.

The delayed form develops insidiously over 12 hours to several days following a CNS insult. It may be precipitated by head or spinal injury, SAH, or intracranial surgery. Hypoxemia, dyspnea, and characteristic chest x-ray findings are seen.

It should be noted that the nature of the CNS condition does not specify the form of NPE; either form can be seen with any variety of CNS insult.

NPE is thought to be the result of neural discharge and catecholamine release leading to systemic and pulmonary microvascular hypertension. Blood is forced into the central circulation, augmenting venous return to the heart and resulting in left ventricular (LV) overload. Intrinsic LV function may be directly compromised by the CNS insult. Increased hydrostatic pressure increases pulmonary capillary permeability, and there may be a permeability defect evoked by the CNS pathology itself. Extravascular lung water increases, resulting in pulmonary edema.

Treatment is supportive and depends on the severity of the clinical situation. Most cases are well tolerated, requiring nothing more than supplemental oxygen and observation. Severe hypoxemia is managed in a similar fashion to the adult respiratory distress syndrome (ARDS): supplemental oxygen, mechanical ventilation if a high inspired fraction of oxygen is required, and positive end expiratory pressure (PEEP). High PEEP (>10 cm H_2O) should be used with caution because it decreases cerebral venous return and may increase ICP [38].

Fluid and Electrolyte Problems

Neurosurgical conditions associated with fluid and electrolyte perturbations have already been discussed. Common problems in the postoperative period include syndrome of inappropriate antidiuretic hormone release (SIADH), cerebral salt wasting, DI, hyponatremia, and hypernatremia.

Syndrome of Inappropriate Antidiuretic Hormone Release. SIADH refers to a release of vasopressin (antidiuretic hormone [ADH]) that is inappropriate to a low serum osmolality. In the face of continued water ingestion, the elevated vasopressin results in water retention, hyponatremia, and hypoosmolality.

The laboratory criteria for the diagnosis of SIADH are [39–41]:

1. Low serum sodium (<135 mEq/L)
2. Low serum osmolality (<280 mOsm/kg)
3. Elevated urinary sodium level (>25 mEq/L)
4. Urine osmolality that is inappropriately high compared to the serum osmolality
5. Absence of clinical evidence of volume depletion or diuretic use and normal thyroid, renal, and adrenal function. Symptoms of hyponatremia include confusion, muscle weakness, seizures, anorexia, nausea and vomiting, stupor, or even coma. Patients with underlying neurologic disease tend to have symptoms at higher sodium levels than those without.

SIADH may accompany numerous medical conditions and administration of drugs. Neurosurgical conditions associated with SIADH include subdural hematomas, SAH, brain tumors, head trauma, CVA, and infections of the CNS [41–43]. Medications of neurosurgical interest associated with the development of SIADH include narcotics, carbamazepine, and barbiturates.

TREATMENT. The treatment of SIADH depends on the severity of the clinical presentation. The first line of treatment, if symptoms are mild, is fluid restriction to 800 to 1000 ml daily. For more rapid correction of hyponatremia, infuse a 3 percent saline solution with or without the administration of diuretics. The following formula provides a guide to calculating the required total sodium requirement (in mEq):

(Desired serum Na (mEq/L) − measured serum Na (mEq/L))

$$\times\ 0.6\ body\ weight\ (kg)$$

Correct the sodium deficit halfway to normal over 6 to 8 hours. One should be careful not to increase the serum sodium concentration more than 12 mEq/L/day or to overcorrect it. Rapid correction of hyponatremia has been associated with the development of central pontine myelinolysis [44, 45].

Sodium replacement may be combined with administration of furosemide (Lasix) to eliminate retained free water. Monitor urine output and losses of sodium, potassium, and chloride. Urea has been advocated for the treatment of SIADH; its action appears to be increased sodium retention coupled with an osmotic diuresis. It may be given in a dose of 40 gm every 8 hours with intravenous infusion of normal saline [46].

Demeclocycline, which interferes with the renal tubular effects of ADH, may be helpful in SIADH [47].

Cerebral Salt Wasting. In this syndrome, the kidney is unable to conserve sodium due to a presumed central deficiency. Another putative culprit is the peptide hormone atriopeptin or atrial natriuretic peptide (ANP), which is synthesized by the cardiac atria and ventricles as well as the brain. It possesses diuretic, natriuretic, and vasorelaxant properties. Studies of serum ADH and ANP levels in patients with serum electolyte features of SIADH have identified subsets of patients with ANP and ADH levels more consistent with a diagnosis of cerebral salt wasting. These patients may have similar laboratory findings to SIADH, however, they have a significant decrease in their total blood volume [48–50]. A determination of blood volume is necessary to make the diagnosis. They do not respond to water restriction. The treatment is blood volume replacement with packed red cells and colloids to correct both sodium and volume deficits [50].

Diabetes Insipidus. The underlying deficit is a lack of free water from a partial or complete deficiency of ADH. Clinical symptoms include polyuria (the diagnosis should be entertained if urine output is greater than 300 ml/hour or 500 ml/2 hours), thirst, dehydration, hypovolemia, and polydipsia. The most commonly encountered form of DI in neurosurgical patients is central or pituitary DI.

Examples include head injury (usually severe), following transsphenoidal surgery to remove a pituitary adenoma (usually transient), cerebrovascular lesions (particularly ruptured aneurysms of the anterior communicating artery), and tumors in the region of the hypothalamus. Less commonly encountered is nephrogenic DI in which the end-organ (renal tubules) does not respond to ADH secretion; this form is associated with chronic kidney disease, hypercalcemia, hypokalemia, and various drugs.

Laboratory criteria for the diagnosis of DI are (1) urine specific gravity of less than 1.005, (2) urine osmolality between 50 and 150 mOsm/kg, and (3) serum sodium greater than 150 mEq/L.

TREATMENT. There are varying degrees of DI. It may present as a mild transient nuisance in the perioperative period following pituitary surgery to a medical emergency in a severely head-injured patient. An important consideration in the management of DI is the patient's level of consciousness.

In *mild DI*, the awake patient with normal thirst mechanisms and a ready supply of water is generally able to maintain a solute and volume status within normal limits, although polyuria and polydipsia continue. Nocturia and polydipsia may curtail sleep, so for the patient's convenience it may be necessary to administer a dose of pitressin or DDAVP, a synthetic analog of the neurohypophyseal nonapeptide arginine vasopressin, at night. Another option is intranasal DDAVP.

However, if the patient is comatose or otherwise unable to satisfy a thirst drive, critical alterations in electrolyte and water balance may result. Accurate fluid and electrolyte measurements must be maintained so that adequate replacement can be given.

In *severe DI*, there is a profound negative fluid balance with tachycardia and hypotension. Treatment is volume (free water) replacement and the administration of DDAVP or aqueous pitressin.

DDAVP is the treatment of choice for central DI. It may be administered intravenously, subcutaneously, or intransally; the typical dose is 0.5 ml

(2.0 μg) to 1.0 ml (4.0 μg) intravenously or subcutaneously daily, usually in two divided doses. It has less pressor activity and a longer duration of action compared with aqueous vasopressin.

Aqueous pitressin is given subcutaneously or intramuscularly in doses of 5 to 10 units every 4 to 6 hours. If the situation is critical, it may be given as a continuous intravenous infusion and titrated according to the therapeutic response. Pitressin is also available as a tannate in oil, which has a longer duration—24 to 72 hours. It may be given in a dose of 2 to 5 units intramuscularly. For patients with some ADH reserve, chlorpropamide releases ADH and facilitates the action of ADH on the kidney. It may be given in a dose of 250 to 500 mg by mouth once a day. Clofibrate also releases ADH from the neurohypophysis and may be used as an alternate to chlorpropamide or in combination with it. It is given in a dose of 500 mg by mouth four times a day.

Hyponatremia. Hyponatremia is due to net water retention or salt loss. Symptoms depend on the rate of fall of the serum sodium and its absolute level and include anorexia, muscle cramps, depression of consciousness, nausea and vomiting, seizures, or even coma. The diagnosis and treatment of hyponatremia is partly a function of the status of the extracellular fluid (ECF) compartment. Hyponatremia without a corresponding fall in serum osmolality or ECF volume contraction may be due to hyperglycemia, hyperproteinemia, hyperlipidemia, azotemia, or mannitol. These osmotically active molecules draw water into the ECF, diluting the serum sodium concentration.

Hyponatremia with ECF expansion and increased total body water (edema) is commonly found with medical conditions such as the nephrotic syndrome, cirrhosis, and congestive heart failure. SIADH and cerebral salt wasting, which are important causes of hyponatremia in neurosurgical patients, have been discussed previously.

Hypernatremia. Hypernatremia may be associated with serum hyperosmolality and dehydration from repeated use of mannitol and diuretics for control of ICP or osmotic diuresis from glycosuria. This results in isotonic or hypotonic urine.

Symptoms include thirst, fever, nausea and vomiting, depressed level of consciousness, seizures, and even coma.

Generally, hypernatremia should be corrected when the serum sodium level is greater than 150 mEq/L or the serum osmolality is greater than 300 mOsm/kg.

The water deficit may be calculated according to the following formula:

Water deficit = calculated ideal body water − actual body water

where

Calculated ideal body water = 0.6 × body weight (kg)

$$\text{Actual body water} = \frac{140 \text{ mEq/L (ideal serum sodium)}}{\text{actual serum sodium (mEq/L)}}$$

$$\times \ 0.6 \times \text{body weight (kg)}$$

Hydration should be commenced with isotonic or hypotonic saline depending on the severity of the hypernatremia. Hypernatremia from central causes is usually the syndrome of DI.

Fever of Cerebral Origin

Neurosurgical procedures in the region of the third ventricle may be associated with a noninfectious fever. Local trauma to temperature-regulating centers, spillage of blood into the CSF, and regional electrolyte disturbances may play a role. Patients with severe head injuries are prone to fevers of this kind. The fevers are usually resistant to antipyretics; cultures are by definition negative.

One should explore all possible causes of infection before making a diagnosis of "central fever," which is a diagnosis of exclusion.

Cardiac Arrhythmias and Myocardial Infarction

These problems are more common in the setting of existing cardiac disease. Patients undergoing carotid endarterectomy and those who have suffered a subarachnoid hemorrhage are examples of neurosurgical patients who commonly have cardiac problems.

Urinary Retention and Urinary Tract Infection

Urologic problems are common in the spinal cord injured patient. Postoperative lumbar laminectomy, especially multiple levels for lumbar spinal stenosis in older patients, may be associated with voiding difficulties in the postoperative period. Most of these problems resolve in a few days.

Gastric (Cushing's) Ulcers

These classically accompany severe intracranial injury or intracranial hypertension. The use of steroids also predisposes to varying degrees of gastric irritation. Treatment is with antacids, H_2-receptor blockers, and carafate (Sucralfate) [51–53].

References

1. Plum F., Posner J. B. *The Diagnosis of Stupor and Coma* (3rd. ed.). Philadelphia: Davis, 1987.
2. Peerless S. J. Pre- and postoperative management of cerebral aneurysms. *Clin. Neurosurg.* 26:209, 1979.
3. Clark K. Complications of aneurysm surgery. *Clin. Neurosurg.* 23:342, 1976.
4. Lazar M. L., Watts C. C., Kilgore B., et al. Cerebral angiography during operation for intracranial aneurysms and arteriovenous malformations. Technical note. *J. Neurosurg.* 34:706, 1971.
5. Lougheed W., Morley T., Tasker R., et al. The results of surgical treatment of ruptured aneurysms. In W. F. Fields and A. L. Sahs (eds.), *Intracranial*

Aneurysms and Subarachnoid Hemorrhage. Springfield, IL: Charles C Thomas, 1965. Pp. 295–314.

6. Heiskanen O., Marttila I. Risk of rupture of a second aneurysm in patients with multiple aneurysms. *J. Neurosurg.* 32:295, 1970.

7. Drake C. G., Allcock J. M. Post-operative angiography and the "slipped" clip. *J. Neurosurg.* 39:683, 1973.

8. Oyesiku N. M., Jones R. K. Migration of a Heifetz aneurysm clip to the cauda equina causing lumbar radiculopathy. *J. Neurosurg.* 65:256, 1986.

9. van Gijn J., Hijdra A., Wijdicks E. F. M., et al. Acute hydrocephalus after aneurysmal subarachnoid hemorrhage. *J. Neurosurg.* 63:355, 1985.

10. Bove E. L., Fry W. J., Gross W. S., et al. Hypotension and hypertension as consequences of baroreceptor dysfunction following carotid endarterectomy. *Surgery* 85:633, 1979.

11. Towne J. B., Bernhard V. M. The relationship of postoperative hypertension to complications following carotid endarterectomy. *Surgery* 88:575, 1980.

12. Watts N. B., Tindall G. T. Rapid assessment of corticotropin reserve after pituitary surgery. *J.A.M.A.* 259:708, 1988.

13. Tindall G. T., Barrow D. L. *Disorders of the Pituitary.* St. Louis: Mosby, 1986.

14. Kornblith P. L., Walker M. Chemotherapy for malignant gliomas. *J. Neurosurg.* 68:1, 1988.

15. Walker M. D., Alexander E. Jr., Hunt W. E., et al. Evaluation of BCNU and/or radiotherapy in the treatment of anaplastic gliomas. A cooperative clinical trial. *J. Neurosurg.* 49:333, 1978.

16. Nelson D. F., Scheonfield D., Weinstein A. S., et al. A randomized comparison of misonidazole sensitized radiotherapy plus BCNU for treatment of malignant glioma after surgery: Preliminary results of an RTOG study. *Int. J. Radiat. Oncol. Biol. Phys.* 9:1143, 1983.

17. Chang C. H., Horton J., Schonfield D., et al. Comparison of postoperative radiotherapy and combined postoperative radiotherapy and chemotherapy in the multidisciplinary management of malignant gliomas. A Joint Radiation Therapy Oncology Group and Eastern Cooperative Oncology Group study. *Cancer* 52:997 1983.

18. Kornblith P. L., Walker M. Chemotherapy for malignant gliomas. *J. Neurosurg.* 68:1, 1988.

19. Bullard D. E., Gillespie G. Y., Mahaley M. S., et al. Immunobiology of human gliomas. *Semin. Oncol.* 13:94, 1986.

20. Nelson D. F., Urtasun R. C., Saunder W. M., et al. Recent and current investigations of radiation therapy of malignant gliomas. *Semin. Oncol.* 13:46, 1986.

21. Morantz R. Radiation therapy in the treatment of cerebral astrocytoma. *Neurosurgery* 20:975, 1987.

22. Bernstein M., Gutin P. H. Interstitial irradiation of brain tumors: A review. *Neurosurgery* 9:741, 1981.

23. Salcman M., Sewchand W., Amin P. P., et al. Technique and Preliminary Results of Interstitial Irradiation for Recurrent Glial Tumors. In M. D. Walker and D. G. T. Thomas (eds.), *Biology of Brain Tumors.* Boston: Martinus Nijhoff, 1986. P. 365.

24. Bakay R. A. E. Brachytherapy. *Contemp, Neurosurg.* 9:1, 1987.

25. Patchell R. A., Murauyama Y., Tibbs P. A., et al. Neutron interstitial brachytherapy for malignant gliomas: A pilot study. *J. Neurosurg.* 68:67, 1988.

26. Sheline G. E., Wara W. M., Smith V. Therapeutic irradiation and brain injury. *Int. J. Radiol. Oncol. Biol. Phys.* 6:1215, 1980.

27. Rawlings C., Wilkins R. H., Gallis H., et al. Postoperative intervertebral space infection. *Neurosurgery* 13:371, 1983.

28. Kopecky K. K., Gilmor R. L., Scott J. A., et al. Pitfalls of computed tomography in diagnosis of discitis. *Neuroradiology* 27:57, 1985.
29. Kalfas I. H., Little J. R. Postoperative hemorrhage: A survey of 4992 intracranial procedures. *Neurosurgery* 23:343, 1988.
30. Joffe S. N. Incidence of postoperative deep vein thrombosis in neurosurgical patients. *J. Neurosurg.* 42:201, 1975.
31. Valladares J. B., Hankinson J. Incidence of lower extremity postoperative deep vein thrombosis in neurosurgical patients. *Neurosurgery* 6:138, 1980.
32. Swann K. W., Black P. McL. Deep venous thrombosis and pulmonary emboli in neurosurgical patients: A review. *J. Neurosurg.* 61:1055, 1984.
33. Powers S. K., Edwards M. S. B. Prophylaxis of thromboembolism in the neurosurgical patient: A review. *Neurosurgery* 10:509, 1982.
34. Skillman J. J., Collins R. E. C., Coe N. P., et al. Prevention of deep venous thrombosis in neurosurgical patients: A controlled, randomized trial of external pneumatic compression boots. *Surgery* 83:354, 1978.
35. Turpie A. G. G., Gallus A. S., Beattie W. S., et al. Prevention of venous thrombosis in patients with intracranial disease by intermittent pneumatic compression of the calf. *Neurology* 27:435, 1977.
36. Barnett H. G., Clifford J. R., Llewellyn R. C. Safety of mini-dose heparin administration for neurosurgical patients. *J. Neurosurg.* 47:27, 1977.
37. Cerrato D., Ariano C., Fiacchino F. Deep venous thrombosis and low-dose heparin prophylaxis in neurosurgical patients. *J. Neurosurg.* 49:378, 1978.
38. Colice G. L. Neurogenic pulmonary edema. *Clin. Chest. Med.* 6:473, 1985.
39. Bartter F. C., Schwartz W. B. The syndrome of inappropriate secretion of antidiuretic hormone. *Am. J. Med.* 42:790, 1967.
40. DeTroyer A., Demanet J. C. Clinical, biological and pathogenic features of the syndrome of inappropriate secretion of antidiuretic hormone. *Q. J. Med.* 45:521, 1976.
41. Lester M. C., Nelson P. B. Neurosurgical aspects of vasopressin release and the syndrome of inappropriate secretion of antidiuretic hormone. *Neurosurgery* 8:735, 1981.
42. Fox J. L., Falik J. L., Shalhoub R. J. Neurosurgical hyponatremia: The role of inappropriate antidiuresis. *J. Neurosurg.* 34:506, 1971.
43. Nelson P. B., Seif S. M., Robinson A. G., et al. Increased secretion of antidiuretic hormone in patients with intracranial aneurysms. *Neurosurgery* (abstr.) 1:66, 1977.
44. Kleinschmidt-DeMasters B. K., Norenberg M. D. Rapid correction of hyponatremia causes demyelination: Relation to central pontine myelinolysis. *Science* 211:1068, 1981.
45. Ayus J. C., Krothapalli R. K., Arieff A. I. Treatment of symptomatic hyponatremia and its relation to brain damage. A prospective study. *N. Engl. J. Med.* 317:1190, 1987.
46. Reeder R. F., Harbaugh R. E. Administration of intravenous urea and normal saline for the treatment of hyponatremia in neurosurgical patients. *J. Neurosurg.* 70:201, 1989.
47. Troyer A. Demeclocycline treatment for syndrome of inappropriate secretion of antidiuretic hormone. *J.A.M.A.* 237:2723, 1977.
48. Diringer M., Ladenson P. W., Borel C., et al. Sodium and water regulation in a patient with cerebral salt wasting. *Arch. Neurol.* 46:928, 1989.
49. Weinand M. E., O'Boynick P. C., Goetz K. L. A study of serum antidiuretic hormone and atrial natriuretic peptide levels in a series of patients with intracranial disease and hyponatremia. *Neurosurgery* 25:781, 1989.
50. Nelson P. B., Seif S. M., Maroon J. C., et al. Hyponatremia in intracranial

disease: Perhaps not the syndrome of inappropriate secretion of antidiuretic hormone (SIADH). *J. Neurosurg.* 55:938, 1981.

51. Cushing H. Peptic ulcers and the interbrain. *Surg. Gynecol. Obstet.* 55:1, 1938.
52. Chan K. H., Mann K. S., Jai E. C. S., et al. Factors influencing the development of gastrointestinal complications after neurosurgery: Results of multivariate analysis. *Neurosurgery* 25:378, 1989.
53. Messer J., Reitman D., Sacko H.S., et al. Association of adrenocorticosteroid therapy and peptic ulcer disease. *N. Engl. J. Med.* 309:21, 1983.

Suggested Reading

Ropper A. H., Kennedy S. K. (eds.). *Neurological and Neurosurgical Intensive Care.* Rockville, MD: Aspen Publishers, 1988.

Horwitz N. H., Rizzoli H. V. *Postoperative Complications of Extracranial Neurological Surgery.* Baltimore: Williams & Wilkins, 1987.

Horwitz N. H., Rizzoli H. V. *Postoperative Complications of Intracranial Neurological Surgery.* Baltimore: Williams & Wilkins, 1982.

Wirth F. P., Ratcheson R. A. (eds.). *Neurosurgical Critical Care.* Baltimore: Williams & Wilkins, 1987.

Index

Index

An italicized page number denotes a figure; the abbreviation *t* denotes a table.